The Herb Society's
COMPLETE
MEDICINAL
HERBAL

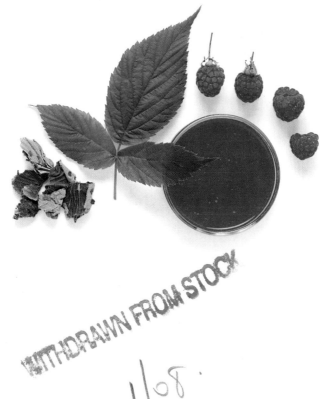

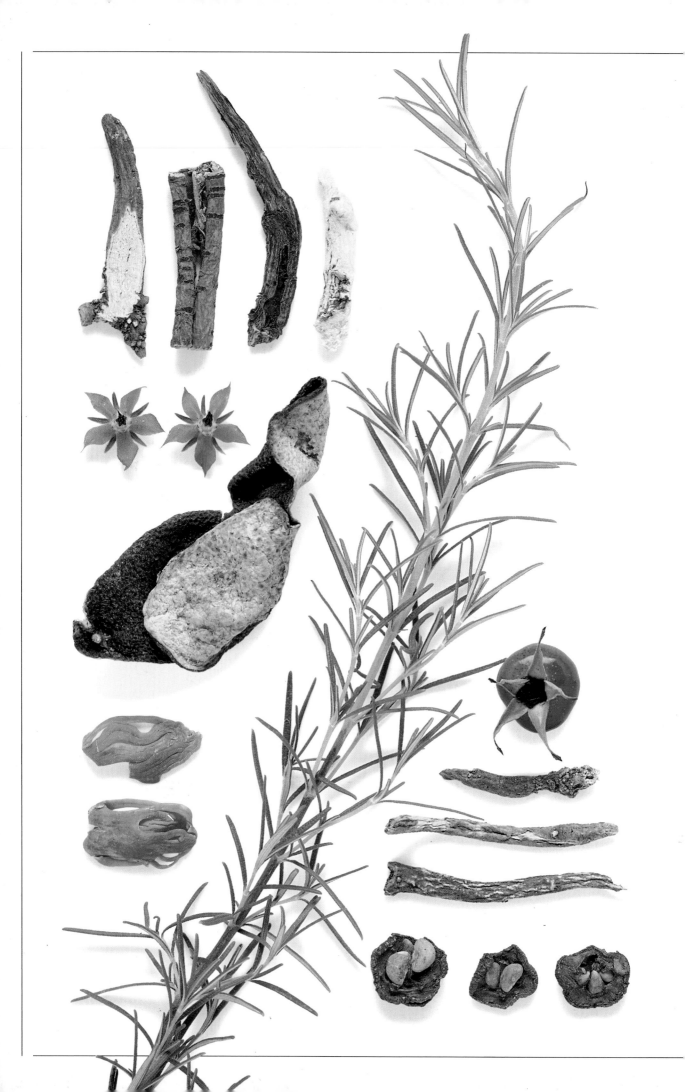

The Herb Society's

COMPLETE
MEDICINAL
HERBAL

PENELOPE ODY MNIMH

DK

DORLING KINDERSLEY

LONDON · NEW YORK · STUTTGART

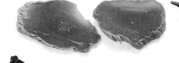

A DORLING KINDERSLEY BOOK

Art editor
Tina Hill

Project editor
Tanya Hines

Assistant designer
Kate Sarluis

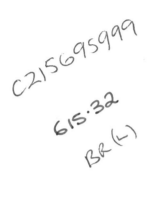

Assistant editor
Blanche Sibbald

Senior managing editor
Daphne Razazan

Managing art editor
Carole Ash

Production manager
Maryann Rogers

Main photographer
Steve Gorton

IMPORTANT NOTICE

The recommendations and information in this book are appropriate in most cases.
However, the advice this book contains is general, not specific to individuals and their particular
circumstances. Any plant substance, whether used as food or medicine, externally or internally, can
cause an allergic reaction in some people. Neither the author nor the publishers can be held responsible
for claims arising from the mistaken identity of any herbs, or the inappropriate use of any remedy or
healing regime. Do not try self-diagnosis or attempt self-treatment for serious or long-term problems
without consulting a medical professional or qualified practitioner. Do not undertake any self-treatment
while you are undergoing a prescribed course of medical treatment without first seeking professional
advice. Always seek medical advice if symptoms persist.

First published in Great Britain in 1993
by Dorling Kindersley Limited,
9 Henrietta Street, London WC2E 8PS

A CIP catalogue record for this book is available from the British Library

ISBN 0 7513 0025 X

Reproduced in Italy by GRB Editrice, Verona
Printed and bound in Italy by New Interlitho, Milan

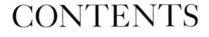

CONTENTS

INTRODUCTION

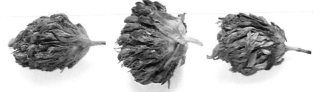

ONE OF THE EARLIEST Chinese herbals – Shen Nong's *Classic of Materia Medica* dating from the first or second centuries AD – lists 365 healing remedies, most of them plants but including a few mineral and animal extracts. The Greek physician Dioscorides, writing in the first century AD, mentions around 400 herbs. Today, the list of plants with known medicinal properties is rather longer: around 5,800 in the Chinese *materia medica*, 2,500 in India, at least 800 regularly collected from the tropical forests of Africa, almost 300 currently detailed for the medical profession in Germany – so far the only Western country with official herbal monographs – and many thousands more known only to traditional healers in the more remote corners of the world. To produce a truly complete medicinal herbal would fill many volumes and be the work of several lifetimes. Yet, despite this bewildering array of healing plants, the average Western herbalist generally finds that a working knowledge of 150 to 200 plants is more than enough to cope with most human ailments.

Herbs may be defined as any plants that can be put to culinary or medicinal use, and include those we associate with orthodox drugs, such as foxglove and opium poppy, as well as everyday plants like garlic or sage. The herbs in this book are a representative cross-section of these potent plants, ranging from exotic Eastern herbs such as *ma huang* and ginseng to more mundane apples and cabbages, as we often forget that many of our familiar foods have significant medicinal properties that we greatly undervalue.

Interest in herbal medicine throughout the world is increasing. In the West, people often cite the risk of side effects from powerful orthodox drugs as a reason for turning to gentler, plant medicines. In the developing world, a lack of hard currency to pay for imported pharmaceuticals is encouraging a reappraisal of traditional folk remedies. This trend towards more natural medicine has gained added impetus from our growing concern with environmental issues, such as the destruction of the rainforests and the loss of rare species.

Although the therapeutic effects of many herbs have not been scientifically proven, research is continually being done to learn more about the way in which these plants work, and to identify the active ingredients that give them their healing properties. Such research, scientists hope, may uncover new active plant ingredients that can then form the basis of drugs to fight cancer or Aids; these drugs will join the many thousands of other widely used synthetic remedies derived originally from medicinal herbs.

And yet, in extracting these chemicals and seeking to turn herbal remedies designed to help the body heal itself into powerful drugs to obliterate symptoms, we forget one of the basic tenets of traditional healing: a belief that one tries to treat the cause of disharmonies and "dis-ease" rather than the effects. We forget, too, that traditional health care has as much to do with preventing disease as with curing it, and that the responsibility for good health rests equally with the patient and the practitioner. The Greek physician Hippocrates urged fresh air, a good diet and exercise; the early founders of Ayurveda, the classical Indian school of medicine, focused as much on personal hygiene and sensible eating as on herbal brews; and in China, early texts are full of comments along the lines that the "good doctor attends to keeping people well, while the inferior only treats those that are sick".

The use of simple herbal remedies can encourage us once again to take responsibility for our own health. Instead of trying to obliterate symptoms when they become severe, we need to be sufficiently in tune with our bodies to recognize those symptoms as they develop and treat likely causes – whether physical, emotional or spiritual – to restore essential energy and balance.

In this book I do not simply aim to give a wealth of detail about a limited number of plants or provide cure-all lists of remedies that can be taken to alleviate symptoms. I have tried instead to look at how a few herbs have been used by the traditional healers of many cultures, and have suggested a therapeutic approach for ailments that focuses on healing the whole person. For some, these suggestions may represent an effective solution. For others, they will only be the starting point for a wider exploration of the healing power of herbs.

Penelope Ody

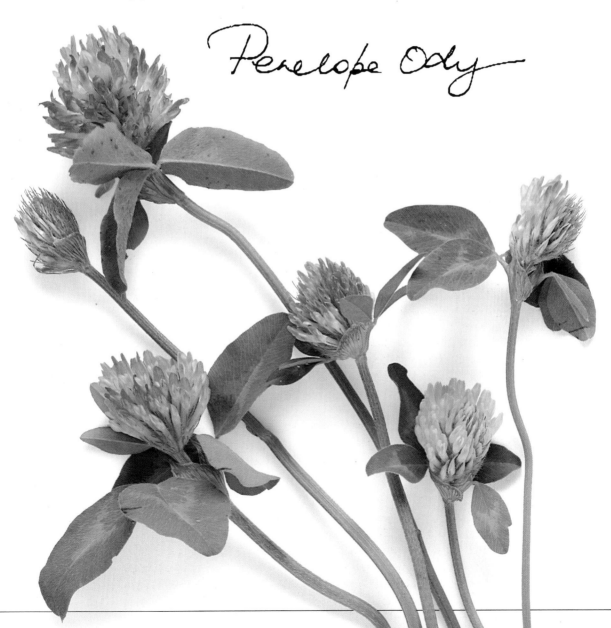

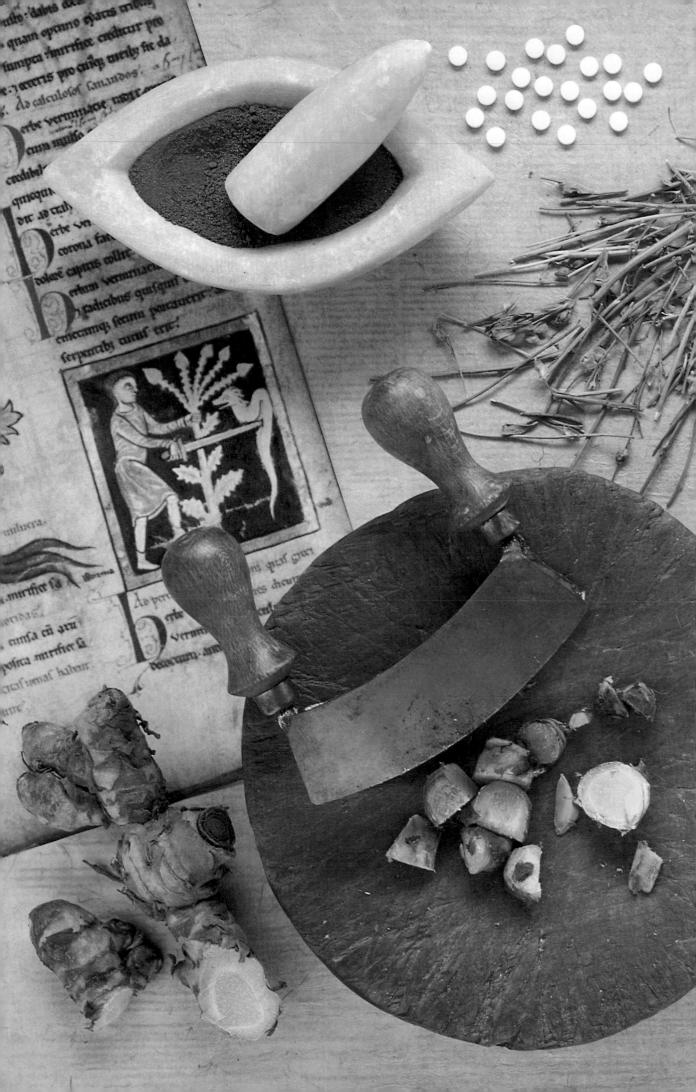

HERBS PAST & PRESENT

From ancient times, herbs have played a vital role in the healing traditions of many cultures. This section looks at the major herbal systems in different parts of the world throughout the ages. Some may seem incomprehensible to us in modern Western society, but the alternative way of looking at health care that they represent can be just as valid today as it was 5,000 years ago.

ORIGINS OF WESTERN HERBALISM

HIPPOCRATES MAY BE KNOWN today as the father of medicine, but for centuries pride of place in medieval Europe was given to Galen, a 2nd-century physician, who wrote extensively about the four "humours" – blood, phlegm, black bile and yellow bile – and classified herbs by their essential qualities: as hot or cold, dry or damp.

These theories were later expanded by 7th-century Arab physicians such as Avicenna, and today Galenical theories continue to dominate *Unani* medicine, practised in the Muslim world and India. Galen's descriptions of herbs as, for example, "hot in the third degree" or "cold in the second" were still being used well into the 18th century.

Ancient Civilizations

HERBS IN PAPYRI
Surviving Egyptian papyri dating back to around 1700 BC record that many common herbs, such as garlic and juniper, have been used medicinally for around 4,000 years. In the days of Ramesses III, hemp was used for eye problems just as it may be prescribed for glaucoma today, while poppy extracts were used to quieten crying children.

THE GREEK CONTRIBUTION
By the time of Hippocrates (468-377 BC), European herbal tradition had already absorbed ideas from Assyria and India, with Eastern herbs such as basil and ginger among the most highly prized, and the complex theory of humours and essential body fluids had begun to be formulated. Hippocrates categorized all foods and herbs by fundamental quality – hot, cold, dry or damp – and good health was maintained by keeping them in balance, as well as taking plenty of exercise and fresh air.

Pedanius Dioscorides wrote his classic text *De Materia Medica* in around AD 60, and this remained the standard textbook for 1,500 years. Dioscorides was reputed to have been either the physician to

The Greek model
Early Greeks saw the world as composed of four elements: earth, air, fire and water. These elements were related to the seasons, to four fundamental qualities, to four bodily fluids or humours, and to four temperaments. In almost all individuals, one humour was thought to dominate, affecting both personality and the likely health problems that would be suffered.

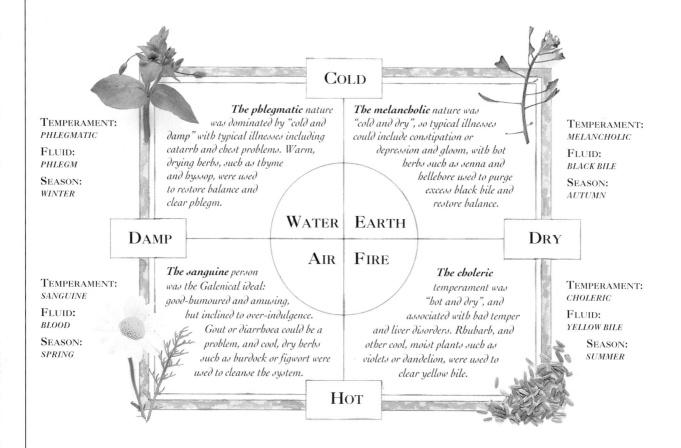

TEMPERAMENT:
PHLEGMATIC

FLUID:
PHLEGM

SEASON:
WINTER

COLD

The phlegmatic nature was dominated by "cold and damp" with typical illnesses including catarrh and chest problems. Warm, drying herbs, such as thyme and hyssop, were used to restore balance and clear phlegm.

The melancholic nature was "cold and dry", so typical illnesses could include constipation or depression and gloom, with hot herbs such as senna and hellebore used to purge excess black bile and restore balance.

TEMPERAMENT:
MELANCHOLIC

FLUID:
BLACK BILE

SEASON:
AUTUMN

WATER   EARTH

DAMP

AIR   FIRE

DRY

TEMPERAMENT:
SANGUINE

FLUID:
BLOOD

SEASON:
SPRING

The sanguine person was the Galenical ideal: good-humoured and amusing, but inclined to over-indulgence. Gout or diarrhoea could be a problem, and cool, dry herbs such as burdock or figwort were used to cleanse the system.

The choleric temperament was "hot and dry", and associated with bad temper and liver disorders. Rhubarb, and other cool, moist plants such as violets or dandelion, were used to clear yellow bile.

TEMPERAMENT:
CHOLERIC

FLUID:
YELLOW BILE

SEASON:
SUMMER

HOT

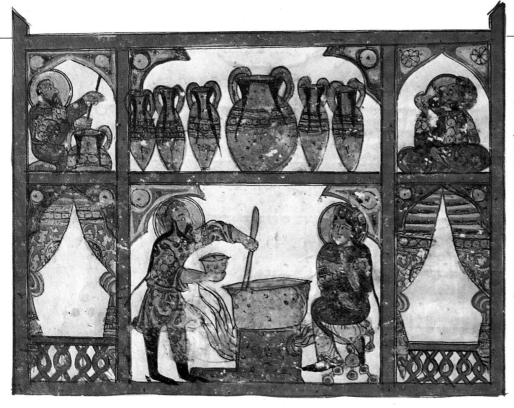

Antony and Cleopatra or, more prosaically, an army surgeon during the reign of the Emperor Nero. Many of the actions Dioscorides describes are familiar today: parsley as a diuretic; fennel to promote milk flow; white horehound mixed with honey as an expectorant.

ROMAN REMEDIES

The Greek theories of medicine reached Rome around 100 BC. As time passed, they became more mechanistic, presenting a view of the body as a machine to be actively repaired, rather than following the Hippocratic dictum of allowing most diseases to cure themselves. Medicine became a lucrative business with complex, highly priced herbal remedies.

Opposing this practice was Claudius Galenus (AD 131-199), who was born in Pergamon in Asia Minor and was a court physician to the Emperor Marcus Aurelius. Galen reworked many of the old Hippocratic ideas and formalized the theories of humours. His books soon became the standard medical texts not only of Rome, but also of later Arab and medieval physicians, and his theories still survive in *Unani* medicine today.

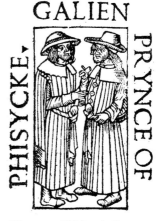

The "Prynce of Phisycke"
Galen's writings were influential for centuries; this woodcut dates from 1542.

Islamic Influences

THE ARAB WORLD

With the fall of Rome in the 5th century, the centre of Classical learning shifted East and the study of Galenical medicine was focused in Constantinople and Persia. Galenism was adopted with enthusiasm by the Arabs, and merged with both folk beliefs and surviving Egyptian learning. It was this mixture of herbal ideas, practice and traditions that was reimported into Europe with the invading Arab armies.

Probably the most important work of the time was the *Kitab al-Qanun*, or Canon of Medicine, by Avicenna. This was based firmly on Galenical principles and by the 12th century had been translated into Latin and imported back into the West to become one of the leading textbooks in Western medical schools.

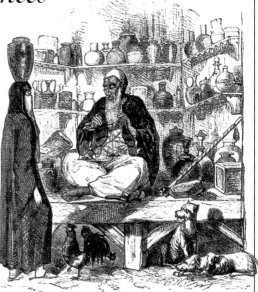

Eastern spices
The Arabs were great traders and introduced many exotic herbs and spices from the East, such as nutmeg, cloves, saffron and senna, to the materia medica of Dioscorides and Galen. Here, a Cairo street trader displays his wares.

A SCIENCE OF LIFE

THE TERM AYURVEDA comes from two Indian words: *ayur*, or life, and *veda*, or knowledge. Ayurvedic medicine is thus described as a "knowledge of how to live", emphasizing that good health is the responsibility of the individual. In Ayurvedic medicine, illness is seen in terms of imbalance, with herbs and dietary controls used to restore equilibrium. The earliest Ayurvedic texts date from around 2500 BC, with successive invaders adding new herbal traditions: the Persians in 500 BC, the Moghuls in the 14th century bringing the medicine of Galen and Avicenna (known as *Unani*), and the British, who closed down the Ayurvedic schools in 1833, but luckily did not obliterate the ancient learning altogether. Tibetan medicine has much in common with Ayurveda, but can be vastly more complicated, having 15 subdivisions for the humours and placing strong emphasis on the effect of past lives – *karma* – on present health.

The Way of the Ayurveda

A WORLD VIEW
As in Ancient Greek and traditional Chinese medicine, the Ayurvedic model links the microcosm of the individual with the cosmos. At the heart of the system are three primal forces: *prana*, the breath of life; *agni*, the spirit of light or fire; and *soma*, a manifestation of harmony, cohesiveness and love. There are also five elements comprising all matter: earth, water, fire, air and ether (a nebulous nothingness that fills all space and was also known to the Ancient Greeks).

BALANCING THE HUMOURS
The five universal elements are converted by *agni*, the digestive fire, into three humours, which influence individual health and temperament and are sometimes called waste products of digestion. If digestion were perfect there would be no humoral imbalance, but because it is not, imbalance and ill health can follow. Air and ether yield *vata* (wind), fire produces the humour *pitta* (fire or bile), while earth and water combine to give *kapha* (phlegm). The dominant humour is seen as controlling the character of the individual: a *vata*-type roughly conforms to Galen's melancholic personality, *pitta* matches the choleric type and a *kapha* person is reminiscent of the phlegmatic. Food, drink, sensual gratification, light, fresh air and spiritual activities are used to "feed" the digestive fire and produce the correct mix of humours.

Crown chakra
Associated with the pineal gland; helped by herbs like gotu kola *and* nutmeg.

Brow chakra (third eye)
Associated with the pituitary gland; supported by sandalwood *and* elecampane.

The chakras
Ayurveda stresses the need to strengthen the chakras, or energy centres, of the body. These may be stimulated by applying particular herbs to the energy points, or strengthened by taking other herbs internally. Modern theorists now link the chakras to various organs and glands.

Throat chakra
Associated with the thyroid gland; strengthened by herbs like cloves and vervain.

Heart chakra
Associated with the thymus gland and heart; helped by herbs like saffron and rose.

Solar plexus chakra
Associated with the liver and adrenal glands; supported by herbs like goldenseal and lemon balm.

Splenic chakra
Associated with the testes and ovaries; strengthened by herbs like coriander and fennel.

Root chakra
Associated with the uterus and prostate gland; strengthened by herbs like ashwagandha or haritaki.

واسهال ببابهند دوالله اعلم
غرب درختی بود که بهای
اوراسپیداد خوانند شیخ ریس
گفته چوب اورا بسوزند
وسبکه سرشت کند ثا ایل را
خشک کند و پوست این درخت
در خضاب سوی داخل شود و
فایده نیک کند برگ اورا بسایند
وبرزخهای تازه کند بصلاح آرد و کشه چون جلو مطبق کسی اوبخنه بابشیش بابک
اوراببابشا سندذا یل کند کل اوتاریکی چشم را نافع بود و صمغ اورا بر نیشتر بیرون آرد از رم
بورق نیک بنا شود مخره در او تاریکی چشم را نافع بود این هم از شیخ رئیس مرویست
فاوانیا درخت عود صلیب بود
بعضی ازان دوسی باشد و بعضی ازان هنگ
شیخ رئیس کفته چوب اونشانهای سیاه
ازبدن دور سازد و نقرس و صرع را نافع کند
تابا وبیتن اوبیز بدهستی چوب اورا بر
صاحب صرع اوبخته بود ند بدا فنیدا یافند
که مرصع را نامع شد بحثیثیته که صرع آمد
آمدة چون آبجوب را از ازاین شخص دور کرد ید

Indian herbal
In Moghul India, Ayurvedic traditions were less valued than Greek or Arab ideas. This herbal is written in Persian.

such as *gotu kola*, *guggal* or myrrh, all designed to dry excess water or phlegm. In Ayurvedic theory, taste is important: pungent, bitter and astringent tastes can help reduce *kapha*, so the diet would favour these over sweet, salty or sour flavours. Treatment might also include massage with warm herbal oils such as eucalyptus, burning pungent incense such as frankincense, and encouraging the sufferer to wear bright, hot reds and yellows instead of cold blues or white.

OTHER PRINCIPLES
Ayurvedic medicine emphasizes a "holistic" approach, treating the whole person with appropriate remedies for the mind, body and spirit. This can include meditation, physical exercises, or herbs that are focused at some particular aspect of being. Problems of the heart, for example, are considered as much a spiritual issue as pathology since the heart is the seat of the *atman* or divine self. Suitable herbs might include *arjuna*, used as a heart tonic, with sandalwood oil as a sedating massage oil to calm and uplift the spirits and encourage joy.

The essential energy of the body (*ojas*, like the Chinese *qi*) can be strengthened with tonic herbs such as *ashwagandha*, *shatavari* or *guduchi*. Like the Chinese *wei qi*, *ojas* is associated with the immune system and herbs to strengthen it tend to be immunostimulants.

A health problem associated with excess phlegm, such as catarrh, oedema or water retention, for example, would be treated with warm, light, dry foods, fasting and avoiding cold drinks that would increase *kapha*. Herbal remedies might include hot spices such as cayenne, pippali and cinnamon; bitters such as aloe or turmeric; pungent tonics such as saffron; and stimulating, mind-clearing herbs

Tibetan Herbalism

RITUAL & RELIGION
Before the Chinese invasion of 1959, medicine in Tibet was largely under the control of the lamas and closely linked with religion. Medical students memorized four complex "tantras", which explained the cause and progression of disease with the aid of "illustrated trees of medicine". Physicians used meditation and mantras to "energize" the medicine and increase its efficacy, and harvesting of herbs was also carefully timed to use any helpful astrological influences.

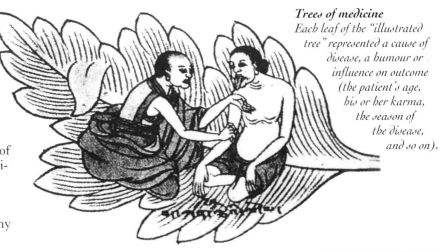

Trees of medicine
Each leaf of the "illustrated tree" represented a cause of disease, a humour or influence on outcome (the patient's age, his or her karma, the season of the disease, and so on).

CHINESE HERBAL MEDICINE

TRADITIONAL CHINESE MEDICINE is an ancient system of healing that can be traced back to around 2500 BC. The texts produced at that time are still studied and followed by practitioners, and while much has been added to the basic philosophy, very little has been taken out. In Chinese medicine, illness is seen as a sign of disharmony within the whole person, so the task of the traditional Chinese practitioner is always to restore harmony and balance, thus enabling the body's natural healing mechanisms to work more efficiently. Herbs are central to treatment, aided by other therapies such as acupuncture or specialist massage. In the past few years, Chinese herbal traditions have become more familiar in the West, and are now used by many qualified practitioners.

The Principles of Chinese Medicine

THE THEORY OF ELEMENTS

As with early Greek philosophy, the Chinese tradition is based on a theory of elements (in this model five, rather than the Greek four), which is used to explain every interaction between man and his environment. These elements, namely wood, fire, earth, metal and water, are seen to be related, with wood encouraging fire, fire resolving to earth, earth yielding up metal, metal producing water (seen as condensation on a cold metal surface), and water giving birth to wood by encouraging the growth of vegetation.

Each element has a number of associations, ranging from parts of the body and emotions to human sounds, the seasons, colours and tastes, all underpinned by a simple logic. Wood, for example, relates to spring and the colour green; fire to summer; and water to the kidneys. For good health to prevail, the elements need to be in harmony; if one element becomes over-dominant, illness may result.

Chinese practitioners often look for the cause of illness in a related element: weakness in the liver (wood), for example, may be due to deficiencies in the kidneys (water). A weak stomach (earth) might be caused by over-exuberant wood (liver) failing to be controlled by deficient metal (lungs).

The five elements

The elements form a network of relationships: the red arrows in the diagram show how one element gives rise to another; the grey arrows indicate how one element controls another. Herbs can be linked to the model in various ways. The taste of the herb, for example, can suggest the bodily organ that the plant might influence.

Shan zhu yu

Wu wei zi

WOOD
SEASON: *SPRING*
TASTE: *SOUR*
EMOTION: *ANGER*
PARTS OF THE BODY: *LIVER, GALL BLADDER, TENDONS, EYES.*

Sour herbs like shan zhu yu and wu wei zi are generally astringent and used for discharges, excessive bleeding, sweating or diarrhoea. Their main action is on the liver and gall bladder.

Hai zao

Qing dai

Jin qian cao

WATER
SEASON: *WINTER*
TASTE: *SALTY*
EMOTION: *FEAR*
PARTS OF THE BODY: *KIDNEYS, BLADDER, EARS, HAIR, BONES.*

Salty herbs such as hai zao, qing dai and jin qian cao generally reduce swellings. They are usually cooling, acting on kidneys and bladder.

YIN, YANG & QI

Complementing the basic model of the five elements is the Chinese theory of opposites – *yin* and *yang*. According to this, everything in the cosmos both contains and is balanced by its own polar opposite. *Yin* is seen as female, dark and cold, while *yang* is characterized as male, light and hot.

In traditional Chinese medicine, *yin* and *yang* need to be in balance to maintain health, and many ills can be attributed to a deficiency or excess of either factor.

Different parts of the body are also described as predominantly *yin* or *yang*: body fluids and blood are mainly *yin*, for example, while *qi*, the vital energy, tends to be *yang*. *Qi* is regarded as flowing in a network of channels, or meridians, through the body and can be stimulated using acupuncture.

ANCIENT CHINESE MEDICINE

The origins of Chinese herbalism are shrouded in myth. There are legendary figures such as Shen Nong, the "divine cultivator", who "invented" agriculture and identified many medicinal plants. Shen Nong was said to have "tasted the flavour of hundreds of herbs and drank the water from many springs and wells so that people might know which were sweet and which were bitter". He supposedly discovered tea drinking, too, when some leaves fell from a tea bush into a bowl of water boiling nearby. An important Chinese herbal from around 200 BC is named after Shen Nong.

The founding father of Chinese medical theory is the Yellow Emperor, who is reputed to have lived around 2500 BC. However, the classic text that bears his name, the *Huang Ti Nei Ching Su Wên* or *Yellow Emperor's Canon of Internal Medicine*, is generally dated to around 1000 BC. It could well represent an older verbal tradition. As in the West, medicine at that time was inseparable from philosophy and religion, and the *Nei Ching* is an important Taoist text, rich in spiritual wisdom.

Historically, there were many different medical philosophies and techniques in China, with a mix of itinerant physicians, village herbalists or native shamans. There were also the Taoist philosopher-doctors, who produced the classic medical texts and who would have been the first choice, in sickness, for the aristocracy.

MODERN CHINESE MEDICINE

By the 19th century, Western mission hospitals had begun to represent a real alternative to the old practices. Chinese medicine survived, but became a national, standard medical system only in the 1960s when Mao Tse-tung founded five colleges of traditional Chinese medicine.

Today, older regional healing styles persist among traditional Korean, Vietnamese and Japanese practitioners; classic styles are also followed by surviving Chinese medical families, many of whom have emigrated to Hong Kong, Singapore and San Francisco.

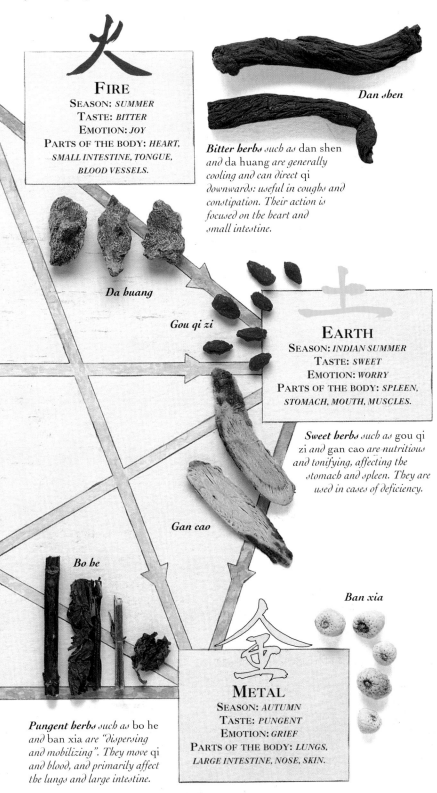

FIRE
SEASON: *SUMMER*
TASTE: *BITTER*
EMOTION: *JOY*
PARTS OF THE BODY: *HEART, SMALL INTESTINE, TONGUE, BLOOD VESSELS.*

Dan shen

Bitter herbs such as dan shen *and* da huang *are generally cooling and can direct* qi *downwards: useful in coughs and constipation. Their action is focused on the heart and small intestine.*

Da huang

Gou qi zi

EARTH
SEASON: *INDIAN SUMMER*
TASTE: *SWEET*
EMOTION: *WORRY*
PARTS OF THE BODY: *SPLEEN, STOMACH, MOUTH, MUSCLES.*

Sweet herbs such as gou qi zi *and* gan cao *are nutritious and tonifying, affecting the stomach and spleen. They are used in cases of deficiency.*

Gan cao

Bo he

Ban xia

METAL
SEASON: *AUTUMN*
TASTE: *PUNGENT*
EMOTION: *GRIEF*
PARTS OF THE BODY: *LUNGS, LARGE INTESTINE, NOSE, SKIN.*

Pungent herbs such as bo he *and* ban xia *are "dispersing and mobilizing". They move* qi *and blood, and primarily affect the lungs and large intestine.*

The Practice of Chinese Medicine

HEATING VERSUS COOLING

Chinese medicine also identifies five tastes which can be characterized as hot or cold: pungent and sweet tastes are both deemed to be heating, while sour, bitter and salty tastes are more cooling. Some herbs combine several different flavours: the name *wu wei zi* (schisandra berries) literally means "five-taste fruit".

These characteristics also influence which part of the body the herb will affect. Hot things rise or float, for example, so pungent and sweet herbs tend to affect the upper and exterior parts of the body. Cold things sink, so the sour, bitter and salty herbs are more effective for the lower half or interior of the body. In the treatment of arthritis, for example, the Chinese will often add *qiang huo* to the mixture if the pain is in the shoulders or arms, while *du huo* is preferred if hips or knees are affected. Both of these herbs would be used if the entire body were affected.

Pungent tastes are also stimulating, sour ones cause contraction, sweet are tonifying, bitter are used to send *qi* downwards, while salty tastes are softening.

Gui zhi, or cinnamon twig, is the Minister or supporting herb, helping to increase sweating, and ease pains in the limbs.

Ma huang is the Emperor, or principal therapeutic herb, which relieves coughs and smooths the flow of qi.

Chinese prescription for ma huang tang
This typical Chinese decoction is used for some types of common cold. Prescriptions always contain particular categories of ingredients that have specific actions. They are assigned "names", or roles to play.

Gan cao, or liquorice root, is the Harmonizer, helping to meld the formula together; here, it also acts as the Messenger, directing the actions of the other herbs to their appropriate meridians.

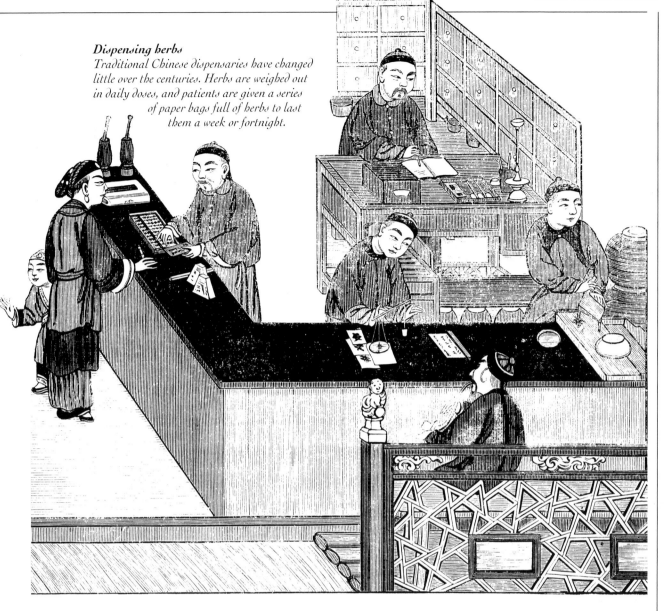

Dispensing herbs
Traditional Chinese dispensaries have changed little over the centuries. Herbs are weighed out in daily doses, and patients are given a series of paper bags full of herbs to last them a week or fortnight.

Xing ren, or apricot seed, acts as the Assistant, helping to ventilate the lungs.

HOW HERBS ARE PRESCRIBED

The Chinese usually prescribe herbs in standard formulae (there are several thousand in regular use), and these may be adjusted slightly depending on the specific condition affecting the patient. The formulae might include just two herbs or as many as twenty, and the interaction between the different plants is just as significant as their individual properties. The result is often a potent brew that can have a dramatic, therapeutic effect, but generally defies any rational scientific explanation.

Herbs are generally given as pills, powders or, most commonly, in the form of decoctions or "soups" which patients brew up at home for an hour or so in special earthenware crocks kept for the purpose. Sometimes the herbs may be cooked with rice to produce a porridge-like therapeutic meal.

HERBS IN HERBALS

In traditional Chinese herbals, the characteristics of a plant always include taste, dominant temperature, and generally an indication of the organ and meridians that it affects. These are sometimes obviously related: Chinese gold thread (*huang lian*), for example, is a very bitter herb; it is cold and linked to the heart – characteristics that can be traced directly to the five-element model. It may be used in conditions associated with too much heat in the heart, which in traditional Chinese medicine would lead to insomnia, palpitations and hot flushes.

Bai shao yao is sour and widely used for liver problems – both of which are aspects of the element wood – while many nutritious herbs, such as rice or oats, and major tonics like ginseng, are characterized as sweet and are good for the stomach and spleen.

OUT OF THE DARK AGES

AFTER THE FALL OF ROME, European herbal traditions were not completely submerged by the ensuing Dark Ages. The "barbarians" brought with them their own herbal healing customs to add to the Roman practices that survived and, with the spread of Christianity, there was considerable exchange of both actual medicines and tried-and-tested remedies. Throughout the Middle Ages, the Church played a significant role both in cultivating physic gardens and in introducing new herbs. With the advent of the printing press, Classical knowledge spread from the confines of the cloister to complement the folk medicine and household herbal remedies passed through the generations.

The Growth of European Herbalism

ANGLO-SAXON HERBALS
Europe's oldest surviving herbal written in the vernacular, *The Leech Book of Bald*, dates from the first half of the 10th century, and includes remedies sent by the Patriarch of Jerusalem to King Alfred. Numerous treatments are described for ailments caused by "flying venom" and "elfshot", thought to be responsible for a wide range of sudden or wasting illnesses. Among the most popular herbs in Saxon times were wood betony, vervain, mugwort, plantain and yarrow, taken in many internal remedies but more often worn as amulets to ward off the evil eye.

Although medical schools spread through Europe (the most famous, at Salerno, was founded in the early 10th century and taught the Hippocratic principles of good diet, exercise and fresh air), healing and herbalism were largely in the hands of the Church, with all monasteries growing physic herbs and tending the sick as part of Christian duty. Healing was as much a matter of prayer as medicine, and early herbals frequently combine religious incantations with infusions, concluding that with "God's help" the patient would be cured.

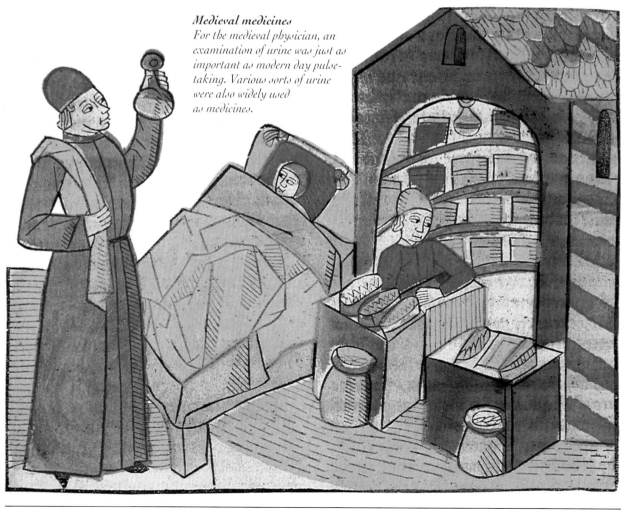

Medieval medicines
For the medieval physician, an examination of urine was just as important as modern day pulse-taking. Various sorts of urine were also widely used as medicines.

PARACELSUS

As learning moved away from the cloister, emphasis was gradually again given to the healing skills and disciplines once taught at the Salerno school. By the 1530s, Paracelsus (born Philippus Theophrastus Bombastus von Hohenheim, near Zürich in 1493) was revolutionizing European attitudes to health care. As much an alchemist as a physician, he insisted on lecturing in German instead of the usual Latin. He regarded most apothecaries and physicians as crooked conspirators intent upon milking the public; condemning the complex and often lethal purgatives and emetics they prescribed, he urged a return to simpler medicines inspired by the Doctrine of Signatures.

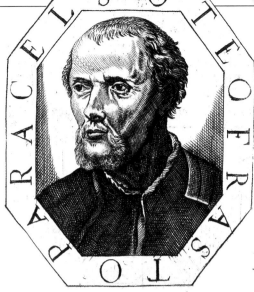

The leaves of lungwort were said to resemble diseased lungs, so the plant was used for bronchitis and tuberculosis.

Many yellow-flowered plants were linked with jaundice, so toadflax, greater celandine and dandelion were used for liver disorders.

Doctrine of Signatures

Paracelsus was a supporter of the Doctrine of Signatures, which maintained that the outward appearance of a plant gave an indication of the ailments it would cure. At times the theory was surprisingly accurate. Similar theories still prevail in Africa.

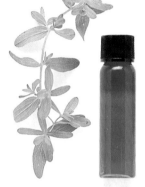

The tiny oil sacs in St. John's wort leaves look like holes, while extracts from the plant are blood-red: signs that it will be good for wounds.

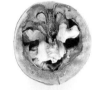

Nutmeg and walnuts were compared to the brain and thought helpful for strengthening mental activity.

The round leaves of lady's mantle were compared to the cervix.

Illustrated Herbals

HERBAL WARFARE

Paracelsus was followed by physicians such as William Turner, who wrote in English so that "the apothecaries and old wives that gather herbs" would understand which plants physicians really meant by their Latin prescriptions, and would not put "many a good man by ignorance in jeopardy of his life". Nicholas Culpeper (1616-54) was later to adopt a similar view, earning the wrath of the newly formed College of Physicians by translating their *Pharmacopoeia* into English so that ordinary people could find herbal medicines in the hedgerows instead of paying vastly inflated apothecaries' bills.

The battles between physicians, apothecaries and "herb wives" raged through the 17th and 18th centuries as medicine came more and more under the control of the academic physicians, with their university training, while dispensing was strictly regulated by the apothecaries. The emphasis was on expensive and complex nostrums using ingredients such as mercury and antimony.

REMEDIES FROM AFAR

By the time that the great herbals of Gerard (1597), Parkinson (1640) and Culpeper (1653) appeared, numerous new herbs were starting to be imported from the East Indies and North America. Plants such as yucca, nasturtium and nutmeg began to appear in the herbals, often accompanied by imaginative applications and claims for their medicinal properties. Tea is a classic example: proclaimed as a cure-all in the 17th century, it is now regarded by many as no more than a popular drink.

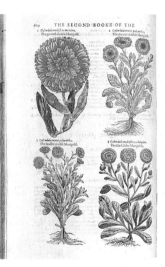

Medicinal marigolds

Gerard describes 10 types of marigold, including the "double globe marigold". He recommended marigold conserve as a preventative "in time of plague".

NORTH AMERICAN TRADITIONS

THE FIRST EUROPEAN SETTLERS arriving in North America brought with them the familiar healing plants from home: heartsease and plantain, also known as "white man's foot" because it was soon found growing wherever the settlers penetrated. They also absorbed some Native American healing traditions, discovering new herbs such as boneset, purple coneflower,

goldenseal and pleurisy root. Several of the American tribes also made great use of sauna-like sweat houses, and the idea of heat as a healing technique was adopted by Samuel Thomson (see below). This melding of traditions bore fruit in the Physiomedical and Eclectic schools, which were later imported into Europe and had a lasting influence on European herbal practices.

Ritual Herbalism

MAGIC & MEDICINE

Native American herbalism was shamanistic – it centred on the activities of the medicine man, or shaman. Through the use of drums and rattles and the smoking of mixtures of tobacco or peyote, the shaman would enter a trance-like state that enabled him to "spirit-travel" and seek out the soul of the sick person in order to rescue and heal it. Today, shamans in South America still use extracts taken from a particular vine – known in Colombia as *yage* and in Peru and Ecuador as *ayahuasca* – in this way, just as Siberian shamans were once able to "travel" by taking fly agaric toadstool or European witches to "fly" with the help of deadly nightshade, henbane, thorn-apple or mandrake.

The Native Americans also made ritual use of the medicine wheel, and assigned animal totems to the four cardinal directions; they also equated these with different personality types, spiritual energies, diseases and plant medicine. Typically, for example, the South was symbolized by the coyote and the energies of growth and compassion, while the eagle and the powers of wisdom and enlightenment were symbols of the East.

The sweat house
In the sauna-like sweat houses of the Native Americans, the ill person was encouraged to perspire to rid the body of toxins and bacteria.

The shaman
The medicine man, or shaman, would "spirit-travel" in the symbolic directions of the medicine wheel to seek the soul of the sick person and find spirit help for healing.

Merging of Practices

PHYSIOMEDICALISM

Before land battles with the plains tribes decimated the indigenous population, the early pioneers and Native Americans shared much of their herbal lore with each other. An early enthusiast was Samuel Thomson, who founded the Physiomedical movement. Born in New Hampshire in 1769, Thomson learned his craft as a child from Widow Benton, a "root and herb doctor" who combined Native American skills with the traditional role of "herb wife".

Thomson believed that parents were responsible for both their own and their children's health, and patented "Thomson's Improved System of Botanic Practice of Medicine", a mixture of handbooks and patent remedies which swept America in the early 19th century. Thomson's principal theory was that "all disease is caused by cold", which in the bitter New England winters may well have been accurate. By the late 1830s, he claimed three million followers.

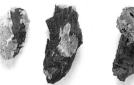

Black root *is used as a relaxant for the liver.*

Indian tobacco *is an important Physiomedical relaxant.*

Fringe tree bark *is relaxing and stimulating for the liver and gall bladder.*

Founder of Physiomedicalism
Samuel Thomson started using herb and sweat-house therapies in his twenties after his mother had been "galloped out of the world in nine weeks" by orthodox treatment. He used many of the Native American herbs shown here.

Cayenne *is classified as a stimulant.*

Black cohosh *is stimulating and relaxing for the nervous system.*

Blue cohosh *is a stimulating relaxant for the female reproductive organs.*

True unicorn root *is a uterine stimulant.*

MAINTAINING BALANCE

Central to the Physiomedical view was the belief that it is possible to strengthen the body's "vital force" by keeping both tissues and nervous state in balance. The key therapeutic treatment involved relaxing or astringing tissues, and then stimulating or sedating nerves. Suitable herbs, classified as either stimulating or sedating, relaxing or astringing, were used to achieve this balance. Irritable bowel syndrome, for example, might be treated with chamomile to sedate the nervous system and relax the digestive tissues, followed by an astringent like agrimony and a stimulant such as ginger in order to encourage the vital force and internal energy levels once more.

ECLECTICISM

Other "botanic" systems followed, among them the Eclectic school founded by Dr. Wooster Beech in the 1830s. Like the Thomsonians, the Eclectics also used herbal remedies and Native American healing practices, but combined these with more orthodox medical techniques in their analysis of disease. At its peak, Eclecticism claimed more than 20,000 qualified practitioners in the United States and was a serious rival to regular medicine. The challenge ended only in 1907 when, following a review of medical training schools, philanthropists Andrew Carnegie and John D. Rockefeller decided to give financial support solely to the orthodox medical schools.

THE MOVEMENT IN EUROPE

Thomsonian Physiomedicalism was brought to Britain in 1838 by Dr. Albert Isaiah Coffin, who set up a similar "system" of patent remedies and do-it-yourself guides to diagnosis. Wooster Beech followed in the 1850s to preach his Eclectic message, and the movement took hold in working-class areas of the country, remaining popular, in the North especially, until well into the 1930s.

In 1864, the various groups merged to form the National Association of Medical Herbalists. The association continues to thrive today as the National Institute of Medical Herbalists – the oldest formalized body of specialist herbal practitioners in Europe.

FROM PLANTS TO PILLS

ALTHOUGH EXTRACTS, such as essential oils, have been prepared from various plants for centuries, traditional herbalism has always combined herbs to modify effects, viewing the whole as greater than the parts. The move to identify the individual active ingredients and use these as single drugs began in the 18th century, and many thousands are now known. These chemicals display quite different properties from the original herbs.

Initially, these drugs could only be obtained from plant extracts but later the chemical structures of many extracts were identified and the drugs are now made synthetically. In the transition from the use of crude plants to clinical pills, modern medicine has lost the art of combining herbs to modify toxicity and of using whole plants, which themselves contain chemical ingredients that can reduce the risk of side effects.

Herbs in Modern Medicine

THE FOXGLOVE CURE

According to tradition, a physician, William Withering, persistently failed to bring about an improvement in a patient suffering from severe dropsy caused by heart failure. Suddenly, the patient started to recover. His relatives admitted administering a herbal brew based on an old family recipe and, in 1775, Dr. Withering began experimenting with the various herbs it contained, identifying foxglove as the most significant. In 1785, he published his *Account of the Foxglove and Some of its Medical Uses.* This detailed 200 cases of dropsy and heart failure that he had successfully treated with the herb, along with research notes on the parts of the plant producing the strongest effects and when to harvest it to achieve these.

Withering also realized that the therapeutic dose of foxglove is very close to the quantity at which toxic side effects develop, so great care was needed in its administration. Further analysis followed, and the cardiac glycosides digoxin and digitoxin were eventually extracted. These are still used in treating heart conditions today.

William Withering
Before publishing his ground-breaking research, Withering spent 10 years studying the side effects of foxglove and identifying the plant's optimum dose.

Foxgloves and pills
The common foxglove is still used to produce digitoxin.

DRUGS FROM PLANTS

One of the first modern drugs to be isolated from a plant was morphine, first identified in 1803 by Friedrich Serturner in Germany. He extracted white crystals from crude opium poppy. Similar techniques soon produced aconitine from monkshood, emetine from ipecacuanha, atropine from deadly nightshade, and quinine from Peruvian bark. All of these compounds, categorized as alkaloids, are extremely potent, and could only be obtained from the raw plants until scientists were able to synthesize them.

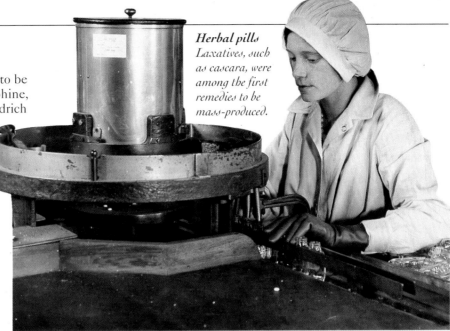

Herbal pills
Laxatives, such as cascara, were among the first remedies to be mass-produced.

SYNTHESIZED SUBSTANCES

The breakthrough came in 1852 when salicin, identified as one of the active ingredients in willow bark, was artificially synthesized for the first time. This was later modified to be less irritant on the stomach, and acetylsalicylic acid was launched in 1899, as aspirin, by the drug company Bayer.

In less than 100 years, plant extracts have filled pharmacists' shelves. There are many ephedrine preparations from *ma huang*, for example, both prescription and over-the-counter, which are mainly used for coughs, catarrh, hay fever or asthma. Pilocarpine, obtained from jaborandi, is used for treating glaucoma; vincristine, from the Madagascar periwinkle, is used for leukaemia; while strophanthin from *Strophanthus kombé*, found in tropical Africa and used to tip poison arrows, is taken for severe heart problems.

CHEMICAL POWER

Extracted chemicals can often be extremely potent, and can cause effects that were unknown when the whole plant was used. Indian snakeroot, *Rauwolfia serpentina*, for example, has been used for centuries in Ayurvedic medicine for a range of ailments including snakebites, anxiety, headaches, fevers and abdominal pains. Mahatma Gandhi reputedly drank snakeroot tea at night if he felt over-stimulated. In the West, snakeroot was valued as a potent tranquillizer and was used for high blood pressure; it was also prescribed in the treatment of schizophrenia and psychosis.

In 1947, CIBA extracted the alkaloid reserpine from snakeroot and began marketing the drug Serpasil as a cure for hypertension. However, resperine has unfortunate side effects that include severe depression and abnormal slowing of the heartbeat. By the 1960s, the herb had been restricted to the status of a prescription-only drug in Britain and its use by herbalists is thus effectively banned. To this day, however, snakeroot continues to be widely used in other parts of Europe and Asia, taken by many as a soothing tranquillizer.

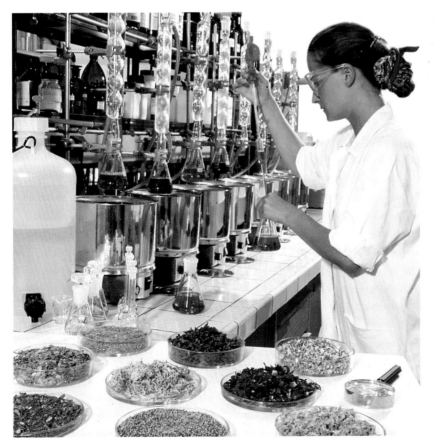

High-tech herbalism
In mainland Europe, herbal remedies are widely used in conventional medicine. Production is as streamlined and clinical as in any modern pharmaceutical plant.

MEDICINAL MEALS

TODAY'S CATEGORIZATION OF PLANTS as herbs, vegetables, fruits and even "weeds" is a recent invention. To the 17th-century cook, cabbage, carrots and cucumbers were all "kitchen herbs" just as marigolds or marjoram were. We often forget, too, that the active constituents, such as alkaloids or saponins, in "herbs" are not confined to the plants we label as such; fruits and vegetables can also be both therapeutic or, in excess, damaging. Past cultures have classified foods by temperature or taste, matched to the body's needs to maintain balance: Hippocrates noted that fresh foods "give more strength" because they are more alive, while Tibetan medicine regards frozen foods as colder and more mucus-forming than their fresh originals.

Galenical Menu-making

"One good old fashion is not yet left off, viz to boil fennel with fish: for it consumes that phlegmatic humour which fish most plentifully afford and annoy the body with, though few that use it know wherefore they do it."
Nicholas Culpeper, 1653.

Classifications of foods
Hippocrates first classified foods into hot, cold, dry or damp categories in around 420 BC. (Some examples are shown below.) Galen and others later expanded these ideas into a complex classification in which many foods were considered to belong to more than one category: apples, for example, were both cold and damp.

THERAPEUTIC FOODS
Galen and his followers labelled not only what we term "herbs" as hot or cold, dry or damp, but "foods" as well. In the Galenical system, meat tended to be heating, fish was damp, fresh beans and apples cold and moist, wheat generally hot and moist, and so on.

Food intake was considered to have a direct action on the four humours: blood, phlegm, yellow bile and black bile. For example, eating too many cold, moist foods would encourage the phlegmatic humour, and this could lead to catarrh. Too many hot, dry foods,

on the other hand, encouraged the choleric humour (yellow bile), with resulting liver or skin problems.

The medieval housewife would automatically balance the character of different ingredients, cooking fish with "hot and dry" fennel, or adding pepper to "cold and moist" beans, and she would have been quite appalled at the thought of serving strawberries in the middle of winter, as we are able to do now: such a cold fruit would inevitably lead to stomach chills if eaten at such a time. Today we have lost sight of this sense of balance, eating foods regardless of climate.

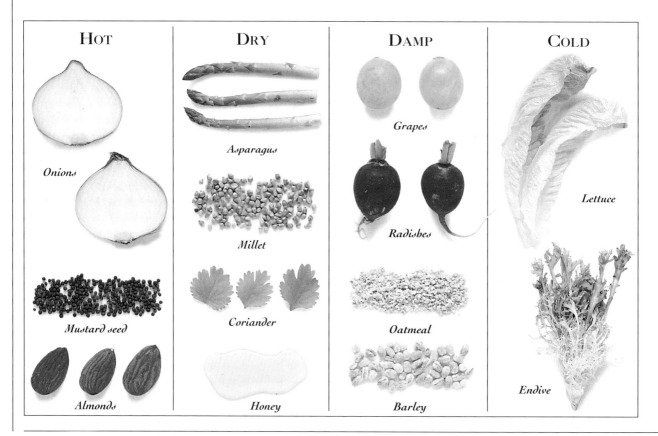

HOT	DRY	DAMP	COLD
Onions	Asparagus	Grapes	Lettuce
Mustard seed	Millet	Radishes	Endive
Almonds	Coriander	Oatmeal	
	Honey	Barley	

The Taste of Health

"From food are born all creatures, which live upon food and after death return to food. Food is the chief of all things. It is therefore said to be the medicine of all diseases of the body."
The Upanishads, *c.* 500 BC.

The six tastes
In Ayurveda, all foods and herbs can be classified in terms of the six tastes. Selected examples for each of the categories are shown below.

BALANCING TASTES
In Ayurvedic medicine, taste is all-important and different foods can be categorized according to the six defined tastes. These are believed to act on the body to increase or decrease the three humours: *kapha* (water or phlegm), *pitta* (fire or bile) and *vata* (air or wind).

The humours are regarded as the waste products of digestion – consequently, if food intake is too heavily biased towards one or other of the humours, imbalance and illness can follow. A healthy diet has to contain a good mixture of the six tastes, while in ill health, particular tastes can be emphasized to restore balance. The correct combination of tastes is also considered so essential for growth and normal development that special herbal pills containing all six tastes are regularly given to children.

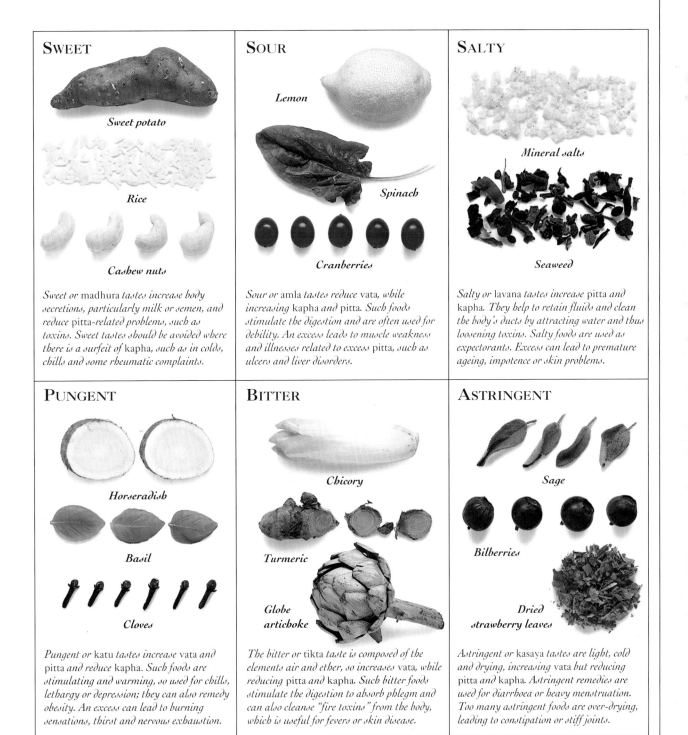

SWEET
Sweet potato

Rice

Cashew nuts

Sweet or madhura *tastes increase body secretions, particularly milk or semen, and reduce* pitta-*related problems, such as toxins. Sweet tastes should be avoided where there is a surfeit of* kapha, *such as in colds, chills and some rheumatic complaints.*

SOUR
Lemon

Spinach

Cranberries

Sour or amla *tastes reduce vata, while increasing* kapha *and* pitta. *Such foods stimulate the digestion and are often used for debility. An excess leads to muscle weakness and illnesses related to excess pitta, such as ulcers and liver disorders.*

SALTY
Mineral salts

Seaweed

Salty or lavana *tastes increase* pitta *and* kapha. *They help to retain fluids and clean the body's ducts by attracting water and thus loosening toxins. Salty foods are used as expectorants. Excess can lead to premature ageing, impotence or skin problems.*

PUNGENT
Horseradish

Basil

Cloves

Pungent or katu *tastes increase* vata *and* pitta *and reduce* kapha. *Such foods are stimulating and warming, so used for chills, lethargy or depression; they can also remedy obesity. An excess can lead to burning sensations, thirst and nervous exhaustion.*

BITTER
Chicory

Turmeric

Globe artichoke

The bitter or tikta taste is composed of the elements air and ether, so increases vata, *while reducing* pitta *and* kapha. *Such bitter foods stimulate the digestion to absorb phlegm and can also cleanse "fire toxins" from the body, which is useful for fevers or skin disease.*

ASTRINGENT
Sage

Bilberries

Dried strawberry leaves

Astringent or kasaya *tastes are light, cold and drying, increasing* vata *but reducing* pitta *and* kapha. *Astringent remedies are used for diarrhoea or heavy menstruation. Too many astringent foods are over-drying, leading to constipation or stiff joints.*

Balancing Yin and Yang

"To take medicine only when you are sick is like digging a well only when you are thirsty – is it not already too late?" Ch'i Po, *c.* 2500 BC.

HARMONIZING ENERGIES

A balanced diet in Chinese terms is not necessarily one with the right amounts of proteins, vitamins, fats or sugars, but one that balances the body's energies and so ensures that the correct relationship between *yin* and *yang* is maintained.

Foods are classified according to the five-element model (see pp. 14-15), with five flavours – sweet, pungent, sour, bitter, and salty – and five temperatures: hot, cold, warm, cool, and neutral. Many foods are also related to particular organs and acupuncture meridians just as Chinese herbs are. Cool, bitter and salty foods are more *yin*

in character, while hot, sweet and pungent foods are more *yang*. Most fruits, for example, are considered very *yin* in character, similar to the "cold and damp" classification in Galenical medicine.

In a hot, dry climate, *yin* can be adversely affected, so eating an adequate quantity of fruit is one way of feeding this type of energy. The tourist from the cold north who heads for the tropics in the depths of winter is a fairly *yin* individual to start with since he or she comes from a cold, damp climate. In the unfamiliar tropical temperatures, such a person may be tempted to "cool off" by eating too many mangos, melons, paw-paws and pomelos, which pushes *yin* energies into excess and results in the cold-moist type of diarrhoea that mars so many holidays.

Just as in the Galenical or the Ayur-vedic systems, the Chinese may categorize people according to their physical constitution – those who are predominantly hot or cold, dry or damp. For example, a "hot" person, who opens windows and walks around in a T-shirt on a cold autumn day, may be thirsty and prone to boils, acne, hot flushes or constipation; he or she should eat more cold, bitter foods (such as celery), and avoid pungent foods (such as onions) that tend to be more heating and drying.

The temperature of foods
The Chinese assign foods to the five temperatures or energies. Hot foods, for example, encourage heat so, while suitable for "cold" individuals, could be contra-indicated for those who tend to be "hot" by nature.

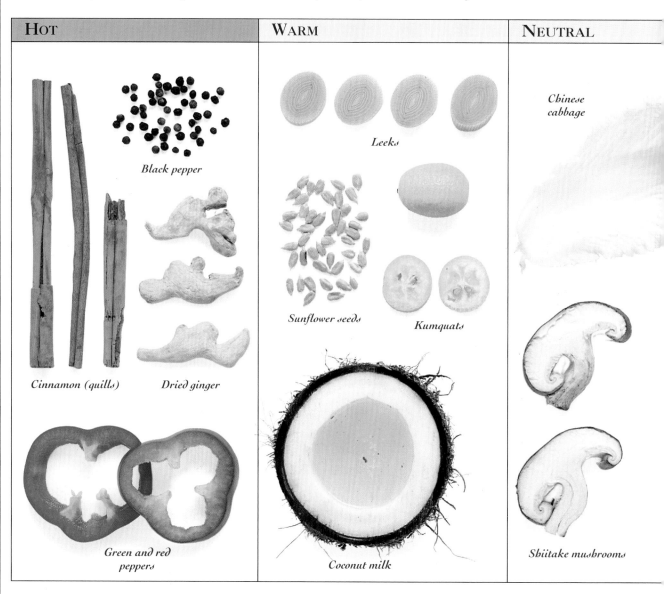

HOT	WARM	NEUTRAL

Black pepper

Cinnamon (quills)   *Dried ginger*

Green and red peppers

Leeks

Sunflower seeds   *Kumquats*

Coconut milk

Chinese cabbage

Shiitake mushrooms

EATING FOR HEALTH

The idea of hot and cold foods still persists in the traditional cookery of China, and therapeutic restaurants, where diners are able to select dishes to balance their own particular energy needs, are found throughout the Far East. The emphasis is upon eating particular food types to maintain balance and prevent disease. Foods are not intrinsically "good" or "bad": what matters is how they affect each individual.

In the West, many fashionable "diets" run a great risk of imbalance as the faddists eliminate entire categories of food from their diet, weakening particular aspects of their vital energies and essence. Too little meat, for example, can weaken *yang* energies, while too much can put *yin* under pressure.

Coffee

Bitter *Associated with the heart; cool and drying; used to reduce fevers and dry excess body fluids.*

Lemon

The five tastes
These are linked to the five-element model. Salt, for example, is associated with the kidneys, water and coldness. Excess increases dampness, while a deficiency leads to dryness and hardening of the tissues. Many foods have more than one taste.

Date

Sour *Associated with the liver; thought to obstruct movement; taken for diarrhoea or excessive sweating.*

Sweet *Associated with the stomach; encourages weight gain; slows down and eases acute symptoms.*

Rock salt

Garlic

Salty *Considered stimulants; used to soften hard swellings, such as enlarged lymph nodes or hardened muscles.*

Pungent *Associated with lungs and skin; used to encourage the circulation of qi (energy), and to increase sweating.*

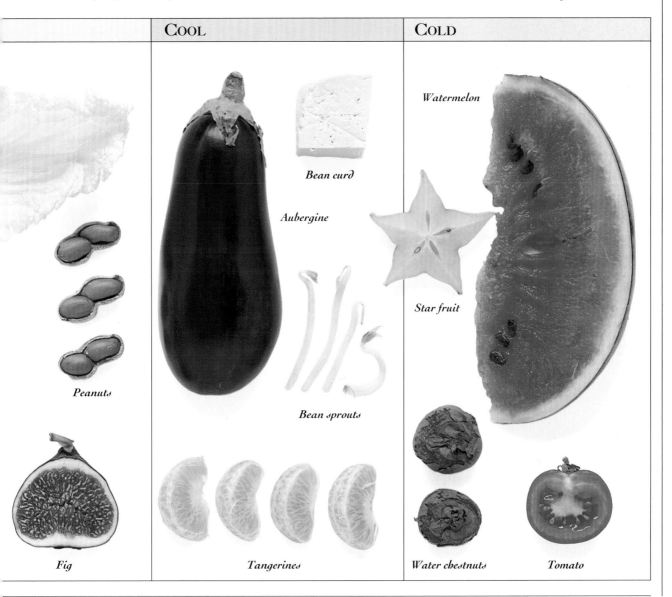

COOL	COLD

Bean curd

Aubergine

Watermelon

Star fruit

Peanuts

Bean sprouts

Fig

Tangerines

Water chestnuts

Tomato

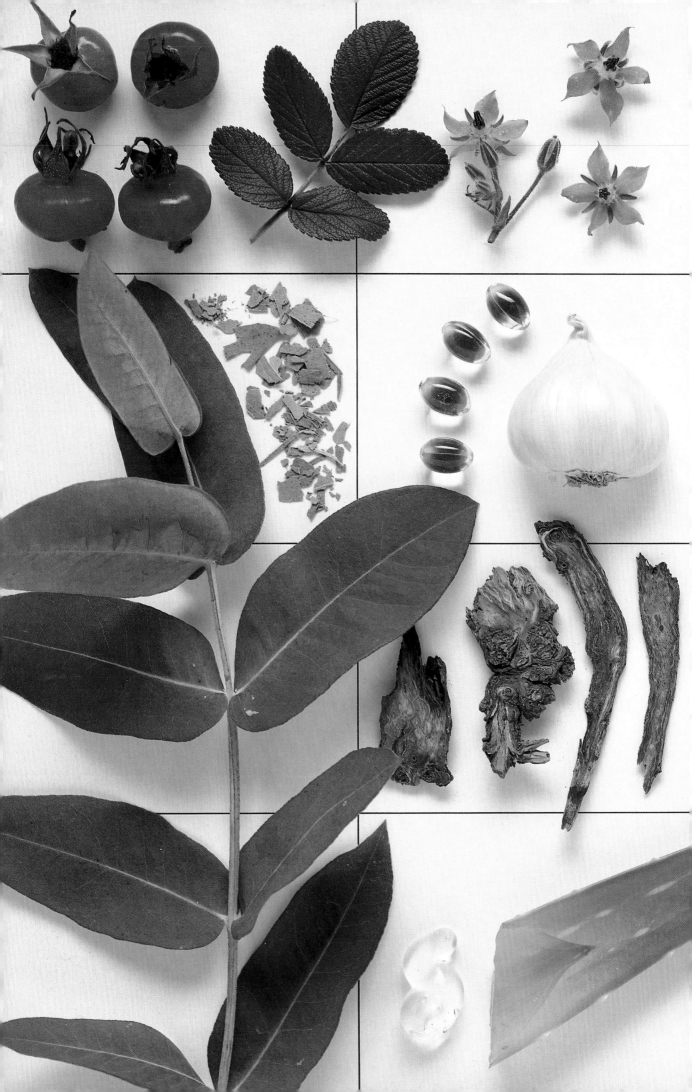

A-Z OF
MEDICINAL
HERBS

The herbs in this index include a representative
selection of the many thousands of plants with
medicinal properties, and show the range of herbal
remedies available. Each entry gives details of the parts
used, actions, active ingredients and character, based on
traditional Western, Ayurvedic (classical Indian) or
Chinese classification. There are also suggested
applications; before using these, refer to the ailment-
by-ailment guides in *Home Remedies* (pp. 128-79) or to
Other Medicinal Herbs (pp. 180-2). All preparations
and dosages are standard (pp. 120-5)
unless otherwise specified. Do not
take essential oils internally
unless directed.

Achillea millefolium
YARROW

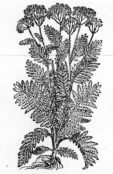

"Most men say, that the leaves chewed, and especially greene, are a remedie for toothach."
John Gerard, 1597.

THE PLANT'S LATIN NAME is derived from the Greek hero Achilles, and during the Trojan wars, yarrow was reputedly used to treat wounds. A folk name, "nosebleed", confirms its traditional first aid use as an emergency styptic to stop bleeding. Today, yarrow is valued mainly for its action in colds and influenza, and also for its effect on the circulatory, digestive and urinary systems. The plant can usually be found growing among grass in meadows.

Character
Cool, dry; sweet, astringent, slightly bitter taste.
Constituents
Volatile oil (inc. proazulenes), isovalerianic acid, salicylic acid, asparagin, sterols, flavonoids, bitters, tannins, coumarins.
Actions
Aerial parts: astringent, promote sweating, relax peripheral blood vessels, digestive stimulant, restorative for menstrual system, febrifuge.
Essential oil: anti-inflammatory, anti-allergenic, antispasmodic.

Parts used

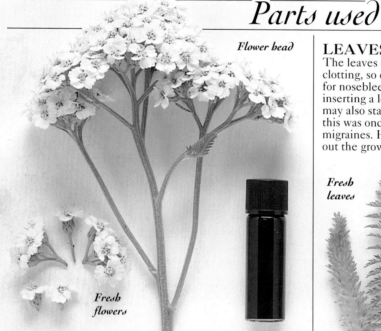

Flower head

Fresh flowers

FLOWERS
Rich in chemicals that are converted by steam into anti-allergenic compounds, the flowers are used for various allergic catarrhal problems, including hay fever. Harvest during summer and autumn.

ESSENTIAL OIL
The dark blue oil, extracted by steam distillation of the flowers, is generally used as an anti-inflammatory or in chest rubs for colds and influenza.

LEAVES
The leaves encourage clotting, so can be used fresh for nosebleeds. However, inserting a leaf in the nostril may also start a nosebleed; this was once used to relieve migraines. Harvest throughout the growing season.

Fresh leaves

Dried aerial parts

AERIAL PARTS
Used for catarrhal conditions, as a bitter digestive tonic to encourage bile flow, and as a diuretic. They act as a tonic for the blood, stimulate the circulation, and can be used for high blood pressure. Also useful in menstrual disorders, and as an effective sweating remedy to bring down fevers. Harvest during flowering.

Applications

FLOWERS

 INFUSION Drink for upper respiratory catarrh or use externally as a wash for eczema.

INHALATION For hay fever and mild asthma, use fresh in boiling water.

ESSENTIAL OIL

MASSAGE OIL For inflamed joints, dilute 5-10 drops yarrow oil in 25 ml infused St. John's wort oil.

CHEST RUB For chesty colds and influenza, combine with eucalyptus, peppermint, hyssop or thyme oils, diluting a total of 20 drops oil in 25 ml almond or sunflower oil.

LEAVES

FRESH To stop a nosebleed, insert a leaf into the nostril.

POULTICE Bind washed, fresh leaves to cuts and grazes.

AERIAL PARTS

 INFUSION Use to reduce fevers and as a digestive tonic.

TINCTURE Use for urinary disorders or menstrual problems. Prescribed for cardiovascular complaints.

COMPRESS Soak a pad in the infusion or dilute tincture to soothe varicose veins.

CAUTIONS
• In rare cases, yarrow can cause severe allergic skin rashes; prolonged use can increase the skin's photosensitivity.
• Avoid large doses in pregnancy as the herb is a uterine stimulant.

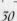

Agrimonia spp.
AGRIMONY

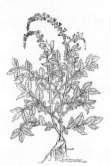

*"If it be leyd under mann's heed,
He shal sleepyn as he were deed,
He shal never drede ne wakyn,
Till fro under his heed it be takyn."*
Medieval medical manuscript.

MAINLY VALUED TODAY as a healing herb for the mucous membranes and for its astringent properties to stop bleeding, *A. eupatoria* has been used since Saxon times for wounds. In the 15th century, it was the prime ingredient of "arquebusade water", a battlefield remedy for gunshot wounds. This healing power is now attributed to the herb's high silica content. A related variety, *A. pilosa*, known as *xian he cao* in China, is used in a similar way.

Character
Cool, drying; bitter, astringent taste.
Constituents
Tannins, silica, essential oil, bitter principle, flavonoids, minerals, vitamins B, K.
Actions
Astringent, diuretic, tissue healer, stops bleeding, stimulates bile flow, some anti-viral activity reported.
A. PILOSA: also antiparasitic and antibacterial.

Parts used

AERIAL PARTS
A. EUPATORIA
A cooling astringent, the aerial parts can be used for "hot" conditions, including diarrhoea, bronchitis and urinary infections; to clear inflammations, phlegm and toxins, and encourage healing. Good for skin inflammations and ulcers, they stem bleeding from cuts. Gather before and during early flowering in summer.

Fresh aerial parts

Dried aerial parts

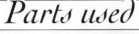

Tincture

Dried aerial parts

AERIAL PARTS
A. PILOSA
As well as stopping bleeding, the Chinese variety has antibacterial and antiparasitic actions and is used for *Trichomonas vaginalis*, tapeworms, dysentery and malaria.

Applications

AERIAL PARTS/LEAVES
A. EUPATORIA

 INFUSION A gentle remedy, ideal for diarrhoea, especially in infants and children. Can be taken by breast-feeding mothers to dose babies.

 TINCTURE More potent and drying than the infusion, and effective if the condition involves excess phlegm or mucus. Use for cystitis, urinary infections, bronchitis and heavy menstrual bleeding.

POULTICE Apply a poultice of the leaves for migraines.

WASH Use the infusion for wounds, sores, eczema and varicose ulcers.

EYEWASH Use a weak infusion (10 g herb to 500 ml water) for conjunctivitis.

GARGLE Use the infusion for sore throats and nasal catarrh.

AERIAL PARTS
A. PILOSA

 DECOCTION Used in China for heavy uterine bleeding, blood in the urine, dysentery and digestive parasites.

COMPRESS Soak a pad in the decoction and use for boils.

DOUCHE Cool and strain the decoction, and use for *Trichomonas vaginalis*.

CAUTION
• As the herb is astringent, do not take if suffering from constipation.

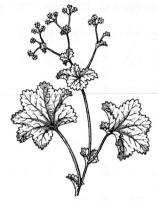

Alchemilla vulgaris
LADY'S MANTLE

REMINISCENT OF THE VIRGIN'S cloak in medieval paintings, the leaves with scalloped edges are reputed to have given lady's mantle its name. Like many herbs with "lady" or "mother" as part of their common name, it is a valuable gynaecological herb, specifically for heavy menstrual bleeding and vaginal itching. Highly astringent and rich in tannins, it was one of the most popular wound herbs on the battlefields of the 15th and 16th centuries.

"It is one of the most singular wound herbs and therefore highly prized and praised, used in all wounds, inwards and outwards."
Nicholas Culpeper, 1653.

Character
Cool, dry; bitter, astringent taste.
Constituents
Tannins, salicylic acid, saponins, phytosterols, volatile oil, bitter principle.
Actions
Astringent, menstrual regulator, digestive tonic, anti-inflammatory, heals wounds.

Parts used

AERIAL PARTS
The astringent aerial parts are good for gastroenteritis and diarrhoea. As well as helping to control heavy periods, they can be used for period pain, to regulate the cycle, and for vaginal discharges. They are cooling, and useful in inflammation and infections. Harvest while flowering in summer.

Fresh aerial parts

Tincture

Dried aerial parts

Ointment

Applications

AERIAL PARTS

 INFUSION Use for gastroenteritis or diarrhoea: take up to five times daily for acute symptoms.

TINCTURE Use for period pain, menstrual irregularities and menopausal problems.

OINTMENT To relieve vaginal itching, combine 50 g ointment base with around 20 ml rosewater and 15 ml of the infusion or tincture, and use night and morning.

WASH Apply the infusion externally for weeping eczema or sores.

MOUTHWASH/GARGLE Use the infusion for sore throats, laryngitis and mouth ulcers.

DOUCHE Use the infusion for vaginal discharges and itching.

 PESSARIES Use for vaginal discharges and itching. Combine 20 drops tincture with 20 g cocoa butter to make 12-16 pessaries, depending on mould size.

CAUTIONS
• Avoid the herb in pregnancy as it is a uterine stimulant.
• Seek professional advice for any sudden or abnormal change in uterine bleeding.

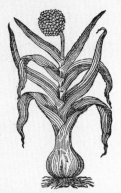

Allium sativum
GARLIC

PRIZED FOR AT LEAST 5,000 years, garlic has long been known to reduce blood cholesterol levels. Even orthodox medicine acknowledges that the plant reduces the risk of further heart attacks in cardiac patients; it is also a stimulant for the immune system and an antibiotic. Garlic's strong odour is largely due to sulphur-containing compounds, which account for most of its medicinal properties; deodorized preparations are significantly less effective.

"...in men oppressed by melancholy it will... send up... many strange visions to the head: therefore, inwardly, let it be taken with great moderation."
Nicholas Culpeper, 1653.

Character
Very hot, dry, pungent.
Constituents
Volatile oil with sulphur-containing compounds (notably allicin, alliin and ajoene); enzymes, B vitamins, minerals, flavonoids.
Actions
Antibiotic, expectorant, promotes sweating, reduces blood pressure, anticoagulant, reduces blood cholesterol levels, reduces blood sugar levels, antihistaminic, antiparasitic.

Parts used

CLOVES
The cloves are used widely for infections, especially chest problems, digestive disorders, and fungal infections such as thrush. They are a good long-term remedy for cardiovascular problems, reducing excessive blood cholesterol levels, atherosclerosis, and the risk of thromboses; they also dilate peripheral blood vessels, lowering blood pressure. Garlic also helps regulate blood sugar levels, and so can be helpful in late-onset diabetes. Topically, the cloves are effective for skin infections and acne. Best used fresh.

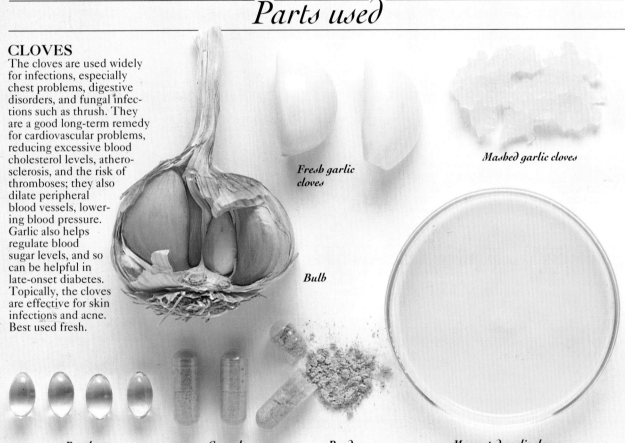

Fresh garlic cloves

Mashed garlic cloves

Bulb

Pearls

Capsules

Powder

Macerated garlic cloves

Applications

CLOVES

FRESH Rub on acne, or mash and use on warts and verrucas, or to draw corns. Add the cloves regularly to the diet as a prophylactic against infection, to reduce high cholesterol levels, to improve the quality of the cardiovascular system and help lower blood sugar levels. Eat crushed cloves (3-6 daily in acute conditions) for severe digestive disorders (gastroenteritis, dysentery, worms), and infections.

JUICE Drink for digestive disorders and infections, or to combat atherosclerosis.

MACERATION Steep 3-4 garlic cloves in water or milk overnight and drink the liquor the next day for intestinal parasites.

CAPSULES Garlic powder can be made into capsules as an aromatic alternative to commercial "pearls". Clinical trials suggest that 2 g powder in capsules daily can prevent further heart attacks in those who have already suffered one attack. Taking the capsules daily can also combat infections, including thrush.

PEARLS Use as an alternative to capsules. The more "deodorized" the pearls, the less effective they are.

CAUTIONS
• Garlic is very heating and can irritate the stomach.
• While culinary quantities are generally safe, do not take garlic in therapeutic doses during pregnancy and lactation; it can cause digestive problems such as heartburn, and babies may dislike the taste in breast milk.
• Garlic's strong aromatic compounds are excreted via the lungs and the skin; eating fresh parsley may eliminate odour on the breath.

Aloe vera
ALOE

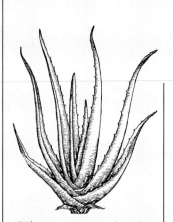

"There are many uses for it, but the chief is to relax the bowels, for it is almost the only laxative that is also a stomach tonic..."
Pliny, AD 77.

THE ALOE ORIGINATES from tropical Africa, where related species are used as an antidote to poison arrow wounds. It was known to the Greeks and Romans, who also used the gel for wounds; one of Pliny's many recommendations was to rub leaves on "ulcerated male genitals". Aloe was a favourite purgative during the Middle Ages. In China, similar uses developed to those in the West, although only the gel is used; in India, the gel is a highly regarded cooling tonic. Aloe reached the West Indies in the 16th century and is widely cultivated there.

Character
Leaves: bitter, hot, moist.
Gel: salty, bitter, cool, moist.
Constituents
Anthraquinone glycosides, resins, polysaccharides, sterols, gelonins, chromones.
Actions
Purgative, promotes bile flow, heals wounds, tonic, demulcent, antifungal, stops bleeding, sedative, expels worms.

Parts used

GEL
The thick mucilaginous gel is an ideal home first-aid cure for burns, wounds and sunburn. It is also useful for any dry skin condition, especially eczema around the eyes and sensitive facial skin, and can be used for treating fungal infections such as ringworm. In Ayurvedic medicine, the gel is an important tonic for excess *pitta* (fire).

Gel

Ointment

The gel *is usually applied fresh: it can be converted into an ointment for long-term use.*

Fresh leaf

LEAVES
A strong purgative, the leaves are good for chronic, stubborn constipation. They stimulate bile flow and the digestion, and can be useful for poor appetite. Extracts of leaves were once used on children's fingers to stop them biting their nails. Aloes can be grown as a houseplant in temperate climates.

Powdered leaf　　*Capsules*

Applications

GEL

 FRESH Apply the split leaf directly to burns, wounds, dry skin, fungal infections and insect bites. Take up to 2 tsp in a glass of water or fruit juice, three times a day, as a tonic.

 OINTMENT Split several leaves to collect a large quantity of gel, and boil it down to a thick paste. Store in clean jars in a cool place and use as the fresh leaves.

TONIC WINE Fermented aloe gel with honey and spices is known as *kumaryasava* in India, and is used as a tonic for anaemia, poor digestive function and liver disorders.

INHALATION Use the gel in a steam inhalation for bronchial congestion.

LEAVES

TINCTURE Use 1-3 ml per dose as an appetite stimulant or for constipation. The taste is unpleasant.

 POWDER Use 100-500 mg per dose or in capsules as a purgative for stubborn constipation and to stimulate bile flow.

CAUTIONS
• Avoid in pregnancy as the anthraquinone glycosides are strongly purgative.
• High doses of the leaves can cause vomiting.

Althaea officinalis
MARSHMALLOW

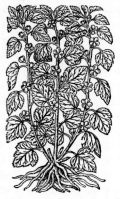

"... whoever swallows daily half a cyathus of the juice of any one of them [the mallows] will be immune to all diseases."
Pliny, AD 77.

TAKING ITS BOTANICAL NAME from a Greek word, *altho*, meaning "to heal", marshmallow has been used since Ancient Egyptian times. The root, rich in sugars, is very mucilaginous and softening for the tissues. The leaves are not as mucilaginous as the root and are used as an expectorant and as a soothing remedy for the urinary system. Both leaves and root have been used as a vegetable. All members of the mallow family have similar properties, with varieties such as garden hollyhocks and common mallow occasionally used medicinally as well.

Character
Cool, moist, sweet.
Constituents
Flowers: mucilage, flavonoids.
Leaves: mucilage, flavonoids, coumarin, salicylic and other phenolic acids.
Root: mucilage, polysaccharides, asparagin, tannins.
Actions
Flowers: expectorant.
Leaves: expectorant, diuretic, demulcent.
Root: demulcent, expectorant, diuretic, heals wounds.

Parts used

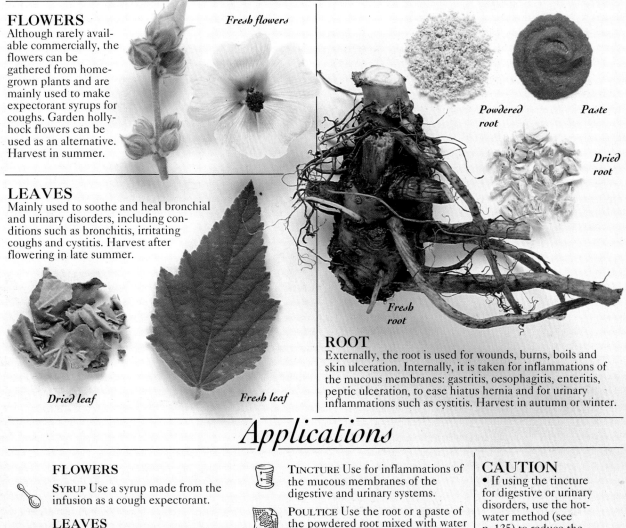

FLOWERS
Although rarely available commercially, the flowers can be gathered from home-grown plants and are mainly used to make expectorant syrups for coughs. Garden hollyhock flowers can be used as an alternative. Harvest in summer.

Fresh flowers

Powdered root   *Paste*

Dried root

LEAVES
Mainly used to soothe and heal bronchial and urinary disorders, including conditions such as bronchitis, irritating coughs and cystitis. Harvest after flowering in late summer.

Fresh root

Dried leaf   *Fresh leaf*

ROOT
Externally, the root is used for wounds, burns, boils and skin ulceration. Internally, it is taken for inflammations of the mucous membranes: gastritis, oesophagitis, enteritis, peptic ulceration, to ease hiatus hernia and for urinary inflammations such as cystitis. Harvest in autumn or winter.

Applications

FLOWERS
SYRUP Use a syrup made from the infusion as a cough expectorant.

LEAVES
INFUSION Use for bronchial and urinary disorders.

ROOT
DECOCTION For inflammations such as oesophagitis and cystitis, use 25 g root to 1 litre water, and boil down to about 750 ml. This may need further dilution.

TINCTURE Use for inflammations of the mucous membranes of the digestive and urinary systems.

POULTICE Use the root or a paste of the powdered root mixed with water for skin inflammations and ulcers.

OINTMENT For wounds, skin ulceration, or to help draw splinters, melt 50 g anhydrous lanolin, 50 g beeswax and 300 g soft paraffin together, then heat 100 g powdered marshmallow root in these liquid fats for an hour over a waterbath. When cool, stir in 100 g powdered slippery elm bark.

CAUTION
• If using the tincture for digestive or urinary disorders, use the hot-water method (see p. 125) to reduce the alcohol.

Angelica spp.
ANGELICA

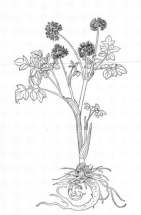

"A water distilled from the root... eases all pains and torments coming of cold and wind…"
Nicholas Culpeper, 1653.

THE LIQUEUR BENEDICTINE derives its distinctive flavour from *A. archangelica*, a tall biennial. The candied stalks and roots were traditionally taken as a tonic to combat infection and improve energy levels. Several other species are used in Eastern medicine, including *A. sinensis* (*dang gui*), one of the most important of the great Chinese tonic herbs, used in many patent remedies as a nourishing blood tonic and to regulate the menstrual cycle. Many over-the-counter preparations based on *dang gui* are available in the West.

Character
Sweet, pungent, warm, generally drying.
Constituents
Volatile oil, bitter iridoids, resin, coumarins, valerianic acid, tannins, bergapten; vitamins A and B also reported in Chinese species.
Actions
A. ARCHANGELICA: carminative, antispasmodic, promotes sweating, topical anti-inflammatory, expectorant, diuretic, digestive tonic, anti-rheumatic, uterine stimulant.
A. SINENSIS: blood tonic, circulatory stimulant, laxative.

Parts used

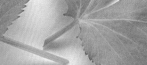

LEAVES
A. ARCHANGELICA
Mainly used for indigestion and bronchial problems, the leaves are generally considered less heating and more gentle than the root. Harvest in summer.

Cream

Fresh leaves

Dried leaves

ROOT
A. ARCHANGELICA
Used for digestive and bronchial problems, to stimulate the appetite and liver, to relieve rheumatism and arthritis, and promote sweating in chills and influenza. As a uterine stimulant, the root has been used in prolonged labour or retention of the placenta. Harvest in the autumn of the first year.

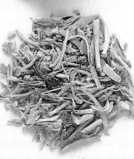

Dried root

ROOT
A. SINENSIS
The root, *dang gui*, is valuable in anaemia, period pain, or as a general tonic after childbirth. It clears liver stagnation (of both energy and toxins), and can relieve constipation, especially in the elderly.

Dried dang gui

Applications

LEAVES
A. ARCHANGELICA

INFUSION Take in standard doses for indigestion.

TINCTURE Take up to 3 ml, three times a day, for bronchitis or flatulent digestion.

CREAM Apply to skin irritations.

ROOT
A. ARCHANGELICA

TINCTURE Take for bronchial catarrh, chesty coughs, digestive disorders or as a liver stimulant.

COMPRESS Soak a pad in the hot diluted tincture or decoction and apply to painful rheumatic or arthritic joints.

MASSAGE OIL Dilute up to 10 drops angelica oil in 25 ml almond or sunflower oil for arthritic or rheumatic pains.

ROOT
A. SINENSIS

DECOCTION Take for anaemia, menstrual irregularities, period pain, liver stagnation, or weakness after childbirth.

CAUTIONS
• Avoid regular or large doses in pregnancy, as it is a uterine stimulant, and in diabetes (because of sugar content).
• Angelica is heating, so can be contraindicated in "hot" conditions.
• The oil can increase photosensitivity, so avoid excess exposure to sunshine if using angelica externally.

Apium graveolens
CELERY

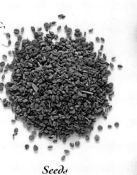

A FAMILIAR AND POPULAR VEGETABLE, celery is also an important medicinal herb. In Eastern medicine, it is categorized as bitter-sweet, making it moist and cooling, and thus good for balancing hot, spicy dishes. The whole plant is gently stimulant, nourishing, and restorative for weak conditions. In the past, celery was grown as a vegetable for winter and early spring; because of its anti-toxic properties, it was a cleansing tonic after the stagnation of winter. A homeopathic extract of the seeds is widely used in France to relieve retention of urine.

"The plant is one of the herbs which is eaten in the spring, to sweeten and purify the blood."
Nicholas Culpeper, 1653.

Character
Slightly cool, moist, bitter-sweet.
Constituents
Volatile oil, glycosides, furanocoumarins, flavonoids.
Actions
Antirheumatic, sedative, urinary antiseptic, increases uric acid excretions, carminative, reduces blood pressure, some anti-fungal activity reported.

Parts used

SEEDS
Mainly used as a diuretic, these help clear toxins from the system, so are especially good for gout, where uric acid crystals collect in the joints, and arthritis. Slightly bitter, they act as a mild digestive stimulant. Harvest after the plant flowers in its second year.

Seeds

ESSENTIAL OIL
Distilled from the seeds, the essential oil is more potent therapeutically. Use with care.

STALK
This shares the medicinal properties of other parts of the plant to a lesser extent. Eating fresh stalks can help stimulate milk flow after birth. Although wild celery is more effective, commercially grown varieties can be used.

ROOT
Rarely used today, the root is an effective diuretic and has been taken for urinary stones and gravel. It also acts as a bitter digestive remedy and liver stimulant.

Tincture

Stalk

Applications

SEEDS
INFUSION For rheumatoid arthritis and gout, combine 2 tsp celery seeds with 1 tsp *lignum vitae*, and add 1/2 tsp to a cup of boiling water.

ESSENTIAL OIL
OIL For painful gout in the feet or toes, add 15 drops oil to a bowl of warm water, and soak the feet.

MASSAGE OIL Dilute 5-10 drops celery oil in 20 ml almond or sunflower oil, and massage into arthritic joints.

ROOT
TINCTURE In the past used mainly as a diuretic in hypertension and urinary disorders, as a component in arthritic remedies, or as a kidney energy stimulant and cleanser.

WHOLE PLANT
JUICE Liquidize the whole fresh plant (seeds, root, stalks and leaves) and drink the juice for joint and urinary tract inflammations, such as rheumatoid arthritis, cystitis or urethritis, for weak conditions and for nervous exhaustion.

CAUTIONS
• Bergapten in the seeds could increase photosensitivity, so do not apply the essential oil externally in bright sunshine.
• Avoid the oil and large doses of the seeds in pregnancy, as they can act as a uterine stimulant.
• Do not buy seeds intended for cultivation, as they are often treated with fungicides.

Arctium lappa
BURDOCK

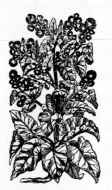

"They are but burs, cousin, thrown upon thee in holiday foolery." As You Like It, William Shakespeare, 1599.

ONCE WIDELY USED in cleansing remedies, burdock is familiar for its hooked burrs, which readily attach themselves to clothing. This property is reflected in the herb's botanical name, from the Greek *arktos*, or bear, suggesting rough-coated fruits, and *lappa*, to seize. Burdock was a traditional blood purifier, often combined in folk brews such as dandelion and burdock wine, and it was once popular for indigestion. In China, the seeds, *niu bang zi*, are used to dispel "wind and heat evils"; they also lower blood sugar levels.

Character
Root/Leaves: cool, drying, bitter; root is slightly sweet.
Seeds: cold, pungent, bitter.
Constituents
Root/Leaves: glycosides, flavonoids, tannins, volatile oil, polyacetylenes, resin, mucilage, inulin, alkaloids, essential oil.
Seeds: essential fatty acids, vitamins A, B$_2$.
Actions
Root: alterative, mild laxative, diuretic, promotes sweating, antirheumatic, antibiotic.
Leaves: mild laxative, diuretic.
Seeds: prevent fever, anti-inflammatory, antibacterial, reduce blood sugar levels.

Parts used

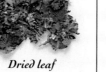

Fresh leaf

ROOT
Western herbalists consider the root the most important part of burdock, and use it as a cleansing, eliminative remedy whenever there is a build-up of toxins leading to skin problems, digestive sluggishness or arthritic pains. Also used externally for skin sores and infections. Harvest in autumn.

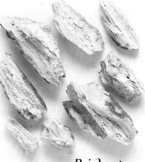

Dried root

SEEDS
American Eclectics (see p. 21) used the seeds for skin diseases and as a diuretic. In China, the seeds are regarded as suitable for common colds characterized by a sore throat and unproductive cough. Harvest when ripe in late summer.

LEAVES
Generally less effective than the root, the large leaves can be used in very similar ways. They are particularly good for stomach problems including indigestion and general digestive weakness. Harvest before or during early flowering.

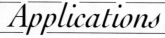

Dried leaf

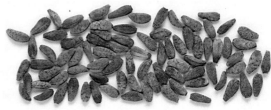

Niu bang zi

Applications

ROOT

 DECOCTION Use for skin disorders, especially persistent boils, sores, and dry, scaling eczema.

 TINCTURE Use in combination with arthritic, digestive herbs such as yellow dock to detoxify the system and stimulate the digestion; also for urinary stones and gravel.

POULTICE Apply to skin sores and leg ulcers.

 WASH Use the decoction for acne and fungal skin infections such as athlete's foot and ringworm.

LEAVES

INFUSION Use for indigestion (take in wine-glass doses before meals) and as a mild digestive stimulant.

POULTICE Apply to bruises and skin inflammations, including acne.

INFUSED OIL Make by the hot infusion method (see p. 122), and use for varicose ulcers.

SEEDS

DECOCTION Take for feverish colds with sore throat and cough. Use with heartsease for skin eruptions.

Artemisia absinthium & A. vulgaris
WORMWOOD & MUGWORT

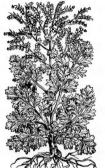

"...eldest of worts... for venom availest, for flying vile things, mighty gainst loathed ones..."
The Lacnunga, 9th century.

THESE TWO RELATED HERBS ARE highly regarded medicinally in both East and West. The Anglo-Saxons listed mugwort as one of the "nine sacred herbs" given to the world by the god Woden. It was also reputedly planted along roadsides by the Romans, who put sprigs in their sandals to prevent aching feet on long journeys. Both herbs are bitter digestive remedies, and many bitter aperitifs such as vermouth contain wormwood as a digestive stimulant. As its name implies, wormwood is also used to expel parasitic worms.

Character
Bitter, pungent, drying, quite cold.
Constituents
Volatile oil (inc. sesquiterpene lactones and thujone), bitter principle, flavonoids, tannins, silica, antibiotic polyacetylenes, inulin, hydroxycoumarins.
Actions
A. ABSINTHIUM: bitter digestive tonic, uterine stimulant, expels worms, antibiotic, bile stimulant, carminative, antiseptic.
A. VULGARIS: bitter digestive tonic, uterine stimulant, stimulating nervine, menstrual regulator, antirheumatic.

Parts used

Fresh aerial parts

Fresh aerial parts

Dried aerial parts

AERIAL PARTS
A. ABSINTHIUM
These expel intestinal worms, stimulate the appetite and liver, and also the uterus, so were traditionally used in childbirth. They contain the potentially addictive thujone, which gave the drink absinthe its notorious reputation. Harvest while in flower in late summer.

Dried aerial parts

AERIAL PARTS
A. VULGARIS
A gentle nervine and menstrual regulator, these can be helpful for menopausal and period problems. A bitter digestive remedy, they can also be used in chills and fevers. In the East, sticks of the dried herb (*ai ye*) are burned at the end of acupuncture needles (moxibustion) to clear "cold" and "dampness". Harvest while flowering in late summer.

Moxa stick

Applications

AERIAL PARTS
A. ABSINTHIUM

INFUSION Take a weak infusion (5-10 g herb to 500 ml water) for sluggish digestion, poor appetite and gastritis. Prescribed for jaundice and hepatitis, and to expel intestinal worms.

TINCTURE Use as the infusion, but do not exceed 3 ml daily.

COMPRESS Soak a pad in the infusion to soothe bruises and bites.

WASH Use the infusion externally for infestations such as scabies.

AERIAL PARTS
A. VULGARIS

INFUSION Take for menopausal syndrome or use as a bitter to cool the digestive tract in fever management.

DECOCTION Combine 5 g with an equal amount of dry ginger to make a warming tea for period pain.

TINCTURE Take for period pain, scanty menstruation and prolonged bleeding. Use as a stimulant in liver stagnation and sluggish digestion. In childbirth it is used for prolonged labour and retained placenta.

CAUTIONS
• Avoid both herbs during pregnancy (they are uterine stimulants, and may cause foetal abnormalities) and if breastfeeding (thujone may be passed to the baby in the mother's milk).
• If using the tincture of either herb for liver or digestive disorders, use the hot-water method (see p. 125) to reduce the alcohol.

Avena sativa
OATS

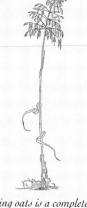

"...taking oats is a complete body overhaul from the inside to the outside."
Peter Holmes, 1989.

THE TRADITIONAL STAPLE of Northern Europe, oats are a warm, sweet food, ideal in a cold climate. Porridge made from oatmeal (the crushed grain) is a nutritious breakfast. For medicinal purposes the whole plant (known as oatstraw) is generally used, and is gathered when the grains are ripe. The herb is a good restorative nerve tonic, ideal for depression and *qi* (energy) deficiency. Recent research has shown that oatbran, and to a lesser extent oatmeal, can help to reduce abnormally high blood cholesterol levels.

Character
Warm, moist, sweet.
Constituents
Saponins, flavonoids, many minerals, alkaloids, steroidal compounds, vitamins B_1, B_2, D, E, carotene, wheat protein (gluten), starch, fat.
Actions
Oatstraw: antidepressant, restorative nerve tonic, promotes sweating.
Grain: antidepressant, restorative nerve tonic, nutritive.
Oatbran: antithrombotic, reduces blood cholesterol levels.

Parts used

OATSTRAW
An excellent tonic for the whole system, used for both physical and nervous debility; it is ideal for depression. Oatstraw can also be used for thyroid and oestrogen deficiency, for degenerative diseases such as multiple sclerosis, and for colds, especially if recurrent or persistent. The crop is harvested when the grain is ripe, and the whole plant dried and chopped.

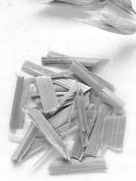

Dried oatstraw

Fresh oats

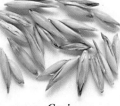

Grain

Oatbran is produced from the coarse husks of the grain; it is particularly good at reducing cholesterol levels.

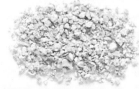

Oatmeal, the ground grains, has a high silica content and can help skin problems if applied externally.

GRAIN
The seeds have very similar properties to the whole plant, and can be used for the same conditions. They are harvested in late summer and milled to produce oatbran and oatmeal.

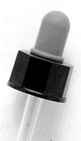

Dr. Bach recommended his Wild Oats flower remedy for times of uncertainty and dissatisfaction.

Applications

OATSTRAW

FLUID EXTRACT Take doses of 2-3 ml for insomnia, anxiety and depression. (The tincture can be used similarly.) Combines well with vervain. Also makes a nutritive addition to remedies for colds and chills to encourage sweating.

DECOCTION Make from the whole dried plant, and use for the same ailments as the fluid extract.

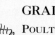
WASH Use the decoction as a healing wash for skin conditions.

GRAIN

POULTICE Use an oatmeal poultice for skin conditions such as eczema, cold sores and shingles.

CAUTION
• For those sensitive to gluten (as in coeliac disease), allow the decoction or tincture to settle, then decant the clear liquid only for use.

Borago officinalis
BORAGE

THE GREAT HERBALIST John Gerard, writing in 1597, quotes the old tag *ego borago gaudia semper ago* ("I, borage, always bring courage"). Modern research has given a new slant to the saying, as the plant is now known to stimulate the adrenal glands, encouraging the production of adrenaline, the "fight or flight" hormone, which gears the body for action in stressful situations. The pretty blue flowers have been added to salads since Elizabethan times to "make the mind glad", a practice that modern cooks can follow.

"...of known virtue to revive the hypochondriac and cheer the hard student."
John Evelyn, 1699.

Character
Cold, moist, slightly sweet.
Constituents
Leaves/Flowers: saponins, mucilage, tannins, vitamin C, calcium, potassium.
Seeds: essential fatty acids, including *cis*-linoleic and γ-linolenic acids.
Actions
Leaves/Flowers: adrenal stimulants, promote lactation, diuretic, febrifuge, anti-rheumatic, promote sweating, expectorant.
Seeds: relieve eczema, anti-rheumatic, relieve irritable bowel syndrome, regulate menstruation.

Parts used

LEAVES
The fleshy, rather coarse leaves can be used as an adrenal tonic for stress or to counter the lingering effects of steroid therapy. They can also be used for dry, rasping coughs and to stimulate milk flow; they may be prescribed in the early feverish stages of pleurisy or whooping cough. Harvest throughout the growing season.

Chopped leaves

Fresh flowers

FLOWERS
Traditionally, these were added to wine to "maketh men merrie", and were also used in cough syrups.

SEEDS
The oil extracted from the seeds is used as an alternative to evening primrose oil for rheumatic or menstrual disorders, and can be applied externally for eczema. It is also available commercially in capsules.

Seeds

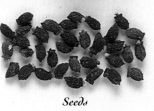

The juice is useful in nervous depression or grief; it also makes a soothing lotion for dry, itching skin.

Seed oil and capsules

Applications

LEAVES

INFUSION Take in the early stages of lung disorders or feverish colds. Lactating mothers may combine it with fennel to stimulate milk.

TINCTURE Take 10 ml, three times a day, as a tonic following steroid therapy and for stress.

JUICE Pulp fresh leaves and drink 10 ml of the juice, three times a day, for depression, grief or anxiety.

LOTION Dilute the juice with an equal volume of water, and use for irritated, dry skin or nervous rashes.

SEEDS

CAPSULES Take 500 mg oil in capsule form daily as a supplement for eczema or rheumatoid arthritis. The oil is also helpful in some cases of menstrual irregularity, for irritable bowel syndrome, or as emergency first aid for hangovers (take 1 g).

FLOWERS

SYRUP Take a syrup made from the infusion as an expectorant for coughs. Can be combined with mullein or marshmallow flowers.

CAUTION
• Restricted herb in Australia and New Zealand.

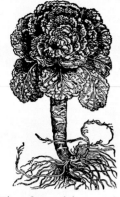

Brassica oleracea
CABBAGE

"The medicine of the poor..."
Dr. Jean Valnet, 1967.

CULTIVATED IN THE WEST since at least 400 BC, cabbage is a valuable medicine. It has been used since Dioscorides' time as a digestive remedy, a joint tonic, and for skin problems and fevers; raw cabbage was eaten by over-indulgent Romans to prevent drunkenness. Known as colewort in folk medicine, cabbage was a standby for all manner of family ills.

Character
Slightly sweet, salty, drying, cool.
Constituents
Minerals, vitamins A, B_1, B_2, C, amino acids, fats.
Actions
Anti-inflammatory, anti-bacterial, antirheumatic, heals tissues by encouraging cells to proliferate, liver decongestant.

Parts used

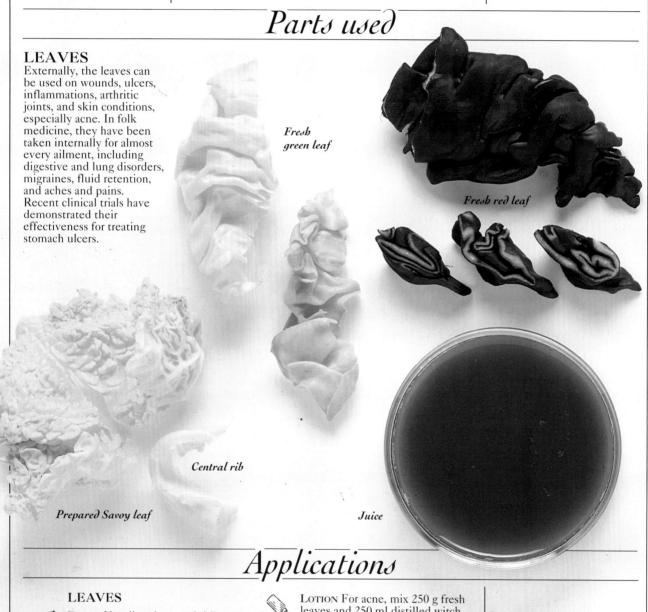

LEAVES
Externally, the leaves can be used on wounds, ulcers, inflammations, arthritic joints, and skin conditions, especially acne. In folk medicine, they have been taken internally for almost every ailment, including digestive and lung disorders, migraines, fluid retention, and aches and pains. Recent clinical trials have demonstrated their effectiveness for treating stomach ulcers.

Fresh green leaf

Fresh red leaf

Central rib

Prepared Savoy leaf

Juice

Applications

LEAVES

FRESH Use directly on arthritic or sprained joints, varicose ulcers and wounds. Strip out the central rib of the leaf first, then beat the leaf gently to soften it slightly and bind on to the area with a bandage. Place prepared leaves in bra cups for mastitis or engorged breasts.

DECOCTION For colitis, boil 60 g leaves in 500 ml water for an hour, and drink in wine-glass doses.

LOTION For acne, mix 250 g fresh leaves and 250 ml distilled witch hazel in a blender. Strain, and add two drops of lemon juice oil: use night and morning.

JUICE Prescribed for gastric or duodenal ulceration.

SYRUP Take a syrup made from the decoction in 10 ml doses for chesty coughs, asthma and bronchitis.

Calendula officinalis
POT MARIGOLD

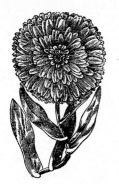

"Somme use it to make theyr here yelow ... not being content with the colour ..."
William Turner, 1551.

THE GOLDEN FLOWERS are a favourite among herbalists. Macer's 12th-century herbal recommends simply looking at the plant to improve eyesight, clear the head and encourage cheerfulness. In Culpeper's day, marigold was taken to "strengthen the heart", and was highly regarded for smallpox and measles. Today, it is widely used in patent homeopathic remedies.

Character
Slightly bitter, pungent, drying, gently cooling.
Constituents
Saponins, flavonoids, mucilage, essential oil, bitter principle, resin, steroidal compounds.
Actions
Astringent, antiseptic, anti-fungal, anti-inflammatory, heals wounds, menstrual regulator, stimulates bile production.

Parts used

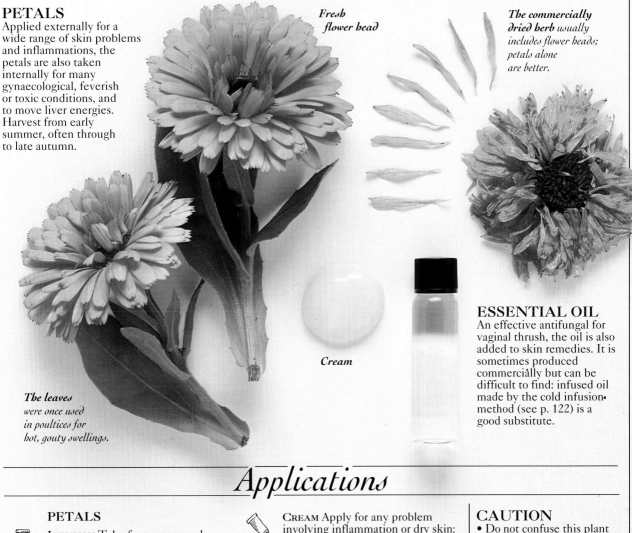

PETALS
Applied externally for a wide range of skin problems and inflammations, the petals are also taken internally for many gynaecological, feverish or toxic conditions, and to move liver energies. Harvest from early summer, often through to late autumn.

Fresh flower head

The commercially dried herb usually includes flower heads; petals alone are better.

Cream

The leaves were once used in poultices for hot, gouty swellings.

ESSENTIAL OIL
An effective antifungal for vaginal thrush, the oil is also added to skin remedies. It is sometimes produced commercially but can be difficult to find: infused oil made by the cold infusion method (see p. 122) is a good substitute.

Applications

PETALS

 INFUSION Take for menopausal problems, period pain, gastritis and for inflammation of the oesophagus.

TINCTURE Take for stagnant liver problems, including sluggish digestion, and also for menstrual disorders, particularly irregular or painful periods.

COMPRESS Apply a pad soaked in the infusion to slow-healing wounds or varicose ulcers.

 MOUTHWASH Use the infusion for mouth ulcers and gum disease.

CREAM Apply for any problem involving inflammation or dry skin: wounds, dry eczema, sore nipples in breastfeeding, scalds and sunburn.

INFUSED OIL Use on chilblains, haemorrhoids and broken capillaries.

ESSENTIAL OIL

PESSARIES Use pessaries containing 2-5 drops each of marigold and tea tree oils, 1-2 times a day, for vaginal thrush.

OIL Add 5-10 drops to bath water for nervous anxiety or depression.

CAUTION
• Do not confuse this plant or its essential oil with preparations made from the French marigold, *Tagetes patula*, and related species. These are used for warts and also as insecticides or weed-killers.

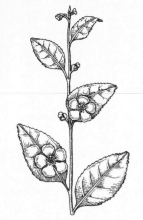

Camellia sinensis
TEA

"Better to be deprived of food for three days, than of tea for one."
Ancient Chinese saying.

KNOWN IN CHINA as *cha*, tea has become such a familiar drink that we forget it is also a potent medicinal herb. The Chinese have been drinking tea since around 3000 BC and regard it as a good stimulant, an astringent for clearing phlegm and a digestive remedy. The three types of tea, green, black and oolong, are made from the leaves of the same plant species. Far Eastern research shows that some green teas appear to reduce the risk of stomach cancer.

Character
Green/Oolong: bitter-sweet, drying, cooling. **Black:** bitter-sweet, drying, warming.
Constituents
Alkaloids (inc. caffeine and theobromine), tannins (polyphenols), catechins, volatile oil, fluoride (in some varieties).
Actions
Stimulant, astringent, antioxidant, antibacterial, diuretic; some varieties reduce blood cholesterol levels; anti-tumour properties reported in green tea.

Parts used

LEAVES
The young, fresh leaves and leaf buds are pan-fried, then rolled or dried to make green tea. The fresh leaves are wilted in sunlight, bruised slightly, then partly fermented for oolong tea. Black tea is a fully fermented variety.

GREEN TEA
Rich in fluoride, green tea can reduce the risk of tooth decay. It is also useful for insect bites and to stem bleeding. The tea has been shown to combat stomach and skin cancers, and to boost the immune system.

OOLONG TEA
Some types, such as *Pu erh*, are especially effective at reducing cholesterol levels after a fatty meal. Japanese research suggests that oolong tea can reduce high blood pressure and limit the risk of arterial disease.

BLACK TEA
Widely drunk in Europe, India and North America, black tea is rich in tannins and highly astringent, so it is a particularly good remedy for diarrhoea.

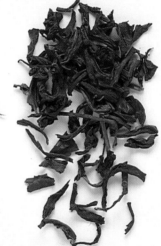
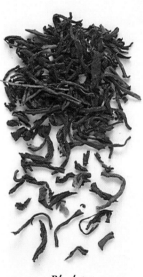

Fresh leaf buds

Fresh leaf

Green tea

Oolong tea

Black tea

Applications

GREEN TEA
INFUSION Drink after meals to help guard against tooth decay.

POULTICE Place damp green tea leaves on insect bites to reduce itching and inflammation.

COMPRESS Use a pad soaked in weak green tea to make an emergency first aid treatment to ease bleeding from cuts and grazes.

OOLONG TEA
INFUSION Drink after fatty meals to reduce cholesterol levels and as a preventative for arterial disease.

BLACK TEA
INFUSION Take a strong infusion of ordinary tea (2 tsp per cup of boiling water, without milk or sugar) for diarrhoea, food poisoning or dysentery. The infusion is also a traditional Cantonese remedy for hangovers.

POULTICE Place used tea bags on tired eyes as a poultice. Damp tea leaves can soothe insect bites.

WASH Use a weak infusion as a cooling wash for sunburn.

CAUTIONS
• Sufferers from an irregular heartbeat, pregnant women and nursing mothers should limit intake to no more than two cups daily, as high levels of caffeine-like alkaloids can lead to increased heart rate.
• People with stomach ulcers should avoid excessive consumption, as the bitter taste can stimulate gastric acid production.

Capsella bursa-pastoris
SHEPHERD'S PURSE

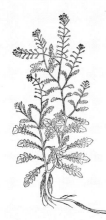

"Few plants possess greater virtues than this, and yet it is utterly disregarded."
Nicholas Culpeper, 1653.

MORE USUALLY CONSIDERED a weed than a medicinal herb, shepherd's purse has its place in both Eastern and Western practice. The heart-shaped seed pods apparently resemble the leather pouches once carried by shepherds, hence the common name; another is "mothers' hearts", a reminder that this is a useful herb for gynaecological conditions. Shepherd's purse is mainly used as a styptic to reduce bleeding; in China, the seeds are said to improve eyesight.

Character
Sweet, dry, cool.
Constituents
Saponins, mustard oil, flavonoids, resin, monoamines, choline, acetylcholine, sitosterol, vitamins A, B, C.
Actions
Astringent, reduces bleeding, urinary antiseptic, circulatory stimulant, reduces blood pressure.

Parts used

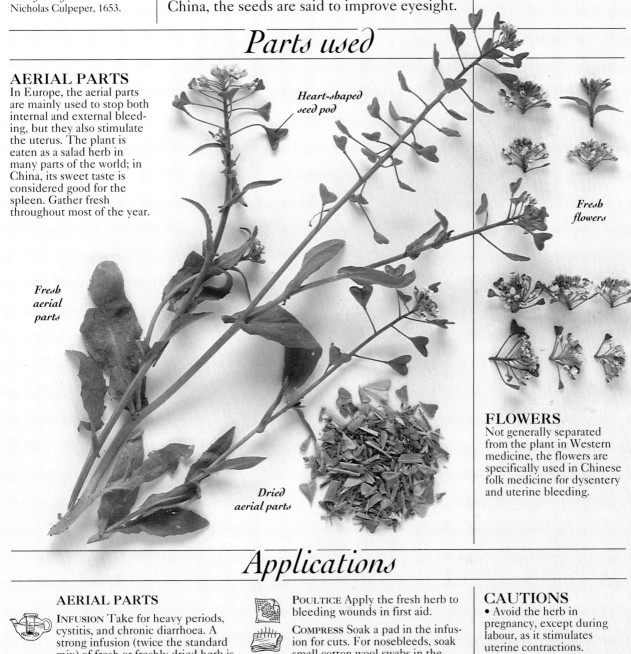

AERIAL PARTS
In Europe, the aerial parts are mainly used to stop both internal and external bleeding, but they also stimulate the uterus. The plant is eaten as a salad herb in many parts of the world; in China, its sweet taste is considered good for the spleen. Gather fresh throughout most of the year.

Heart-shaped seed pod

Fresh flowers

Fresh aerial parts

Dried aerial parts

FLOWERS
Not generally separated from the plant in Western medicine, the flowers are specifically used in Chinese folk medicine for dysentery and uterine bleeding.

Applications

AERIAL PARTS
INFUSION Take for heavy periods, cystitis, and chronic diarrhoea. A strong infusion (twice the standard mix) of fresh or freshly dried herb is best. Sip a hot infusion in labour to stimulate contractions, and after delivery to ease post-partum bleeding.

TINCTURE Take up to 10 ml, three times a day, for heavy periods, cystitis, and diarrhoea.

POULTICE Apply the fresh herb to bleeding wounds in first aid.

COMPRESS Soak a pad in the infusion for cuts. For nosebleeds, soak small cotton wool swabs in the tincture, and insert in the nostril.

CAUTIONS
• Avoid the herb in pregnancy, except during labour, as it stimulates uterine contractions.
• If there is any sudden change in menstrual flow or blood in the urine, seek professional advice before attempting self-medication.

Capsicum frutescens
CAYENNE

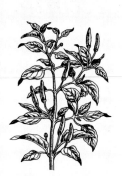

"…it hath in it a malitious qualitie, whereby it is an enemie to the liver and other of the entrails… it killeth dogs."
John Gerard, 1597.

THE HOT RED CAYENNE CHILLI arrived in the West from India in 1548, and was known as Ginnie pepper. Gerard describes it as "extreme hot and dry, even in the fourth degree", and recommends it for scrofula, a prevalent lymphatic throat and skin infection commonly known as the King's Evil. Cayenne was popular with the 19th-century Physiomedicalists (see pp. 20-1), who used its warming properties for chills, rheumatism and depression.

Character
Very hot, pungent, drying.
Constituents
Alkaloids, fatty acids, flavonoids, vitamins A, B_1, C, volatile oil, sugars, carotene pigment.
Actions
Circulatory stimulant, promotes sweating, gastric stimulant, carminative, antiseptic, antibacterial, stimulating nerve tonic. Topical: counter-irritant, increases blood flow to an area.

Parts used

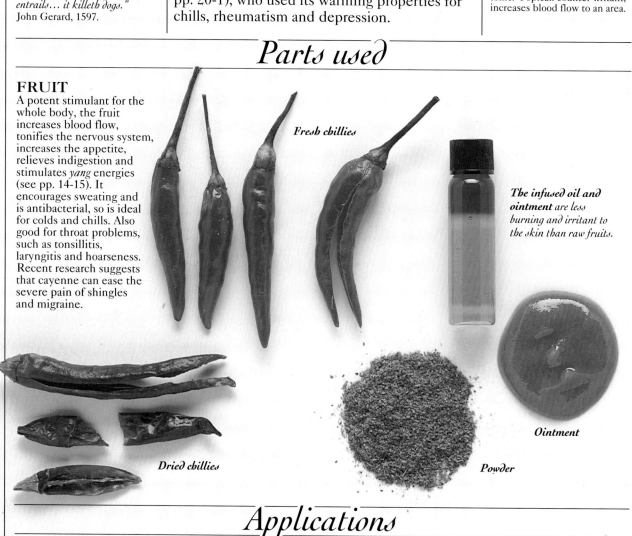

FRUIT
A potent stimulant for the whole body, the fruit increases blood flow, tonifies the nervous system, increases the appetite, relieves indigestion and stimulates *yang* energies (see pp. 14-15). It encourages sweating and is antibacterial, so is ideal for colds and chills. Also good for throat problems, such as tonsillitis, laryngitis and hoarseness. Recent research suggests that cayenne can ease the severe pain of shingles and migraine.

Fresh chillies

The infused oil and ointment are less burning and irritant to the skin than raw fruits.

Ointment

Dried chillies

Powder

Applications

FRUIT

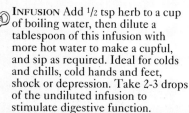

INFUSION Add ¹/₂ tsp herb to a cup of boiling water, then dilute a tablespoon of this infusion with more hot water to make a cupful, and sip as required. Ideal for colds and chills, cold hands and feet, shock or depression. Take 2-3 drops of the undiluted infusion to stimulate digestive function.

TINCTURE Dilute 5-10 drops in half a cup of hot water, and take as a circulatory stimulant and tonic.

COMPRESS Soak a pad in the infusion, and use for rheumatic pains, sprains and bruising.

OINTMENT Use on chilblains, as long as the skin is not broken.

GARGLE Dilute 5-10 drops of tincture in half a tumbler of warm water, and take for throat problems; this is especially useful in weak and deficient conditions.

INFUSED OIL Add 25 g powder to 500 ml sunflower oil, and heat over a waterbath for 2 hours. Apply a little to the skin around a varicose ulcer (not on the ulcer) to encourage blood flow away from the area.

MASSAGE OIL Use the infused oil as a warming massage oil for rheumatism, lumbago and arthritis.

CAUTIONS
• The seeds can be toxic, so do not use them.
• Follow dosages carefully; excessive consumption of cayenne can lead to gastro-enteritis and liver damage.
• Avoid therapeutic doses of cayenne in pregnancy and while breastfeeding.
• Do not leave a compress on the skin for long periods, especially on very sensitive skin, or blistering may occur.
• Avoid touching the eyes or any cuts after handling fresh chillies.

Chamaemelum nobile & Chamomilla recutita
CHAMOMILE

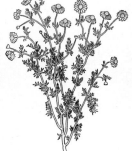

CALLED "GROUND APPLE" by the Ancient Greeks because of its smell, chamomile was "maythen" to the Anglo-Saxons, one of nine sacred herbs given to the world by the god Woden. The two species used medicinally – Roman chamomile (*C. nobile*) and German chamomile (*C. recutita*) – have virtually identical properties and applications. German chamomile used to be known as "matricaria", referring to its role as a gynaecological herb.

"Chamomylle …is very agreeing unto the nature of man, and … is good against weariness…"
William Turner, 1551.

Character
Bitter, mainly warm, moist.
Constituents
Volatile oil (inc. azulenes), flavonoids (inc. rutin), valerianic acid, coumarins, tannins, salicylates, cyanogenic glycosides.
Actions
Anti-inflammatory, anti-spasmodic, bitter, sedative, prevents vomiting.

Parts used

FLOWERS
One home-dried flower can give more flavour than a tea-bag of commercial offerings. Medieval herbalists developed double-flowered varieties to increase the yield of usable parts. Harvest throughout the summer; dry quickly, so that the flowers retain their rich pungent scent for months.

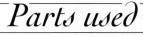

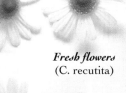
Fresh flowers
(C. recutita)

ESSENTIAL OIL
Distilled from fresh flowers since medieval times, the oil is used for a wide range of complaints including eczema and asthma. True chamomile oil is extremely expensive and is a deep blue because of the azulenes it contains.

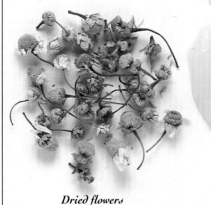

Dried flowers

Ointment

Homeopathic
Chamomilla *tablets or diluted tincture can be helpful for teething and colic in babies, for painful periods or during labour.*

Tincture

Applications

FLOWERS

 INFUSION Take for irritable bowel syndrome, poor appetite and indigestion. Drink a cup at night for insomnia, anxiety and stress. Add 200-400 ml strained infusion to a baby's bath water at night to encourage sleep.

TINCTURE Use for irritable bowel, insomnia and tension.

OINTMENT Use for insect bites, wounds, itching eczema, and for anal or vulval irritation.

MOUTHWASH Use the infusion for mouth inflammations.

EYEWASH Dissolve 5-10 drops of tincture in warm water, and use for conjunctivitis or strained eyes.

INHALATION Add 2 tsp flowers to a basin of boiling water for catarrh, hay fever, asthma or bronchitis.

ESSENTIAL OIL

LOTION For eczema, use 5 drops chamomile oil to 50 ml distilled witch hazel.

INHALATION For bad nasal catarrh, asthma or (under medical super-vision) whooping cough, put 2-3 drops in a saucer of warm water and leave in the room at night.

CAUTIONS
• Do not exceed stated doses of the herb and avoid the oil completely in pregnancy, as it is a uterine stimulant.
• Chamomile can cause contact dermatitis, particularly if sunbathing on damp chamomile lawns.

Cinnamomum spp.
CINNAMON

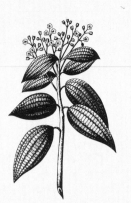

"...there is a tale of cinnamon growing around marshes under the protection of a terrible kind of bats ... invented by the natives to raise the price." Pliny, AD 77.

PUNGENT AND WARMING, cinnamon is good for all sorts of "cold" conditions, from the common cold and stomach chills to arthritis and rheumatism. In the West, we generally use the bark of *C. zeylanicum*, which is sold rolled as the familiar cinnamon sticks. The Chinese prefer the native variety, *C. cassia*, and make use of both the bark (*rou gui*) and the twigs (*gui zhi*). Traditionally, the bark was believed best for the torso, the twigs for the fingers and toes. Research has highlighted hypoglycaemic properties, useful in diabetes.

Character
Bark: pungent, sweet, very hot.
Twigs: pungent, sweet, less hot.
Constituents
Volatile oil, tannins, mucilage, gum, sugars, coumarins.
Actions
Bark & twigs: carminative, promote sweating, warming digestive remedy, antispasmodic, antiseptic, tonic, uterine stimulant.
Essential oil: potent antibacterial, antifungal, uterine stimulant.

Parts used

BARK
In the West, the inner bark is used mainly for digestive upsets: indigestion, general sluggishness, colic and diarrhoea. In China, *rou gui* is considered very warming and tonifying for the kidneys, a good energizing herb for conditions that can be linked to weak kidney *qi* (energy): asthma and menopausal syndrome, for example. The inner bark promotes sweating and can be used for "cold" conditions.

Sticks of inner bark

Gui zhi

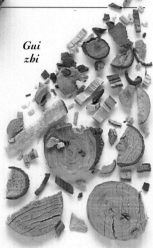

Powdered bark

ESSENTIAL OIL
Distilled from the bark, the oil is used in many parts of the world for a wide range of chronic infections.

TWIGS
Gui zhi can be used as a circulatory stimulant to warm cold hands and feet. It also promotes sweating and is ideal for "cold" conditions.

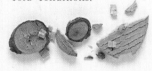

Applications

BARK

 DECOCTION Use for chronic diarrhoea or complaints related to weakened kidney *qi* (energy). Can be used for "cold" conditions.

 TINCTURE Dilute up to 5 ml in a little hot water for colds and chills.

POWDER/CAPSULES Use for "cold" conditions affecting the kidneys and digestion.

ESSENTIAL OIL

 INHALATION Dissolve 5 drops oil in boiling water and inhale the steam for coughs and respiratory irritation.

 MASSAGE OIL Dilute 10 ml cinnamon oil in 25 ml almond or sunflower oil and use for abdominal colic, stomach chills or diarrhoea.

TWIGS

DECOCTION Take for colds, stomach chills, and as a circulatory stimulant. Combines well with ginger.

TINCTURE Dilute up to 5 ml in a little hot water and use as the decoction.

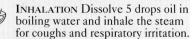 **COMPRESS** Soak a pad in the decoction or diluted tincture to relieve arthritic and rheumatic pain.

CAUTIONS
• Avoid therapeutic doses of cinnamon in pregnancy, especially the essential oil, as the herb is a potential uterine stimulant.
• Use the herb with care in over-heated or feverish conditions.

Citrus spp.
ORANGE

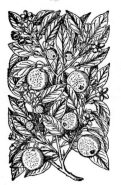

A VALUABLE MEDICINAL HERB, the orange originated in China, and by the Middle Ages was a favourite with Arabian physicians. In the 16th century, an Italian princess named Anna-Marie de Nerola reputedly discovered an oil extracted from the flowers, which she used to scent her gloves; today neroli oil, as it became known, is prohibitively expensive. The Chinese remain the greatest enthusiasts of medicinal oranges: the bitter Seville orange (*C. aurantium*) and sweeter tangerines and satsumas (*C. reticulata*) are mainly used.

"The sweet varieties increase bronchial secretion, and the sour promote expectoration. They quench thirst, and are stomachic and carminative."
Li Shi Zhen, 16th century.

Character
C. AURANTIUM: sour, bitter, slightly cold.
C. RETICULATA: warm, pungent, bitter.
Constituents
Volatile oil, vitamins A, B, C, flavonoids, bitters.
Actions
C. AURANTIUM: carminative, digestive stimulant, nervine, increases blood pressure, diuretic, expectorant, energy tonic.
NEROLI OIL: sedative, tonic, antiseptic, antispasmodic, antidepressant.
C. RETICULATA: diuretic, digestive remedy, expectorant.

Parts used

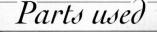

FRUIT
C. AURANTIUM
In China, both the ripe and unripe fruit are used medicinally, although unripe bitter orange (*zhi shi*) is more potent than ripe (*zhi ke*). The fruit stimulates the digestion, so can help constipation, move stagnant *qi* (energy), and make a cooling expectorant for coughs, especially where the phlegm is thick and yellow. It also calms the nerves, so is useful for insomnia and shock.

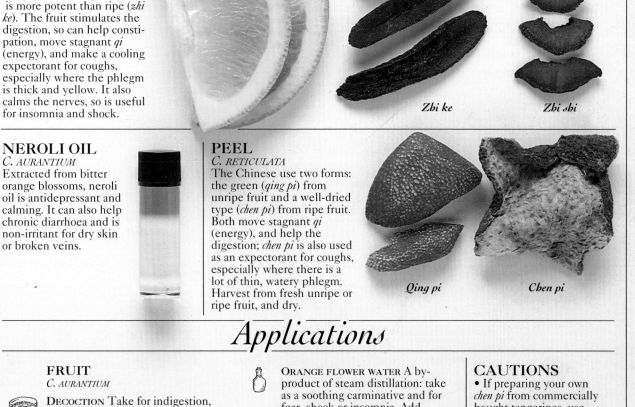

Ripe bitter orange

Zhi ke

Zhi shi

NEROLI OIL
C. AURANTIUM
Extracted from bitter orange blossoms, neroli oil is antidepressant and calming. It can also help chronic diarrhoea and is non-irritant for dry skin or broken veins.

PEEL
C. RETICULATA
The Chinese use two forms: the green (*qing pi*) from unripe fruit and a well-dried type (*chen pi*) from ripe fruit. Both move stagnant *qi* (energy), and help the digestion; *chen pi* is also used as an expectorant for coughs, especially where there is a lot of thin, watery phlegm. Harvest from fresh unripe or ripe fruit, and dry.

Qing pi

Chen pi

Applications

FRUIT
C. AURANTIUM

 DECOCTION Take for indigestion, constipation, or coughs. Combine with *dang gui* for period pain.

TINCTURE Take in drop doses for fear, shock or insomnia.

NEROLI OIL
C. AURANTIUM

CREAM Add 1-2 drops to skin cream and apply to any skin condition.

MASSAGE OIL Add 1-2 drops to 10 ml almond oil for nervous conditions and digestive upsets.

 ORANGE FLOWER WATER A by-product of steam distillation: take as a soothing carminative and for fear, shock or insomnia. Add 5-10 ml to a baby's feed for colic or sleeplessness.

PEEL
C. RETICULATA

DECOCTION Use both types of peel for indigestion and abdominal bloating. Take *chen pi* for coughs.

SYRUP Take 2-4 ml syrup made from *chen pi* for coughs.

CAUTIONS
• If preparing your own *chen pi* from commercially bought tangerines, use organic fruit to minimize pesticide contamination.
• Use bitter orange with caution in pregnancy; it can cause contractions.

Commiphora molmol
MYRRH

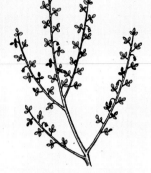

> "The marvellous effects that it worketh in newe and greene wounds, were heere to long to set downe..."
> John Gerard, 1597.

AN OLEO-GUM RESIN collected from the stems of bushy shrubs growing in Arabia and Somalia, myrrh has been regarded as one of the treasures of the East for millennia. The ancient Egyptian housewife burned myrrh in pellets to rid her home of fleas. In folk tradition, myrrh was used for muscular pains and in rheumatic plasters. Called *mo yao* in China, it has been used since at least the Tang Dynasty (AD 600), primarily as a wound herb and blood stimulant.

Character
Hot, dry, acrid, bitter.
Constituents
Volatile oil, resin, gums.
Actions
Antifungal, antiseptic, astringent, immune stimulant, bitter, expectorant, circulatory stimulant, anticatarrhal.

Parts used

RESIN
The stems are cut, exuding a thick pale yellow liquid. As it dries, this hardens to a reddish-brown solid, which can be dissolved in tinctures and oils. Astringent, the resin has been used extensively for wounds, and is also excellent for sore throats and mouth ulcers. Research suggests that it can lower blood cholesterol levels. In China, it is taken to "move" blood and relieve painful swellings. Myrrh tastes particularly unpleasant.

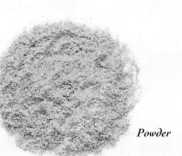
Powder

ESSENTIAL OIL
Distilled from the resin, myrrh oil has been used since Ancient Greek times to heal wounds. It is generally considered *yang* in character but is anti-inflammatory rather than heating. It makes a good expectorant, used in chest rubs for bronchitis and catarrhal colds.

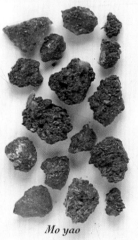

Mo yao   *Solid resin*   *Capsules*   *Tincture*

Applications

RESIN

TINCTURE Use for infectious, feverish conditions, from head colds to glandular fever. It is ideal for upper respiratory catarrh, and can be added to expectorant mixtures. Take up to 5 ml a day in 1-2 ml doses, well diluted with water.

CAPSULES Use as a more palatable alternative to the tincture; take one 200 mg capsule up to 5 times a day.

GARGLE/MOUTHWASH Use 1-2 ml tincture in half a tumbler of water for sore throats and mouth ulcers.

DOUCHE Use the diluted tincture for thrush.

POWDER In China, myrrh (3-9 g) is used as an analgesic, powdered with safflowers for abdominal pain associated with blood stagnation, as in period pain.

ESSENTIAL OIL

OIL Dilute 10 drops in 25 ml water, shake well, and use externally on wounds and chronic ulcers, or in lotions for haemorrhoids.

CHEST RUB Use 1 ml oil in 15 ml almond or sunflower oil for bronchitis and colds with thick phlegm.

PESSARIES Add 10 drops oil to 30 g melted cocoa butter; allow to set in a 24-pessary mould. Use for thrush.

CAUTION
• Avoid in pregnancy, as it is a uterine stimulant.

Crataegus spp.
HAWTHORN

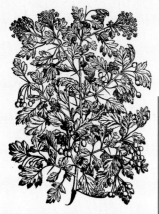

"Crataegus has quickly become one of the most widely used heart remedies."
Rudolf Weiss, 1985.

TRADITIONALLY VALUED for its astringency, hawthorn was used for diarrhoea, heavy menstrual bleeding, and in first aid to draw splinters. Over the past century, the plant's considerable tonic action on the heart has been identified; today, it is one of the most popular cardiac herbs. The species generally used in the West are *C. oxycantha* and *C. monogyna*. In China, the berries of *C. pinnatifida* are taken as a digestive and circulatory stimulant.

Character
Flowering tops: cool; astringent taste.
Berries: sour, slightly sweet, warm.
Constituents
Flavonoid glycosides, procyanidins, saponins, tannins, minerals.
Actions
Relaxes peripheral blood vessels, cardiac tonic, astringent.

Parts used

FLOWERING TOPS
C. OXYCANTHA &
C. MONOGYNA
The flowers are widely used as a heart tonic. Their precise action is still being researched, but it seems that they improve the coronary circulation, reducing the risk of angina attacks and helping to normalize blood pressure. Large doses given by injection have been used successfully for highly irregular heartbeats. Harvest in early summer.

BERRIES
C. OXYCANTHA &
C. MONOGYNA
Research suggests that the berries contain fewer cardiac-influencing constituents than the flowers, although both are prescribed by Western herbalists. The berries can also be used for diarrhoea. Harvest when ripe in late summer or early autumn.

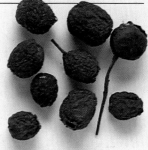

Dried berries

BERRIES
C. PINNATIFIDA
In China, the berries, called *shan zha*, are mainly taken for symptoms of "food stagnation", which can include abdominal bloating, indigestion and flatulence. They are believed to "move" blood, and are used to relieve stagnation, especially after childbirth. Partially charred berries are a standby for diarrhoea.

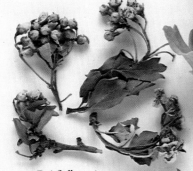

Dried flowering tops

Fresh flowering tops

Dried shan zha

Charred shan zha

Applications

FLOWERING TOPS
C. OXYCANTHA/C. MONOGYNA

INFUSION Use to improve poor circulation and as a tonic for heart problems. Combine with yarrow or *ju hua* for hypertension.

TINCTURE Prescribed with other cardiac herbs for angina, hypertension and related disorders.

BERRIES
C. OXYCANTHA/C. MONOGYNA

DECOCTION Use 30 g berries to 500 ml water and decoct for 15 minutes only. Take for diarrhoea, or with *ju hua* and *gou qi zi* for hypertension.

JUICE Use juice from the fresh berries as a cardiac tonic; also for diarrhoea, poor digestion, or as a general digestive tonic.

BERRIES
C. PINNATIFIDA

DECOCTION Use 10-20 g in 500 ml water with *zhi ke* for abdominal bloating, or combine with *dan shen* and *dang gui* for period and post-partum pain.

CAPSULES Use the powdered berries with *san qi* powder for abdominal pain due to blood stagnation, or for the pain of angina.

Dioscorea spp.
YAM

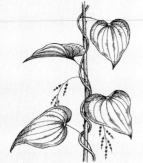

"...wild yams contain diosgenin, a precursor in the synthesis of progesterone, and are the only known available source."
Rudolf Weiss, 1985.

USED TO MAKE THE ORIGINAL contraceptive pills when synthetic hormone production was not a commercial proposition, Mexican wild yam (*D. villosa*) contains hormonal substances very similar to progesterone. It also relaxes smooth muscle; hence another of its common names, colic root. Many other yams are used as a starter material to produce hydrocortisones for orthodox eczema creams. Several related species are popular in China: *D. hypoglauca* is used for urinary disorders, while *D. opposita* is an important spleen and stomach tonic.

Character
Neutral, generally drying, bitter (most species) or sweet (*D. opposita*).
Constituents
Alkaloids, steroidal saponins, tannins, phytosterols, starch.
Actions
D. VILLOSA: relaxant for smooth muscle, antispasmodic, promotes bile flow, anti-inflammatory, promotes sweating.
D. OPPOSITA: expectorant, digestive stimulant, kidney tonic.
D. HYPOGLAUCA: antibacterial, anti-inflammatory, soothes urinary tract infections.

Parts used

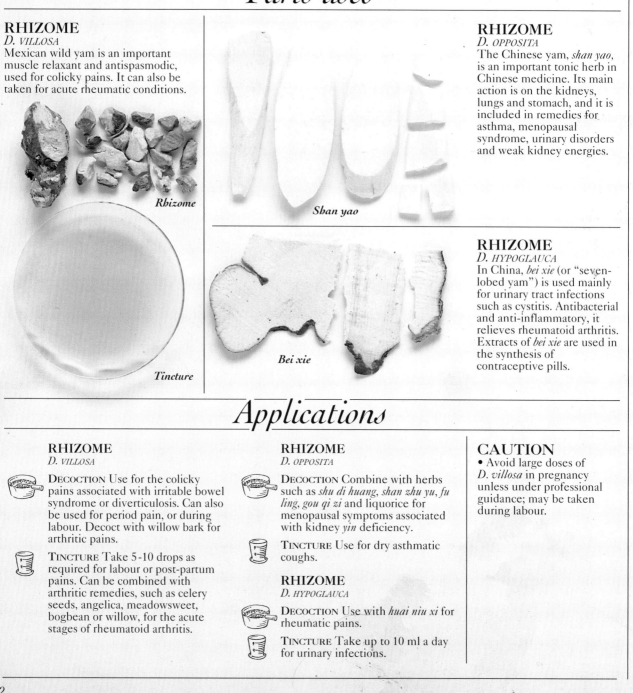

RHIZOME
D. VILLOSA
Mexican wild yam is an important muscle relaxant and antispasmodic, used for colicky pains. It can also be taken for acute rheumatic conditions.

Rhizome

Tincture

RHIZOME
D. OPPOSITA
The Chinese yam, *shan yao*, is an important tonic herb in Chinese medicine. Its main action is on the kidneys, lungs and stomach, and it is included in remedies for asthma, menopausal syndrome, urinary disorders and weak kidney energies.

Shan yao

RHIZOME
D. HYPOGLAUCA
In China, *bei xie* (or "seven-lobed yam") is used mainly for urinary tract infections such as cystitis. Antibacterial and anti-inflammatory, it relieves rheumatoid arthritis. Extracts of *bei xie* are used in the synthesis of contraceptive pills.

Bei xie

Applications

RHIZOME
D. VILLOSA

DECOCTION Use for the colicky pains associated with irritable bowel syndrome or diverticulosis. Can also be used for period pain, or during labour. Decoct with willow bark for arthritic pains.

TINCTURE Take 5-10 drops as required for labour or post-partum pains. Can be combined with arthritic remedies, such as celery seeds, angelica, meadowsweet, bogbean or willow, for the acute stages of rheumatoid arthritis.

RHIZOME
D. OPPOSITA

DECOCTION Combine with herbs such as *shu di huang, shan zhu yu, fu ling, gou qi zi* and liquorice for menopausal symptoms associated with kidney *yin* deficiency.

TINCTURE Use for dry asthmatic coughs.

RHIZOME
D. HYPOGLAUCA

DECOCTION Use with *huai niu xi* for rheumatic pains.

TINCTURE Take up to 10 ml a day for urinary infections.

CAUTION
• Avoid large doses of *D. villosa* in pregnancy unless under professional guidance; may be taken during labour.

Echinacea spp.
PURPLE CONEFLOWER

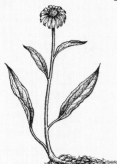

"It has proved a useful drug in improving the body's own resistance in infectious conditions of all kinds..."
Rudolf Weiss, 1985.

THE NATIVE AMERICANS used purple coneflower to treat snakebite, fevers and old, stubborn wounds. The early settlers soon adopted the plant as a home remedy for colds and influenza, and it became popular with the 19th-century Eclectics (see pp. 20-1). In the past 50 years, it has achieved worldwide fame for its antiviral, antifungal and antibacterial properties, and it has also been used in Aids therapy. Cultivated purple coneflower is usually *E. purpurea*, although *E. angustifolia* is considered more potent by some practitioners.

Character
Cool, dry, mainly pungent.
Constituents
Volatile oil, glycosides, amides, antibiotic polyacetylenes, inulin.
Actions
Antibiotic, immune stimulant, anti-allergenic, lymphatic tonic.

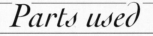
Parts used

ROOT
Generally used in tinctures or powders for almost any type of infection or inflammation; it can be especially useful for recurring kidney infections, as well as more common catarrh and colds. Harvest after flowering; wash, chop and dry.

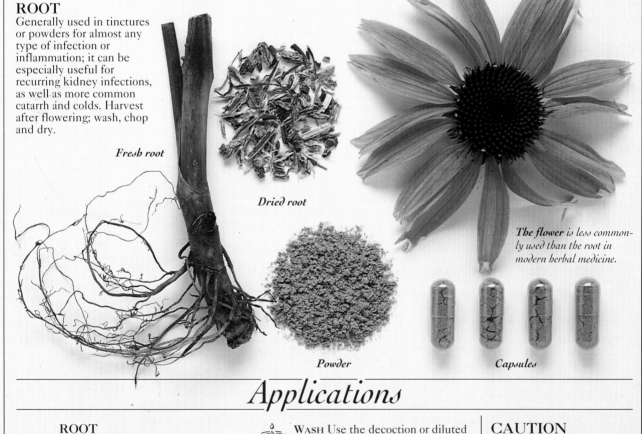

Fresh root

Dried root

Powder

Capsules

The flower is less commonly used than the root in modern herbal medicine.

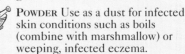
Applications

ROOT

DECOCTION Take 10 ml doses every 1-2 hours for the acute stage of infections.

TINCTURE Take 2-5 ml doses every 2-3 hours for influenza, chills and urinary tract infections, during the first couple of days of acute symptoms. For more chronic conditions, use standard doses and combine with other suitable herbs, such as buchu and couchgrass for kidney infections, or cleavers for glandular fever. May be used in 10 ml doses for food poisoning or snakebites.

WASH Use the decoction or diluted tincture for infected wounds. Bathe the affected area frequently.

GARGLE Use 10 ml tincture in a glass of warm water for sore throats.

POWDER Use as a dust for infected skin conditions such as boils (combine with marshmallow) or weeping, infected eczema.

CAPSULES Take three 200 mg capsules up to three times a day at the onset of acute infections, such as colds, influenza, and kidney or urinary tract infections.

CAUTION
• High doses can occasionally cause nausea and dizziness.

Ephedra sinica
MA HUANG

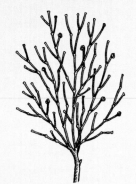

"As a wise man I have taken soma, the sweet draught that gives strength, lending immortal power and freedom to the gods."
The *Rig Veda, c.* 1000 BC.

IN CHINA, MA HUANG has been used as an anti-asthmatic for at least 5,000 years. The alkaloid ephedrine, extracted from the plant, was first identified by Chinese scientists in 1924; two years later the pharmaceutical company Merck produced a synthetic version, still used to treat asthma. The Indian variety, *E. gerardiana*, is thought to have been the prime ingredient of *soma*, a potent tonic and elixir of youth.

Character
Twigs: pungent, bitter, warm.
Root: pungent, neutral.
Constituents
Alkaloids (inc. ephedrine), saponins, volatile oil.
Actions
Twigs: antispasmodic, febrifuge, promote sweating, diuretic; antibacterial and antiviral properties identified in the essential oil.
Root: antihydrotic.

Parts used

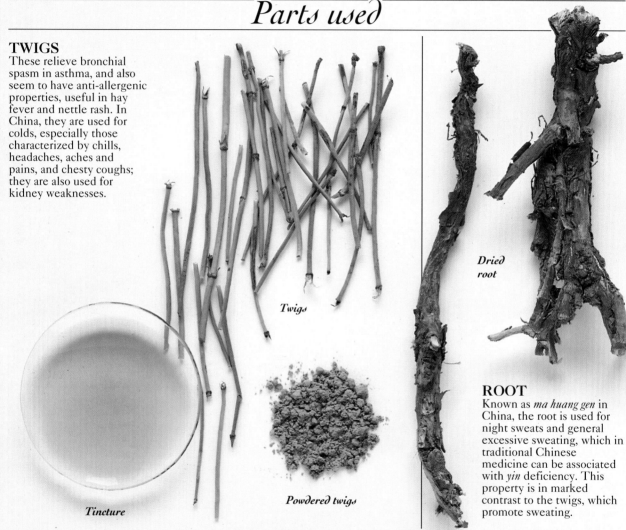

TWIGS
These relieve bronchial spasm in asthma, and also seem to have anti-allergenic properties, useful in hay fever and nettle rash. In China, they are used for colds, especially those characterized by chills, headaches, aches and pains, and chesty coughs; they are also used for kidney weaknesses.

Dried root

Twigs

Tincture

Powdered twigs

ROOT
Known as *ma huang gen* in China, the root is used for night sweats and general excessive sweating, which in traditional Chinese medicine can be associated with *yin* deficiency. This property is in marked contrast to the twigs, which promote sweating.

Applications

TWIGS
TINCTURE Prescribed for asthma, hay fever or severe chills. Combined with cowslip root and thyme tinctures for bronchial asthma, emphysema, whooping cough and other severe chest conditions. In the UK, the maximum permitted dose by law is 2.5 ml of a 1:4 tincture, three times a day.

DECOCTION Prescribed for common colds, coughs, asthma and hay fever; also used as a diuretic in kidney weakness. In China up to 6 g may be used per dose; the maximum legal dose in the UK is 600 mg.

ROOT
DECOCTION The Chinese use the decoction where *yin* or *qi* (energy) weakness leads to uncontrolled sweating.

CAUTIONS
• Restricted in the UK under the 1968 Medicine Act for use by practitioners only; restricted herb in Australia and New Zealand.
• Not to be used by patients taking MAO inhibitors as anti-depressants.
• Should be avoided in more severe cases of glaucoma, hypertension and coronary thrombosis.

Equisetum spp.
HORSETAIL

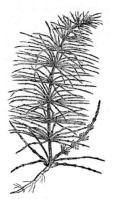

"So wonderful is its nature, its mere touch staunches a patient's bleeding."
Pliny, AD 77.

A PREHISTORIC BOTANICAL RELIC, horsetail is a close relative of the trees that grew on earth 270 million years ago in the Carboniferous period, and are the source of our modern coal seams. Its brittle jointed stems are rich in healing silica, and since the time of the Ancient Greeks, horsetail has been used for wounds. It is now considered an invasive weed. The Chinese use *E. hiemale*, or *mu zei*.

Character
Cold, dry, slightly bitter.
Constituents
Silica, alkaloids (inc. nicotine), saponins, flavonoids, bitter principle, minerals (inc. potassium, manganese, magnesium), phytosterols, tannins.
Actions
Astringent, stops bleeding, diuretic, anti-inflammatory, tissue healer.

Parts used

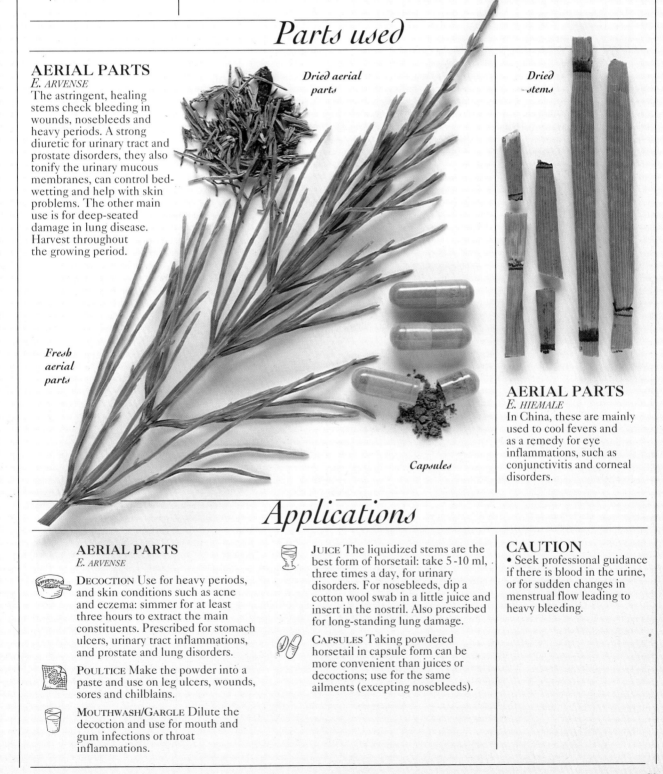

AERIAL PARTS
E. ARVENSE
The astringent, healing stems check bleeding in wounds, nosebleeds and heavy periods. A strong diuretic for urinary tract and prostate disorders, they also tonify the urinary mucous membranes, can control bed-wetting and help with skin problems. The other main use is for deep-seated damage in lung disease. Harvest throughout the growing period.

Dried aerial parts

Dried stems

Fresh aerial parts

Capsules

AERIAL PARTS
E. HIEMALE
In China, these are mainly used to cool fevers and as a remedy for eye inflammations, such as conjunctivitis and corneal disorders.

Applications

AERIAL PARTS
E. ARVENSE

DECOCTION Use for heavy periods, and skin conditions such as acne and eczema: simmer for at least three hours to extract the main constituents. Prescribed for stomach ulcers, urinary tract inflammations, and prostate and lung disorders.

POULTICE Make the powder into a paste and use on leg ulcers, wounds, sores and chilblains.

MOUTHWASH/GARGLE Dilute the decoction and use for mouth and gum infections or throat inflammations.

JUICE The liquidized stems are the best form of horsetail: take 5-10 ml, three times a day, for urinary disorders. For nosebleeds, dip a cotton wool swab in a little juice and insert in the nostril. Also prescribed for long-standing lung damage.

CAPSULES Taking powdered horsetail in capsule form can be more convenient than juices or decoctions; use for the same ailments (excepting nosebleeds).

CAUTION
• Seek professional guidance if there is blood in the urine, or for sudden changes in menstrual flow leading to heavy bleeding.

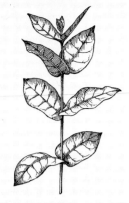

Eucalyptus globulus
EUCALYPTUS

A TRADITIONAL ABORIGINAL fever remedy,
eucalyptus was introduced to the West in the
19th century by the director of the Melbourne
Botanical Gardens, and cultivation of the tree
spread in southern Europe and North America.
The properties of oils from different species
vary slightly, but all are very antiseptic. Russian
research suggests that some species counteract
influenza viruses; others are antimalarial or
highly active against bacteria.

*"For every kind of wound made,
father used eucalyptus leaves as
taught by the blacks."*
May Gilmore, quoted in Bill
Wannan, *Folk Medicine.*

Character
Cool, moist, pungent, bitter.
Constituents
Volatile oil, tannins, aldehydes,
bitter resin.
Actions
Antiseptic, antispasmodic,
stimulant, febrifuge,
expectorant, reduces blood
sugar levels, expels worms.

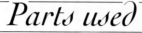

Parts used

LEAVES
In traditional Aboriginal medicine,
these were used in poultices for any
type of wound or inflammation, and
various decoctions were also taken
internally, although this is not
recommended for home use today.

Fresh leaves

*Dried
leaves*

ESSENTIAL OIL
Made by steam distillation
of the leaves, the oil is one
of the most antiseptic
essences in the herbal
repertoire, used in a wide
range of infections, such
as scarlet fever, influenza,
measles and typhoid. It is
available commercially,
but infused oil, which has
a similar but less potent
action, can be made at
home (see p. 122).

Applications

LEAVES

 INHALATION Pour boiling water
over a few leaves, and inhale the
steam for chest infections.

ESSENTIAL OIL

 COMPRESS Soak a pad in 2 ml oil
well dispersed in 100 ml water, and
apply to inflammations, painful
joints and burns.

GARGLE Dilute 5 drops oil in a glass
of water, mix well, and gargle for
throat infections.

CHEST RUB Dilute 0.5-2 ml oil in
25 ml almond oil for colds,
bronchitis, asthma and influenza.

INHALATION Add 10 drops oil to a
little hot water, and inhale the
steam for chest infections.

OIL Dilute 2 drops oil in 10 ml
sunflower oil or ointment base, and
apply to cold sores.

MASSAGE OIL Combine 10-20 drops
eucalyptus oil with 10-20 drops
rosemary oil in 20 ml infused
bladderwrack oil or almond oil for
rheumatic or arthritic pain.

Eupatorium spp.
GRAVELROOT

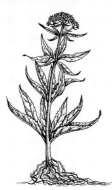

"For a cough, bruise hemp agrimony in a mortar and mix the juice with boiling milk, strain and use."
Remedy of the Physicians of Myddfai, Wales, 13th century.

A FAVOURITE WITH NATIVE Americans, gravelroot (*E. purpureum*) was known as Joe-Pye weed after a New England medicine man who used it to cure typhus. Boneset (*E. perfoliatum*) was similarly used for "boneset fever"; today, it is often given for influenza. A related European species, hemp agrimony (*E. cannabium*), has undergone a revival as immunostimulant constituents, which increase resistance in viral infections, have been identified in the herb.

Character
Bitter, pungent, drying; cool or cold depending on species.
Constituents
Tannins, bitter principle, flavonoids, sesquiterpene lactones.
Actions
E. CANNABIUM: febrifuge, diuretic, prevents scurvy, laxative, tonic, promotes bile flow, expectorant, promotes sweating, anti-rheumatic, immune stimulant.
E. PURPUREUM: diuretic, antirheumatic, promotes menstruation.

Parts used

AERIAL PARTS
E. CANNABIUM
Considered a remedy for feverish colds, the aerial parts were also used externally for putrid sores. Recent research has identified a compound called eupatoriopicrin, believed to have an anti-tumour action. Harvest while flowering in autumn.

ROOT
E. PURPUREUM
"Gravelroot" describes the main action: as a diuretic, useful for clearing urinary stones. It is also taken for prostate problems, for some types of period pain and to ease childbirth. Harvest in autumn.

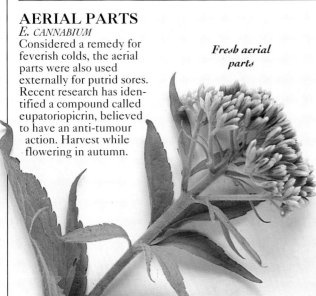

Fresh aerial parts

Dried aerial parts

Fresh root

Dried root

Applications

AERIAL PARTS
E. CANNABIUM

INFUSION Drink for rheumatic pains and arthritis. A stronger infusion is purgative for liver stagnation and some types of constipation.

TINCTURE Take 5 drops as required for feverish colds and influenza. Add to anticatarrhal mixtures, with herbs such as elderflower and ground ivy.

ROOT
E. PURPUREUM

DECOCTION Use for period pain, or sip during labour. Also has a cleansing effect for persistent urinary infections.

TINCTURE Take 2-3 ml, three times a day, for urinary disorders such as cystitis and gravel, or discharges caused by infection. Use with white deadnettle for prostate problems.

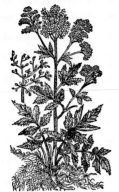

Filipendula ulmaria
MEADOWSWEET

A POPULAR ELIZABETHAN "strewing herb", meadowsweet was also used to ease fever and pains. Anti-inflammatory chemicals called salicylates were first extracted from it in the 1830s. Some 60 years later, the pharmaceutical company Bayer produced acetylsalicylate, a similar substance, artificially. They called this new "wonder drug" aspirin, after *Spiraea ulmaria*, the old botanical name for this herb.

"... the flowers boiled in wine and drunke, do take away the fits of a quartaine fever..."
John Gerard, 1597.

Character
Cold, astringent taste; both moist and drying.
Constituents
Salicylates, flavonoids, tannins, volatile oil, citric acid, mucilage.
Actions
Anti-inflammatory, anti-rheumatic, soothing digestive remedy, diuretic, promotes sweating.

Parts used

AERIAL PARTS
The cooling aerial parts reduce inflammations and fevers, protect the digestive tract and modify the action of salicylic acid; long use of aspirin can lead to gastric ulceration and bleeding, but meadowsweet does not show these side effects, and is actually a gentle digestive remedy for acidity and some types of diarrhoea. Harvest while flowering in summer.

Dried aerial parts

Fresh aerial parts

Tincture

Applications

AERIAL PARTS

INFUSION Take for feverish colds or rheumatic pains. Also soothing for children's stomach upsets.

TINCTURE Generally has a stronger action than the infusion. Add to remedies for gastric ulceration or excess acidity, such as liquorice. Use with herbs such as angelica or willow for arthritis.

 COMPRESS Soak a pad in the dilute tincture, and apply to painful arthritic and rheumatic joints, or use for neuralgia.

 EYEWASH Cool and strain the infusion, and use for conjunctivitis and other eye complaints.

CAUTIONS
• Avoid the herb in cases of salicylate sensitivity.
• If using the tincture for gastric ulceration or excess acidity, use the hot-water method (see p. 125) to reduce the alcohol.

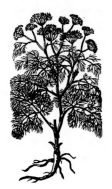

"...both the seeds, leaves and root of our Garden Fennel are much used in drinks and broths for those that are grown fat..."
William Coles, 1650.

Foeniculum officinale
FENNEL

THE ROMANS BELIEVED that serpents sucked the juice of the plant to improve their eyesight, and Pliny recommends the herb for "dimness of human vision". Fennel was also regarded as an early slimming aid, its Greek name *marathron* reputedly derived from a verb meaning "to grow thin". In medieval times, chewing the seeds was a favourite way to stop gastric rumbles during church sermons.

Character
Warming, dry, pungent, sweet.
Constituents
Volatile oil (inc. estragole, anethole), essential fatty acids, flavonoids (inc. rutin), vitamins, minerals.
Actions
Carminative, circulatory stimulant, anti-inflammatory, promotes milk flow, mild expectorant, diuretic.

Parts used

SEEDS
Soothing for the digestion, the seeds also promote milk flow in breastfeeding. When the infusion is taken by nursing mothers, it can also relieve colic in babies. In Chinese medicine, the seeds (*hui xiang*) are thought tonifying for the spleen and kidneys, and are used for urinary and reproductive disharmonies. Harvest in autumn when ripe.

ESSENTIAL OIL
The oil distilled from the seeds is mainly prescribed for digestive problems and, as a mild expectorant, for coughs and respiratory complaints.

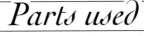

Tincture

Seeds

ROOT
Not as effective as the seeds, the root was once used in similar ways. Today it is mainly taken for urinary disorders. Harvest in late autumn, when the bulbous stems are collected as a vegetable.

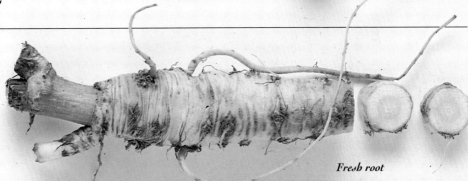

Fresh root

Applications

SEEDS

 INFUSION A useful and palatable digestive remedy: drink after meals for flatulence, indigestion, colic and other digestive upsets. Can also be taken by nursing mothers to increase milk flow or to relieve a baby's colic.

 DECOCTION Used in Chinese medicine for abdominal pain, colic and stomach chills.

 TINCTURE Use for digestive problems; combine with laxatives such as rhubarb root or senna to prevent griping.

 MOUTHWASH/GARGLE Use the infusion for gum disorders, loose teeth, laryngitis or sore throats.

ESSENTIAL OIL

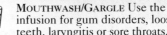 CHEST RUB Dissolve a total of 25 drops thyme, eucalyptus and fennel oils in 25 ml sunflower or almond oil for chest complaints.

ROOT

DECOCTION Use for urinary problems, such as gravel, or disorders associated with high uric acid content.

CAUTION
• Fennel is a uterine stimulant, so avoid high doses of the herb in pregnancy; small amounts used in cooking are safe.

Fragaria vesca
WILD STRAWBERRIES

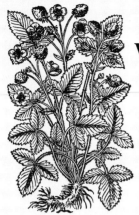

THE BERRIES, LEAVES AND ROOT of the wild or "alpine" strawberry have all been used medicinally in the past. The root was once a popular household remedy for diarrhoea, and the stalks were used for wounds. The berries were considered cooling; according to Gerard, they "quench thirst, cooleth heate of the stomicke and inflammation of the liver". However, eating them in winter or on a "cold stomicke" was thought to risk an increase in phlegmatic humours and digestive upsets.

"...water distilled from the berries is good for the passions of the heart caused by perturbation of the spirits."
John Parkinson, 1640.

Character
Cool, moist, sweet and sour.
Constituents
Tannins, mucilage, sugars, fruit acids, salicylates, minerals, vitamins B, C, E.
Actions
Astringent, heals wounds, diuretic, laxative, liver tonic, cleansing.

Parts used

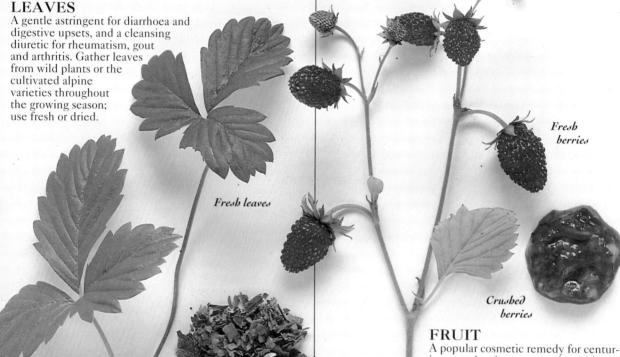

LEAVES
A gentle astringent for diarrhoea and digestive upsets, and a cleansing diuretic for rheumatism, gout and arthritis. Gather leaves from wild plants or the cultivated alpine varieties throughout the growing season; use fresh or dried.

Fresh leaves

Dried leaves

Fresh berries

Crushed berries

FRUIT
A popular cosmetic remedy for centuries, strawberries were used to whiten the complexion and remove freckles. Crushed berries make an emergency treatment for mild sunburn. The berries are also a liver tonic. Strawberry juice shows antibacterial properties, and was used in typhoid epidemics in the past. Harvest ripe fruit in summer.

Applications

LEAVES
INFUSION Take for diarrhoea, for gastric inflammations and infections, and for jaundice; use also as an appetite stimulant. Combine with meadowsweet and St. John's wort for mild arthritic pains, or with celery seed for gout.

FRUIT
FRESH Eat strawberries for gastritis and as a liver tonic: they are good during convalescence after hepatitis. They are also useful in feverish conditions: they are both cooling and unlikely to cause fermentation in the stomach.

POULTICE Apply crushed berries to areas of sunburn or other skin inflammations.

TONIC WINE Steep the berries in wine to make a traditional remedy for "reviving the spirits and making the hart merrie".

Fucus vesiculosis
BLADDERWRACK

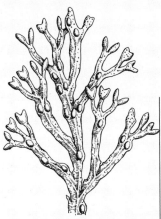

SEVERAL VARIETIES OF THIS SEAWEED have been used therapeutically. In the 18th century, iodine was isolated by distilling the long ribbons, or thalli, and bladderwrack became this element's main source for more than 50 years. The herb was used extensively to treat goitre, a swelling of the thyroid related to lack of iodine. In the 1860s it was claimed that bladderwrack, as a thyroid stimulant, could counter obesity by increasing the metabolic rate. Since then, it has featured in numerous slimming remedies.

"...another trial resulted in the cure of some sick horses fed on seaweed, while others fed on oats remained out of health."
Maud Grieve, 1931.

Character
Salty, cool, moist.
Constituents
Mucilage, iodine and other minerals, mannitol, volatile oil.
Actions
Metabolic stimulant, nutritive, thyroid tonic, antirheumatic, anti-inflammatory.

Parts used

THALLI
As a gentle metabolic stimulant, the thalli are useful in debility and convalescence. They also show antirheumatic properties when taken internally and applied topically. Bladderwrack is rich in iodine which, if lacking in the diet, can lead to thyroid deficiency. Collect from the sea in a healthy, live state rather than gathering from beaches.

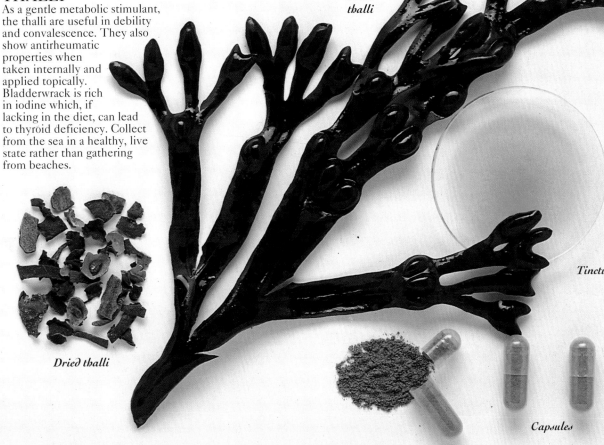

Fresh thalli

Dried thalli

Tincture

Capsules

Applications

THALLI

 TINCTURE Take for thyroid deficiency, as a gentle metabolic stimulant, or for rheumatic conditions.

 INFUSION Take as the tincture. Can be used as part of a weight-reducing programme, especially if obesity is linked to a slow metabolism, but it should not be regarded as an easy method for losing weight.

TABLETS/CAPSULES Take 3-6 a day as a metabolic stimulant. Can help reduce obesity related to thyroid underactivity.

INFUSED OIL Macerate 500 g dried bladderwrack overnight in 500 ml sunflower oil. Heat in a waterbath for two hours and strain. Use the oil externally for arthritic joint pains or rheumatism.

CAUTION
• Like many sea creatures, bladderwrack is at risk from heavy metal pollution. Do not collect where levels of cadmium and mercury are known to be high.

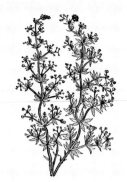

Galium aparine
CLEAVERS

A POPULAR HERB in folk medicine throughout the centuries, cleavers or goosegrass is a vigorously growing weed that twines through hedgerows or garden shrubberies producing long sticky stems. The young shoots are among the first of the weeds to appear in spring, and make an excellent cleansing tonic, a remedy widely used in central Europe and the Balkans.

"Women do usually make pottage of clevers... to cause lanknesse and keepe them from fatnes."
John Gerard, 1597.

Character
Cold, slightly dry, salty.
Constituents
Coumarins, tannins, glycosides, citric acid.
Actions
Diuretic, lymphatic cleanser, mild astringent.

Parts used

AERIAL PARTS
Best used fresh, the aerial parts are a potent diuretic and lymphatic cleanser, effective in many cases involving swollen or enlarged lymph glands. Often described as a blood purifier, they are used for skin problems and other conditions where the body is failing to rid itself of toxins. They can also be cooked as a vegetable, gently sweated in the pan like spinach. Harvest from spring to autumn.

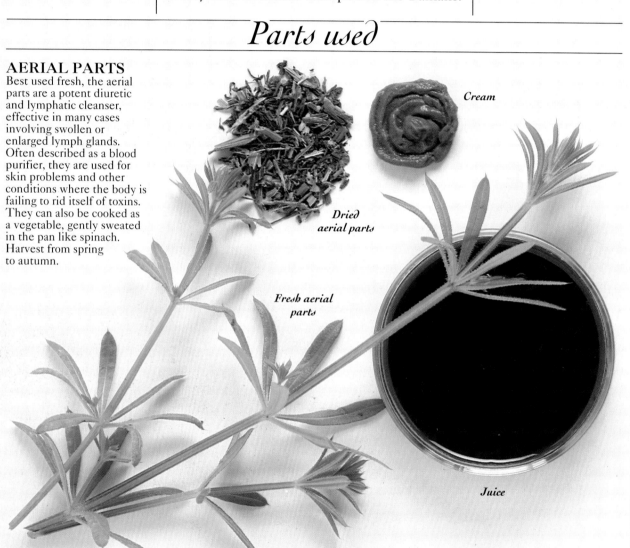

Cream

Dried aerial parts

Fresh aerial parts

Juice

Applications

AERIAL PARTS

JUICE Liquidize or pulp the fresh plant to make an effective diuretic and lymphatic cleanser for a range of conditions, including glandular fever, tonsillitis and prostate disorders.

INFUSION Generally less strong than the juice. Use for urinary problems such as cystitis and gravel; also take as a cooling drink in fevers.

TINCTURE Use for the same ailments as the infusion. Can be combined with other lymphatic and detoxifying herbs such as dried pokeroot or *lian qiao*.

COMPRESS Soak a pad in the infusion and use for burns, grazes, ulcers and other skin inflammations.

CREAM Use regularly to relieve psoriasis.

HAIR RINSE Use the infusion for dandruff or scaling scalp problems.

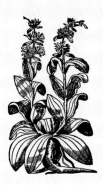

Gentiana spp.
GENTIAN

THE HERB REPUTEDLY TAKES its name from a king of Illyria who discovered its ability to reduce fevers. In medieval times, gentian was an ingredient of the alchemical brew *theriac*, a cure-all made to a highly secret recipe. *G. lutea* is used in the West, while the Chinese usually use either the large-leaved gentian, *G. macrophylla* (*qin jiao*), or *G. scabra* (*long dan cao*).

"It is reported to be good for... such as have evill livers and bad stomackes."
John Gerard, 1597.

Character
Very bitter, cold, astringent, drying.
Constituents
Bitter glycosides, alkaloids, flavonoids.
Actions
Bitter, tonic, appetite and gastric stimulant, anti-inflammatory, febrifuge.

Parts used

ROOT
G. LUTEA
A strong bitter digestive stimulant, the root is effective for conditions involving poor appetite or sluggish digestion. It is also used in fevers, cooling the system and maintaining digestive function, so that stomach contents do not stagnate, leading to further health problems. Harvest in late summer and autumn.

ROOT
G. MACROPHYLLA & G. SCABRA
Bitter remedies, these roots are used for digestive and feverish conditions. In Chinese medicine, they are usually described as clearing "heat and damp", and may be prescribed for some types of hypertension related to heat in the liver, or for urinary infections and rheumatic disorders.

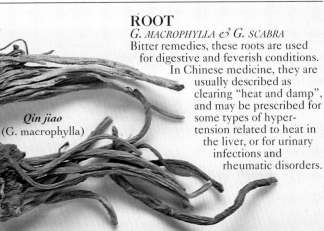

Qin jiao
(G. macrophylla)

Dried root

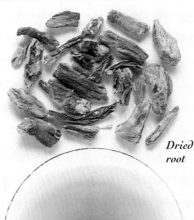

Long dan cao
(G. scabra)

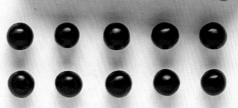

Tincture

Long dan xie gan wan is a patent Chinese remedy, used to clear liver and gall bladder heat, where symptoms can include sore eyes, headaches and constipation.

Applications

ROOT
G. LUTEA

 DECOCTION Use 10 g herb to 500 ml water and decoct for 20 minutes. Take before meals for fullness and stomach pains.

TINCTURE Take up to 2 ml three times a day as a digestive stimulant, or in drop doses to allay cravings for sweet foods. Prescribed for liver disease, including hepatitis, gall bladder inflammations, and where jaundice is a symptom.

ROOT
G. MACROPHYLLA

 DECOCTION Use in combination with other herbs, such as *du huo* and cinnamon, for rheumatic pains, fevers and allergic inflammations.

ROOT
G. SCABRA

DECOCTION Use in combination with other herbs, such as *chai hu*, *zhi zi* and *huang qin*, for liver disorders, hypertension and urinary infections.

Ginkgo biloba
MAIDENHAIR TREE

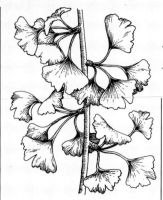

"Significant improvement in mental states, emotional lability, memory, and tendency to tire easily, have been reported..."
Rudolf Weiss, 1985.

DATING BACK AT LEAST 200 million years, the maidenhair tree has probably been extinct in the wild for centuries, but survived in Far Eastern temple gardens. A deciduous conifer with separate male and female forms, the tree was introduced into Europe in 1730 and became a favourite ornamental. Since the 1980s, Western medical interest in the plant has grown dramatically as its potent actions on the cardiovascular system have been identified.

Character
Sweet, bitter, astringent, neutral.
Constituents
Leaves: flavone glycosides (including ginkgolide), bioflavones, sitosterol, lactones, anthocyanin.
Seeds: fatty acids, minerals, bioflavones.
Actions
Leaves: relax blood vessels, circulatory stimulant.
Seeds: astringent, antifungal, antibacterial.

Parts used

LEAVES
Part of the herbal repertoire only since the 1980s, the leaves are used for circulatory diseases; they are particularly good at improving blood flow to the brain. Research has shown that ginkgolide can be as effective as standard pharmaceutical drugs in treating severely irregular heartbeats. The leaves are also used for varicose veins haemorrhoids and leg ulcers. Harvest in summer.

SEEDS
In China, the seeds, called *bai gou*, are considered to act on the lung and kidney acupuncture meridians, and are traditionally used for asthmatic disorders and chesty coughs with thick phlegm. They also have a tonifying effect on the urinary system, so are used for incontinence and excessive urination.

Fresh leaves

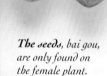

The seeds, bai gou, are only found on the female plant.

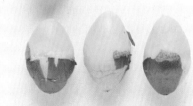

Tincture

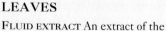

Dried leaves

Applications

LEAVES

 FLUID EXTRACT An extract of the fresh leaves is marketed in Europe for treating cerebral arteriosclerosis in the elderly and for diseases of the peripheral circulation.

 TINCTURE Combine with other cardiovascular herbs, such as greater periwinkle and limeflower, for circulatory problems, or with king's clover for venous disorders.

INFUSION Make with 50 g dried leaves to 500 ml water, and take for arteriosclerosis and varicose conditions. Use as a wash for varicose ulcers or haemorrhoids.

SEEDS

DECOCTION Combine with herbs such as *ma huang** (prescription only), elecampane or mulberry leaves for asthma and severe or persistent coughs: 3-4 seeds are enough for three doses.

CAUTIONS
• Do not exceed the stated dose of the seeds, as this can lead to skin disorders and headaches.
• Cases of contact dermatitis with the fruit pulp (not used medicinally) have been recorded.

**Restricted herb in Australia and New Zealand.*

Glycyrrhiza spp.
LIQUORICE

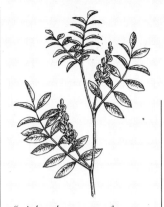

"...it has the property of quenching thirst if one holds it in the mouth..."
Theophrastus of Lesbos, *c.* 310 BC.

LIQUORICE HAS BEEN USED medicinally since at least 500 BC, and still features in official pharmacopoeia as a "drug" for stomach ulcers. *G. glabra* originates in the Mediterranean and the Middle East, and has been cultivated in Europe since at least the 16th century. In China, *G. uralensis* or *gan cao* is used; it is called the "great detoxifier", and is thought to drive poisons from the system. It is also an important tonic, often called "the grandfather of herbs".

Character
Very sweet, neutral, moist.
Constituents
Saponins, glycosides (inc. glycyrrhizin), oestrogenous substances, coumarins, flavonoids, sterols, choline, asparagine, volatile oil.
Actions
Anti-inflammatory, anti-arthritic, tonic stimulant for adrenal cortex, lowers blood cholesterol levels, soothes gastric mucous membranes, possibly anti-allergenic, cooling, expectorant.

Parts used

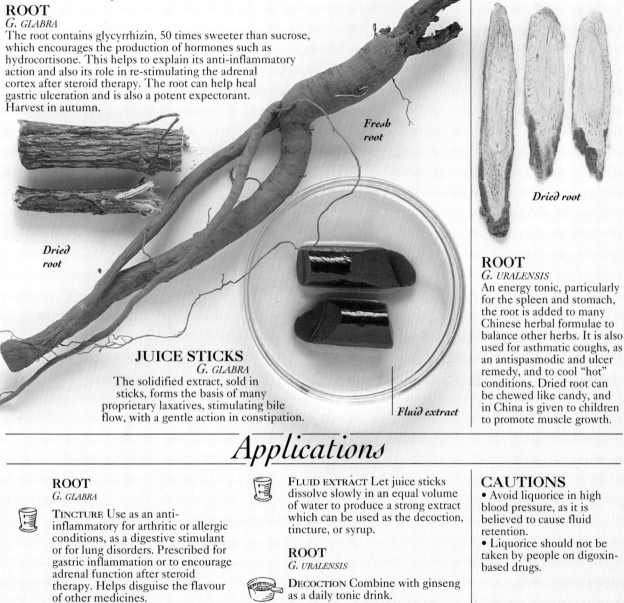

ROOT
G. GLABRA
The root contains glycyrrhizin, 50 times sweeter than sucrose, which encourages the production of hormones such as hydrocortisone. This helps to explain its anti-inflammatory action and also its role in re-stimulating the adrenal cortex after steroid therapy. The root can help heal gastric ulceration and is also a potent expectorant. Harvest in autumn.

Dried root

Fresh root

Dried root

JUICE STICKS
G. GLABRA
The solidified extract, sold in sticks, forms the basis of many proprietary laxatives, stimulating bile flow, with a gentle action in constipation.

Fluid extract

ROOT
G. URALENSIS
An energy tonic, particularly for the spleen and stomach, the root is added to many Chinese herbal formulae to balance other herbs. It is also used for asthmatic coughs, as an antispasmodic and ulcer remedy, and to cool "hot" conditions. Dried root can be chewed like candy, and in China is given to children to promote muscle growth.

Applications

ROOT
G. GLABRA

 TINCTURE Use as an anti-inflammatory for arthritic or allergic conditions, as a digestive stimulant or for lung disorders. Prescribed for gastric inflammation or to encourage adrenal function after steroid therapy. Helps disguise the flavour of other medicines.

DECOCTION Prescribed to reduce stomach acidity in ulceration.

SYRUP Take a syrup made from the decoction as a soothing expectorant for asthma and bronchitis.

FLUID EXTRACT Let juice sticks dissolve slowly in an equal volume of water to produce a strong extract which can be used as the decoction, tincture, or syrup.

ROOT
G. URALENSIS

DECOCTION Combine with ginseng as a daily tonic drink.

TONIC WINE Macerate a piece of root in gin or vodka for a few weeks to produce a tonic wine: drink in small doses after meals.

CAUTIONS
• Avoid liquorice in high blood pressure, as it is believed to cause fluid retention.
• Liquorice should not be taken by people on digoxin-based drugs.

Humulus lupulus
HOPS

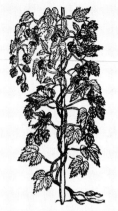

"Hops... preserves the drink, but repays the pleasure in tormenting diseases and a shorter life."
John Evelyn, 1670.

USED IN BREWING IN EUROPE since at least the 11th century, hops were never included in traditional English ale. Initially, they were thought to encourage the melancholic humour, and too many hops in German-style beer was, as Gerard records, "ill for the head". Hops were believed, however, to purge excess choleric and sanguine humours, and beer was regarded as a more "physicall drinke to keep the body in health" than English ale. Hops contain a high proportion of oestrogen and, as a result, too much beer can lead to loss of libido in men.

Character
Cold, dry, bitter, slightly pungent.
Constituents
Volatile oil, valerianic acid, oestrogenic substances, tannins, bitter principle, flavonoids.
Actions
Sedative, anaphrodisiac, restoring tonic for nervous system, bitter digestive stimulant, diuretic.

Parts used

STROBILES
The flowers on the female plant, known as strobiles, are used medicinally. The character of the plant changes significantly with age as the constituents oxidize. The strobiles are best used fresh for insomnia, and the dried hops used in pillows for sleeplessness should be replaced every few months, because old dried strobiles can be stimulating.

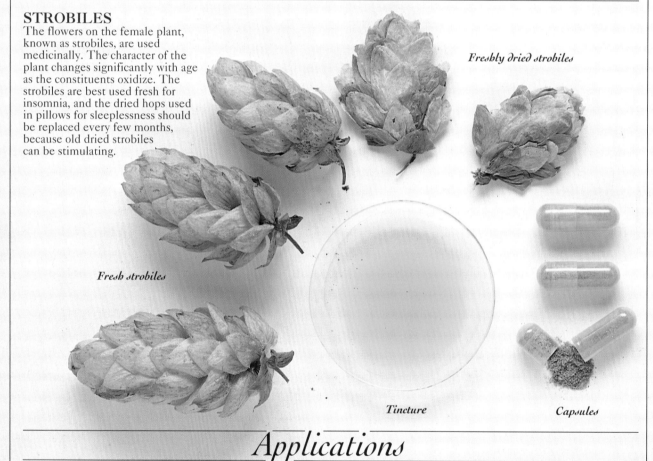

Freshly dried strobiles

Fresh strobiles

Tincture

Capsules

Applications

STROBILES

INFUSION For insomnia, add 2 tsp fresh hops to a cup of boiling water, and infuse for five minutes. Freshly dried or freeze-dried hops can also be used.

TINCTURE Take up to 2 ml, three times a day, as a sedative for nervous tension and anxiety. Combine with other digestive herbs, such as marshmallow, plantain, chamomile and peppermint for irritable bowel syndrome. Take 1.5 ml on a sugar lump for nervous

stomach. Prescribed for some sexual problems, including premature ejaculation.

COMPRESS Use a pad soaked in the infusion or dilute tincture on varicose ulcers.

WASH Use an infusion of fresh or freshly dried hops for chronic ulcers, skin eruptions and wounds.

CAPSULES Available commercially; take two before meals as an appetite stimulant. Do not use continuously for more than a few days.

CAUTIONS
• Hops act as a mild depressant on the higher nerve centres and should be avoided in depression. Do not exceed the stated doses.
• The growing plant can cause contact dermatitis.

Hydrastis canadensis
GOLDENSEAL

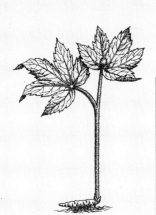

"I am informed that the Cheerake cure it [cancer] with a plant which is thought to be the Hydrastis canadensis."
Benjamin Smith Barton, 1798.

A TRADITIONAL HEALING HERB of Native Americans that has entered the European herbal repertoire, goldenseal was used by the Cherokee for indigestion, local inflammations and to improve the appetite, while the Iroquois used it for whooping cough, liver disorders, fevers and heart problems. The herb was introduced into Europe in 1760. During the 19th century, it became a favourite with Thomsonian and Eclectic practitioners (see pp. 20-1) and was listed in the United States *Pharmacopoeia* until 1926.

Character
Bitter, astringent, dry, predominantly cold.
Constituents
Alkaloids, volatile oil, resin.
Actions
Astringent, tonic, digestive and bile stimulant, anticatarrhal, laxative, healing to gastric mucous membranes, raises blood pressure.

Parts used

RHIZOME
An excellent drying anticatarrhal remedy for the gastric, upper respiratory tract and vaginal mucous membranes, useful for conditions including mucous colitis, nasal inflammations or ear infections. It is good for gynaecological problems, can help reduce menopausal symptoms, and can ease period pain or PMS symptoms linked with stagnation. Popularly taken in patent remedies as a general tonic. Harvest in autumn.

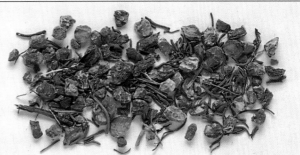

Dried rhizome

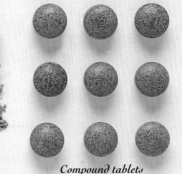

Tincture

Capsules

Compound tablets

Applications

RHIZOME

 TINCTURE Take 0.5-2 ml three times a day (larger doses are more laxative) for any catarrhal condition: nasal catarrh, mucous colitis, gastroenteritis and vaginal discharge. Also use as a liver tonic for sluggish digestion and for digestive problems associated with food sensitivity and alcohol excess. Add to remedies for PMS or heavy menstrual bleeding.

WASH Use 5 ml tincture in 100 ml water to bathe irritant skin inflammations, eczema and measles.

MOUTHWASH/GARGLE Use 2-3 ml tincture in a tumbler of warm water for mouth ulcers, gum disease, sore throats and catarrhal conditions.

DOUCHE Use the dilute tincture (2-3 ml in water) for vaginal discharges and infections, including thrush. For vaginal itching, use 5 ml tincture in 100 ml rosewater.

CAPSULES Take one 200 mg capsule, three times a day, for catarrh and gastric or respiratory infections. Combine with chaste-tree berry powder to relieve menopausal flushes and sweats, and with eyebright for hay fever.

EARDROPS Use 10 ml tincture in 100 ml water for "glue ear", catarrhal congestions and "blocked" ears.

COMPOUND TABLETS Some commercially available tablets may be used for digestive upsets.

CAUTIONS
• Goldenseal is a uterine stimulant, so avoid in pregnancy.
• The herb is hypertensive, so avoid in cases of high blood pressure.
• Do not use eardrops if there is a risk that the ear drum is perforated.
• Eating the fresh plant can cause ulceration of the mucous membranes.

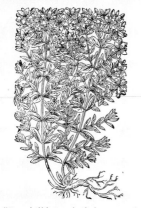

"For chilblains: boil the roots of tutsan and pour upon curds. Pound with old lard and apply as a plaster..."
Remedy of the Physicians of Myddfai, Wales, 13th century.

Hypericum perforatum
ST. JOHN'S WORT

IT IS SAID THAT ST. JOHN'S WORT takes its name from the Knights of St. John of Jerusalem, who used it to treat wounds on Crusade battlefields. It was also believed to dispel evil spirits – which is why the insane were often compelled to drink its infusions. Being yellow, the herb was associated with "choleric" humours and used for jaundice and hysteria. Old herbals often refer to tutsan (*H. androsaemum*), from the French *toutsain* or heal-all, which was also used to treat injuries and inflammations.

Character
Bitter-sweet, cool, drying.
Constituents
Glycosides, flavonoids (inc. rutin), volatile oils, tannins, resins.
Actions
Astringent, analgesic, anti-inflammatory, sedative, restorative tonic for the nervous system.

Parts used

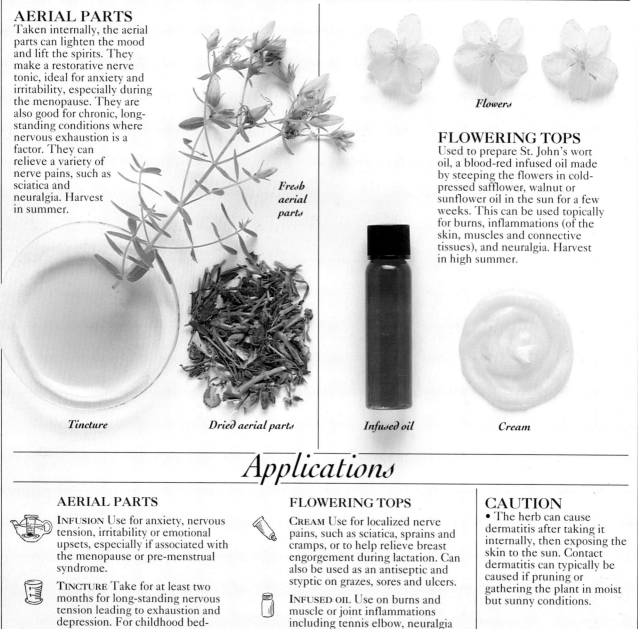

AERIAL PARTS
Taken internally, the aerial parts can lighten the mood and lift the spirits. They make a restorative nerve tonic, ideal for anxiety and irritability, especially during the menopause. They are also good for chronic, long-standing conditions where nervous exhaustion is a factor. They can relieve a variety of nerve pains, such as sciatica and neuralgia. Harvest in summer.

Flowers

FLOWERING TOPS
Used to prepare St. John's wort oil, a blood-red infused oil made by steeping the flowers in cold-pressed safflower, walnut or sunflower oil in the sun for a few weeks. This can be used topically for burns, inflammations (of the skin, muscles and connective tissues), and neuralgia. Harvest in high summer.

Fresh aerial parts

Tincture

Dried aerial parts

Infused oil

Cream

Applications

AERIAL PARTS
INFUSION Use for anxiety, nervous tension, irritability or emotional upsets, especially if associated with the menopause or pre-menstrual syndrome.

TINCTURE Take for at least two months for long-standing nervous tension leading to exhaustion and depression. For childhood bed-wetting, give 5-10 drops at night.

WASH Use the infusion to bathe wounds, skin sores and bruises.

FLOWERING TOPS
CREAM Use for localized nerve pains, such as sciatica, sprains and cramps, or to help relieve breast engorgement during lactation. Can also be used as an antiseptic and styptic on grazes, sores and ulcers.

INFUSED OIL Use on burns and muscle or joint inflammations including tennis elbow, neuralgia and sciatica. Add a few drops of lavender oil for burns, or yarrow oil for joint inflammations.

CAUTION
• The herb can cause dermatitis after taking it internally, then exposing the skin to the sun. Contact dermatitis can typically be caused if pruning or gathering the plant in moist but sunny conditions.

Hyssopus officinalis
HYSSOP

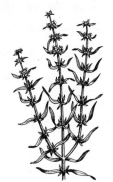

"The brethe or vapor of hisop driveth away the winde that is in the ears if they be holden over it."
William Turner, 1562.

PRESCRIBED BY HIPPOCRATES for pleurisy, hyssop, together with rue, was recommended by Dioscorides for asthma and catarrh. Its name derives from the Greek word *azob*, or holy herb, although the "hyssop" in the Bible seems more likely to have been a local variety of marjoram. Hyssop is one of the more important of the 130 herbs flavouring the liqueur Chartreuse.

Character
Bitter, pungent, dry, slightly warming.
Constituents
Volatile oil, flavonoids, tannins, bitter substance (marrubin).
Actions
Expectorant, carminative, relaxes peripheral blood vessels, promotes sweating, anticatarrhal, topical anti-inflammatory, antiviral (*Herpes simplex*), antispasmodic.

Parts used

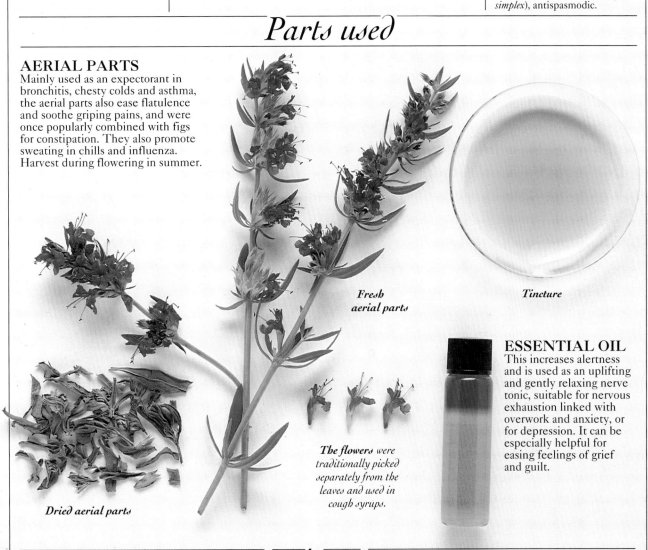

AERIAL PARTS
Mainly used as an expectorant in bronchitis, chesty colds and asthma, the aerial parts also ease flatulence and soothe griping pains, and were once popularly combined with figs for constipation. They also promote sweating in chills and influenza. Harvest during flowering in summer.

Fresh aerial parts

Tincture

ESSENTIAL OIL
This increases alertness and is used as an uplifting and gently relaxing nerve tonic, suitable for nervous exhaustion linked with overwork and anxiety, or for depression. It can be especially helpful for easing feelings of grief and guilt.

The flowers were traditionally picked separately from the leaves and used in cough syrups.

Dried aerial parts

Applications

AERIAL PARTS

INFUSION Drink hot during the early stages of colds and influenza. Also take for digestive upsets and nervous stomach.

TINCTURE Combine with other expectorant herbs, such as liquorice, elecampane and anise, for bronchitis and stubborn coughs.

SYRUP For coughs, use a syrup made from an infusion of either the aerial parts or the flowers. Combine with mullein flowers or liquorice

for stubborn coughs and lung weakness.

ESSENTIAL OIL

CHEST RUB Dilute 10 drops hyssop oil in 20 ml almond or sunflower oil for bronchitis and chesty colds. Combines well with thyme and eucalyptus.

OIL Add 5-10 drops to bath water for nervous exhaustion, melancholy or sorrows.

CAUTION
• The essential oil contains the ketone pino-camphone, which in high doses can cause convulsions. Do not take more than the recommended dose.

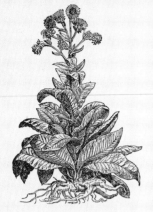

Inula spp.
ELECAMPANE

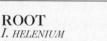

"Inula campana reddit praecordia sana (elecampane will the spirits sustain)."
Traditional Latin saying.

ONE OF THE MOST IMPORTANT herbs to the Greeks and Romans, elecampane (*I. helenium*) was regarded as almost a cure-all for ailments as diverse as dropsy, digestive upsets, menstrual disorders and sciatica. The Anglo-Saxons used the herb as a tonic, for skin disease and leprosy. By the 19th century, it was used to treat skin disease, neuralgia, liver problems and coughs; today it is used almost solely for respiratory problems. In China, *I. japonica* is used.

Character
I. HELENIUM: bitter and slightly sweet, warm, dry.
I. JAPONICA: salty, warm.
Constituents
Mucilage, bitter principle, volatile oil (inc. azulenes), inulin, sterols, possible alkaloids.
Actions
Tonic, stimulating expectorant, promotes sweating, anti-bacterial, antifungal, anti-parasitic, digestive stimulant.

Parts used

ROOT
I. HELENIUM
An excellent tonic, especially for weakness following influenza or bronchitis, the root shifts stubborn phlegm and can help coughs and congestion, particularly in children. It contains inulin, which has been used as a sugar sub-stitute in diabetes. Har-vest in autumn, wash, and chop into small pieces before drying.

Fresh root

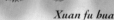

Xuan fu hua

Tincture

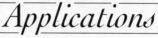
Dried root

FLOWERS
I. JAPONICA
In China, the flowers, *xuan fu hua*, are recommended for asthma and bronchitis with excessive phlegm, and also for vomiting and acid reflux. Chinese research has demonstrated mild antibacterial properties and also a stimulant effect on the nervous system, digestion and adrenal cortex.

Applications

ROOT
I. HELENIUM

DECOCTION Use for bronchitis, asthma, upper respiratory catarrh, or to ease hay fever symptoms. Take regularly as a general tonic or for long-standing chronic respiratory complaints. Also acts as a digestive tonic and liver stimulant.

TINCTURE Take as a tonic in debility and chronic respiratory complaints.

WASH Use the decoction or diluted tincture for eczema, rashes and varicose ulcers.

SYRUP Take a syrup made with the decoction for coughs.

FLOWERS
I. JAPONICA

DECOCTION Take for nausea, vomiting or coughs with copious phlegm. Alternatively, combine 10 g flowers with 10 g fresh ginger root, 10 ml *ban xia* and 5 ml liquorice root, and use for excess phlegm in the stomach with nausea, abdominal distension, flatulence, and vomiting of mucus.

SYRUP Take a syrup made with the infusion in 10-20 ml doses for coughs.

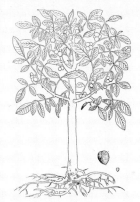

Juglans spp.
WALNUT

ACCORDING TO LEGEND, when the gods walked upon the earth, they lived on walnuts; hence the name *Juglans* or *Jovis glans*, Jupiter's nut. The tree has been cultivated in Europe since Roman times for its nuts; these yield an important oil containing essential fatty acids, such as α-linolenic, which are vital for healthy cell function and prostaglandin development. The white walnut, or butternut (*J. cinerea*), from eastern North America is a useful laxative.

"The oyle of walnuts... maketh smooth the hands and face, and taketh away... black and blew marks that come of bruses."
John Gerard, 1597.

Character
Bitter, astringent, mostly warm, drying; the fresh rind is cooling.
Constituents
Quinones, oils, tannins; nuts contain essential fatty acids, including *cis*-linoleic and α-linolenic.
Actions
J. REGIA: astringent, expels intestinal worms, anti-spasmodic, digestive tonic; the nut rind is anti-inflammatory.
J. CINEREA: purgative, astringent, promotes bile flow.

Parts used

LEAVES
J. REGIA
In Europe, walnut leaves are a popular home remedy for both eczema and blepharitis (eyelid inflammation) in children. Recent research suggests antifungal properties, as well as an antiseptic action; the leaves are also used for intestinal worms and as a digestive tonic. Harvest throughout the growing season.

Fresh leaves

Walnut Bach flower remedy is recommended for times of change, such as the menopause or moving home.

INNER BARK
J. CINEREA
The quills or inner bark are one of the few potent laxatives that are safe to use in pregnancy. Harvest in early summer.

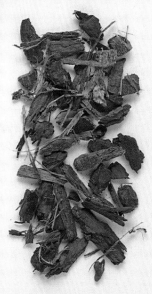

NUT & CASING
J. REGIA
The fleshy green outer casing of the nut is rich in fruit acids and minerals. Traditionally, infusions of this rind were used to darken the hair. The oil extracted from the nut contains essential fatty acids vital for many body processes. Harvest in late summer.

Walnut and casing

Fresh outer rind

Dried inner bark

Applications

LEAVES
J. REGIA

INFUSION Use for skin problems and eye inflammations, and as a digestive tonic for poor appetite.

WASH Use the infusion for eczema or for wounds and grazes.

EYEWASH Use either a well-strained infusion or 5 drops tincture in an eyebath of water for conjunctivitis and blepharitis.

OUTER NUT RIND
J. REGIA

 INFUSION Use for chronic diarrhoea or as a tonic in anaemia.

 HAIR RINSE Use the infusion as a rinse for hair loss.

NUT
J. REGIA

OIL Take 2 tsp unrefined walnut oil daily as a dietary supplement for menstrual dysfunction or for dry, flaky eczema.

INNER BARK
J. CINEREA

 DECOCTION Use for constipation, sluggish digestion, as a liver stimulant and for skin diseases.

 TINCTURE Take up to 5 ml daily for the same ailments as the decoction.

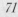

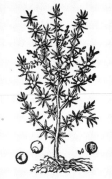

Juniperus communis
JUNIPER

LONG ASSOCIATED with ritual cleansing, juniper was burned in temples as a part of regular purification rites. Several medicinal recipes survive in Egyptian papyri dating to 1550 BC. In central European folk medicine, the oil extracted from the berries was regarded as a cure-all for typhoid, cholera, dysentery, tape worms and other ills associated with poverty.

"A remedy to treat tapeworm: juniper berries 5 parts, white oil 5 parts is taken for one day." Egyptian, c. 1550 BC.

Character
Pungent, slightly bitter-sweet, hot, dry.
Constituents
Volatile oil, flavonoids, sugars, glycosides, tannins, podophyllotoxin (an anti-tumour agent), vitamin C.
Actions
Urinary antiseptic, diuretic, carminative, digestive tonic, uterine stimulant, anti-rheumatic.

Parts used

BERRIES
The ripe, blue berries are mainly used for urinary infections and prescribed to clear acid wastes from the system in arthritis and gout. They reduce colic and flatulence, stimulate the digestion and encourage uterine contractions in labour. Pick after they have turned from green to purplish-blue; this process can take two years.

ESSENTIAL OIL
Made by steam distillation of ripe berries, the oil is a popular external remedy for arthritic and muscle pains. Internally, the oil increases the filtering of waste products by the kidneys, and is effective against many bacteria.

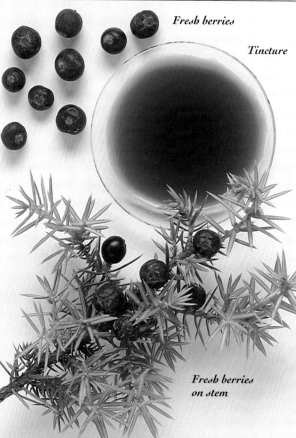
Fresh berries
Tincture
Fresh berries on stem

CADE OIL
Made by dry distillation of the heartwood of various types of juniper tree, cade oil is also known as juniper tar oil. It contains phenol and has a mild disinfectant action. Applied externally, it is non-irritant and is mainly used for chronic skin conditions, such as scaling eczema and psoriasis.

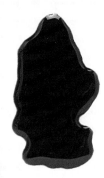
Cade oil

Applications

BERRIES
 INFUSION Sip a weak infusion (15 g berries to 500 ml water) for stomach upsets and chills or period pain.

TINCTURE Take 2 ml, three times a day, for urinary infections, such as cystitis, or to stimulate digestion.

ESSENTIAL OIL
LOTION Add 5 drops of oil to 50 ml equal parts rosewater and witch hazel for oily skin and acne.

CHEST RUB Dilute 10 drops juniper oil and 10 drops thyme oil in 20 ml almond oil, and rub into the chest for stubborn coughs.

OIL Add 5 drops to bath water for arthritic, gout or muscle pains.

MASSAGE OIL Dilute 10 drops juniper oil in 5 ml almond oil, and massage into arthritic joints.

CADE OIL
OINTMENT Add 10 drops to 20 ml melted ointment base. Allow to cool, and apply to chronic, scaling eczema or psoriasis.

 HAIR RINSE For psoriasis affecting the scalp, add 10 drops to 500 ml hot water and mix well. Leave on the hair for at least 15 minutes, then rinse thoroughly.

CAUTIONS
• Avoid the herb in pregnancy, as it is a uterine stimulant; may be taken during labour.
• Juniper may irritate the kidneys in long-term use, so do not take internally for more than six weeks without a break, or at all if there is already kidney damage.

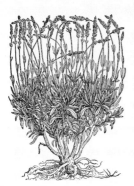

Lavandula spp.
LAVENDER

"...especiall good use for all griefes and paines of the head and brain."
John Parkinson, 1640.

ONE OF THE MOST POPULAR medicinal herbs since ancient times, lavender derives its name from the Latin *lavare*, to wash. In Arab medicine, lavender is used as an expectorant and antispasmodic, while in European folk tradition it is regarded as a useful wound herb, and a worm remedy for children. Species used medicinally include *L. angustifolia* or *L. spica*.

Character
Bitter, dry, mainly cooling.
Constituents
Volatile oil, tannins, coumarins, flavonoids, triterpenoids.
Actions
Relaxant, antispasmodic, circulatory stimulant, tonic for the nervous system, anti-bacterial, analgesic, carminative, promotes bile flow, antiseptic.

Parts used

FLOWERS
LESS potent than the essential oil, the flowers are useful for nervous exhaustion, headaches, or colic and indigestion. Harvest towards the end of flowering, when the petals have begun to fade. Dry in small bunches covered with paper bags to collect the florets as they fall.

Fresh flowers

Dried flowers

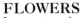

Tincture

Cream

ESSENTIAL OIL
One of the most popular aromatic oils, lavender oil can be used to treat a huge variety of ailments, and is an essential component of any household first aid box.

Applications

FLOWERS

INFUSION Take for nervous exhaustion, tension headaches or during labour; also for colic and indigestion. Give a weak infusion (25% normal strength) to babies for colic, irritability and excitement.

TINCTURE Take up to 5 ml, twice a day, for headaches and depression.

MOUTHWASH Use for halitosis.

ESSENTIAL OIL

CREAM Add a few drops of oil to chamomile cream for eczema.

LOTION Add a few drops of oil to a little water for sunburn or scalds.

CHEST RUB Add 1 ml oil and 5 drops chamomile oil to 10 ml carrier oil for asthmatic and bronchitic spasm.

HAIR RINSE Dilute 5-10 drops of oil in water for lice, or use a few drops of neat oil on a fine comb for nits.

MASSAGE OIL Dilute 1 ml lavender oil in 25 ml carrier oil, and massage into painful muscles. Dilute 10 drops in 25 ml carrier oil and massage into the temples and nape of the neck for tension headaches or at the first hint of a migraine.

OIL Apply neat to insect bites and stings. Dilute 10 drops oil in 25 ml carrier oil for sunstroke or to help prevent sunburn. (Note: this is not an effective sunblock.)

CAUTION
• Avoid high doses of the herb during pregnancy, as it is a uterine stimulant.

Leonurus spp.
MOTHERWORT

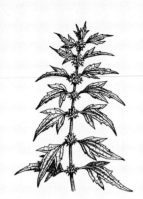

"There is no better herb to take melancholy vapours from the heart, to strengthen it, and make a merry, cheerful, blithe soul."
Nicholas Culpeper, 1653.

AN IMPORTANT HEART HERB since Roman times, motherwort, or *Leonurus cardiaca*, derives the *Leonurus* part of the botanical name from a Greek word meaning lion's tail, describing the shaggy shape of the leaves. Its common name also suggests a medicinal application for, in Gerard's words, "them that are in hard travell with childe". Early herbals also recommend the plant for "wykked sperytis". Chinese herbalists use the related species *L. heterophyllus*, mainly for menstrual disorders.

Character
Pungent, bitter, drying, cool.
Constituents
Alkaloids (inc. stachydrine), bitter glycosides, volatile oil, tannins, vitamin A.
Actions
Uterine stimulant, relaxant, cardiac tonic, carminative.

Parts used

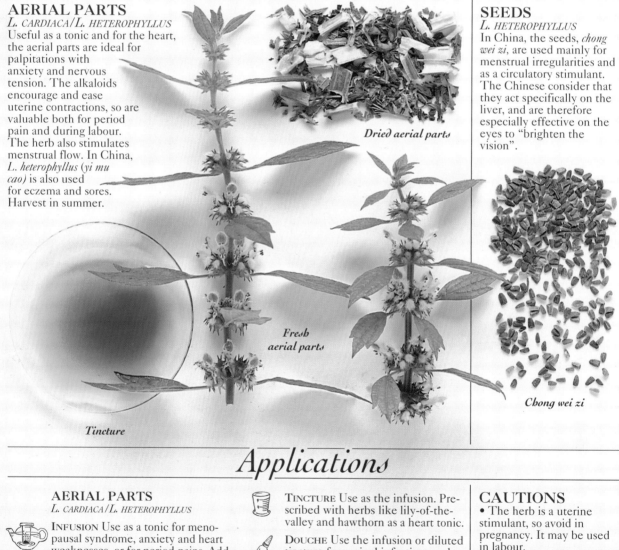

AERIAL PARTS
L. CARDIACA/L. HETEROPHYLLUS
Useful as a tonic and for the heart, the aerial parts are ideal for palpitations with anxiety and nervous tension. The alkaloids encourage and ease uterine contractions, so are valuable both for period pain and during labour. The herb also stimulates menstrual flow. In China, *L. heterophyllus* (*yi mu cao*) is also used for eczema and sores. Harvest in summer.

Dried aerial parts

Fresh aerial parts

Tincture

SEEDS
L. HETEROPHYLLUS
In China, the seeds, *chong wei zi*, are used mainly for menstrual irregularities and as a circulatory stimulant. The Chinese consider that they act specifically on the liver, and are therefore especially effective on the eyes to "brighten the vision".

Chong wei zi

Applications

AERIAL PARTS
L. CARDIACA/L. HETEROPHYLLUS

INFUSION Use as a tonic for menopausal syndrome, anxiety and heart weaknesses, or for period pains. Add 2-3 cloves and drink during labour. Take after childbirth to help restore the uterus and reduce the risk of post-partum bleeding.

SYRUP The infusion is traditionally made into a syrup to disguise the flavour. Use in similar ways.

TINCTURE Use as the infusion. Prescribed with herbs like lily-of-the-valley and hawthorn as a heart tonic.

DOUCHE Use the infusion or diluted tincture for vaginal infections and discharges.

SEEDS
L. HETEROPHYLLUS

DECOCTION Use for menstrual problems.

EYEWASH Use a weak decoction for conjunctivitis, or sore or tired eyes.

CAUTIONS
• The herb is a uterine stimulant, so avoid in pregnancy. It may be used in labour.
• Seek professional advice for all heart conditions.

Linum spp.
FLAX

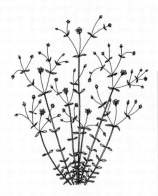

"Wherever flax seeds become a regular food item among the people, there will be better health." Mahatma Gandhi.

AS THE SOURCE OF LINEN FIBRE, *L.usitatissimum* has been cultivated since at least 5000 BC; today it is just as likely to be grown for its oil. The medicinal properties of the seeds, or linseed, were known to the Greeks: Hippocrates recommended them for inflammations of the mucous membranes. In 8th-century France, Charlemagne passed laws requiring the seeds to be consumed, to keep his subjects healthy. The related *L. catharticum* was once popular as a purgative but is little used today.

Character
Moist, warm, sweet; the oil is drying.
Constituents
Mucilage, cyanogenic glycosides, bitter principle; linseed oil contains *cis*-linoleic and α-linolenic acids, vitamins A, B, D, E, minerals and amino acids.
Actions
L. USITATISSIMUM: demulcent, soothing anti-tussive, antiseptic, anti-inflammatory, laxative.
L. CATHARTICUM: laxative, antirheumatic, diuretic.

Parts used

LINSEED
L. USITATISSIMUM
The ripe seeds can be used as a relaxing expectorant, a bulking laxative and extensively in poultices; they are also soothing for gastritis and sore throats. Linseed oil contains *cis*-linoleic and α-linolenic acids, needed for the production of hormone-like prostaglandins, vital for many bodily functions. Harvest when ripe.

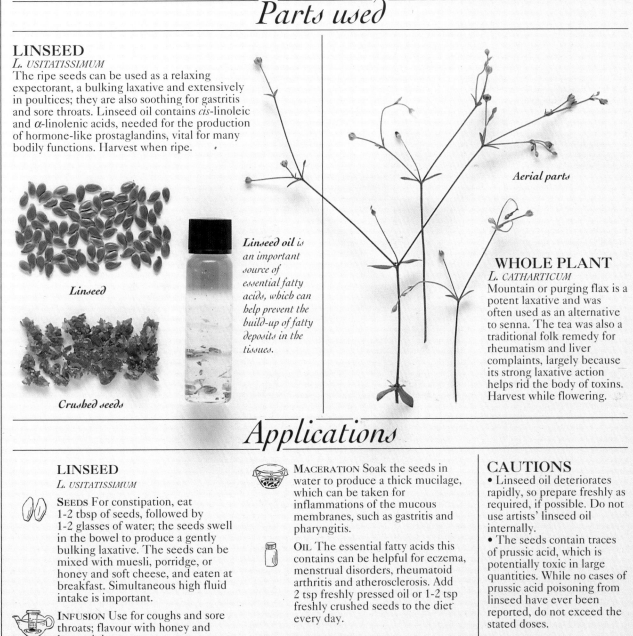

Linseed

Crushed seeds

Linseed oil is an important source of essential fatty acids, which can help prevent the build-up of fatty deposits in the tissues.

Aerial parts

WHOLE PLANT
L. CATHARTICUM
Mountain or purging flax is a potent laxative and was often used as an alternative to senna. The tea was also a traditional folk remedy for rheumatism and liver complaints, largely because its strong laxative action helps rid the body of toxins. Harvest while flowering.

Applications

LINSEED
L. USITATISSIMUM

SEEDS For constipation, eat 1-2 tbsp of seeds, followed by 1-2 glasses of water; the seeds swell in the bowel to produce a gently bulking laxative. The seeds can be mixed with muesli, porridge, or honey and soft cheese, and eaten at breakfast. Simultaneous high fluid intake is important.

INFUSION Use for coughs and sore throats; flavour with honey and lemon juice.

POULTICE Crush the seeds, and apply to boils, abscesses and ulcers; apply locally for pleurisy pain.

MACERATION Soak the seeds in water to produce a thick mucilage, which can be taken for inflammations of the mucous membranes, such as gastritis and pharyngitis.

OIL The essential fatty acids this contains can be helpful for eczema, menstrual disorders, rheumatoid arthritis and atherosclerosis. Add 2 tsp freshly pressed oil or 1-2 tsp freshly crushed seeds to the diet every day.

WHOLE PLANT
L. CATHARTICUM

INFUSION Take the fresh herb for constipation, liver congestion and rheumatic pain.

CAUTIONS
• Linseed oil deteriorates rapidly, so prepare freshly as required, if possible. Do not use artists' linseed oil internally.
• The seeds contain traces of prussic acid, which is potentially toxic in large quantities. While no cases of prussic acid poisoning from linseed have ever been reported, do not exceed the stated doses.

Lonicera spp.
HONEYSUCKLE

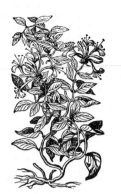

"I know of no better cure for the asthma than this..."
Nicholas Culpeper, 1653.

WOODBINE OR EUROPEAN honeysuckle (*L. periclymenum*) was once widely used for asthma, urinary complaints and in childbirth. Pliny recommended it to be taken in wine for spleen disorders. Today, Chinese honeysuckle (*L. japonica*, or *jin yin*) is more likely to be used medicinally. This was first listed in the *Tang Ben Cao*, written in AD 659, and is one of the most important Chinese herbs for clearing heat and poisons from the body.

Character
Sweet, cold.
Constituents
Tannin, flavonoids, mucilage, sugars; salicylic acid reported in European species.
Actions
L. PERICLYMENUM: diuretic, antispasmodic, expectorant, laxative, promotes vomiting.
L. JAPONICA: antibacterial, reduces blood pressure, anti-inflammatory, mild diuretic, antispasmodic.

Parts used

FLOWERS
L. PERICLYMENUM
Woodbine flowers were traditionally made into a syrup, which was taken as an expectorant for bad coughs and asthma, and as a diuretic. They are still used for coughs today. Harvest in summer.

Fresh flowers

FLOWER BUDS
L. JAPONICA
Known as *jin yin hua*, the flowers are widely used in feverish conditions, especially those attributed to "summer heat". They clear the toxins or "fire poisons" that in traditional Chinese theory cause conditions such as boils and dysentery. To treat some types of diarrhoea, the Chinese warm the buds slightly by stir-frying. Harvest in summer.

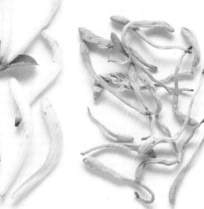

Fresh buds   *Dried buds*

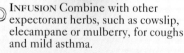

Fresh leaves

STEMS
L. JAPONICA
Called *jin yin teng* and *ren dong teng*, the stems and branches are generally used to remove heat from the acupuncture meridians, by stimulating the circulation of *qi* (energy). They are also used to treat feverish colds and dysentery, and as a cooling remedy in combination with other herbs for the acute stages of rheumatoid arthritis.

Fresh stems

Applications

FLOWERS
L. PERICLYMENUM

INFUSION Combine with other expectorant herbs, such as cowslip, elecampane or mulberry, for coughs and mild asthma.

SYRUP Take a syrup made with the infusion for coughs. Can be combined with other expectorant flowers, such as mullein or marshmallow.

FLOWER BUDS
L. JAPONICA

DECOCTION Take in the early stages of a feverish cold characterized by a headache, thirst and sore throat.

Use 10-15 g herb to 600 ml water. Add *huang lian* and *huang qin* for high fevers.

TINCTURE Use for diarrhoea or gastroenteritis related to food poisoning.

STEMS
L. JAPONICA

DECOCTION Make with 15-30 g herb to 600 ml water and use as the flower bud decoction, especially if there are painful joints, as in influenza. Combine with other cooling herbs, such as *luo shi teng* or *shi hu*, for inflammatory diseases, for example, rheumatoid arthritis.

CAUTIONS
• Do not use honeysuckle berries, as they are toxic.
• If using the tincture for digestive upsets, use the hot-water method (see p. 125) to reduce the alcohol.

Malus spp.
APPLES

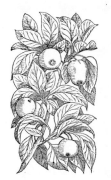

"Their syrup is a good cordial in faintings, palpitations, and melancholy."
Nicholas Culpeper, 1653.

DESPITE THE ADAGE that "an apple a day keeps the doctor away", the apple's medicinal properties are often forgotten. The fruits of *M. communis* have been cultivated since Roman times, with ripe apples used as laxatives and unripe ones to counter diarrhoea. In Galenical medicine (see p. 24), most apples were cool and moist; juices and infusions were prescribed for fevers and eye infections. A 1983 study showed that apples can reduce blood cholesterol levels.

Character
Ripe fruit: cool, moist, generally sweet.
Unripe fruit & some cultivated varieties: cool, moist, sour.
Constituents
Sugars, fruit acids, pectin, vitamins A, B₁, C, minerals.
Actions
Tonic, digestive and liver stimulant, diuretic, anti-rheumatic, laxative, antiseptic.

Parts used

RAW FRUIT
Fresh apples are cleansing for the system, especially if eaten in the morning, while in the evening, they have a more laxative action. They have also been traditionally used in poultices for skin inflammations.

Fresh slices

Stewed apple

STEWED FRUIT
Traditionally used for diarrhoea and dysentery, stewed apples can be especially helpful for babies and small children. They can also be soothing in gastric ulceration or ulcerative colitis.

The peel has been used in France in preparations for rheumatism and gout, and as a diuretic in urinary disorders.

Fresh apple

Applications

RAW FRUIT

 FRESH Eat ripe apples for constipation associated with an overheated stomach. Eat sour apples as a diuretic in cystitis and other urinary infections. Apples are also a good source of minerals and vitamins in anaemia and debility.

 INFUSION Take an infusion of the fresh, raw fruit as a warming drink for rheumatic pains and intestinal colic, and as a cooling remedy for feverish colds.

JUICE Use neat juice or juice mixed with olive oil as a household standby for cuts and grazes.

STEWED FRUIT

FRESH Use for diarrhoea, gastro-enteritis and intestinal infections.

 POULTICE Apply to skin infections, such as scabies.

CAUTION
• Apples are a "cold" fruit, so eating too many or eating them on a chilled stomach can lead to digestive upsets and wind.

Melissa officinalis
LEMON BALM

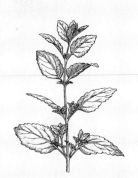

"Balm is sovereign for the brain, strengthening the memory and powerfully chasing away melancholy."
John Evelyn, 1679.

BALM AND BEES have been linked since ancient times. *Melissa* comes from the Greek for "honey bee", and lemon balm has the same healing and tonic properties as honey and royal jelly. Gerard said that the herb "comforteth the hart and driveth away all sadnesse", and it was a favourite in medieval "elixirs of youth"; the alchemist Paracelsus made a preparation called *primum ens melissae*, and even in the 18th century, it was still thought to "renew youth".

Character Cold, dry, sour, slightly bitter.
Constituents Volatile oil (inc. citronellal), polyphenols, tannins, bitter principle, flavonoids, rosmarinic acid.
Actions Sedative, anti-depressant, digestive stimulant, relaxes peripheral blood vessels, promotes sweating, relaxing restorative for nervous system, antiviral (possibly due to polyphenols and tannins), antibacterial, carminative, antispasmodic.

Parts used

LEAVES
Good for depression and tension, the leaves are also carminative, so are ideal for anyone who suffers from digestive upsets when worried or anxious. Lemon balm is cooling, so the leaves are good in feverish colds; fresh leaves make a refreshing lemon tea in summer. Externally, the herb can be used on sores or painful swellings. Harvest before flowering.

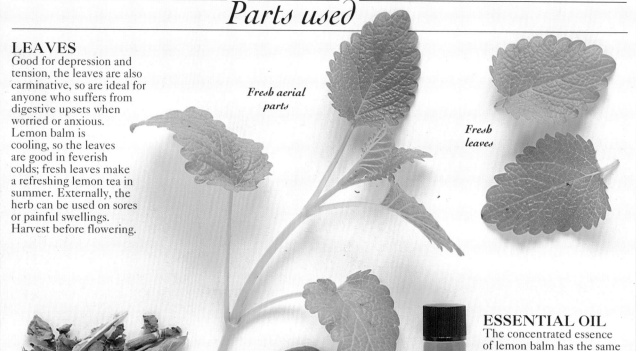

Fresh aerial parts

Fresh leaves

Dried leaves

Ointment

ESSENTIAL OIL
The concentrated essence of lemon balm has the same properties as the leaves, but is far more potent: a few drops make an excellent antidote to depression. Pure essential oil is difficult to obtain commercially; it is often adulterated with lemon or lemongrass oils.

Applications

LEAVES

 INFUSION Take for depression, nervous exhaustion, indigestion, nausea and the early stages of colds and influenza. Best made with fresh leaves.

 TINCTURE Has a stronger but similar action to the infusion. Best made from fresh leaves. Small doses (5-10 drops) are usually more effective.

 COMPRESS Use a pad soaked in the infusion to relieve painful swellings, such as gout.

OINTMENT Use for sores, insect bites or to repel insects.

INFUSED OIL Use hot infused oil as the ointment or as a gentle massage oil for depression, tension, asthma and bronchitis.

ESSENTIAL OIL

OINTMENT Combine 5 ml oil with 100 g ointment base for insect bites or to repel insects.

MASSAGE OIL Dilute 5-10 drops oil in 20 ml almond or olive oil, and use for tension or chest complaints.

Mentha spp.
MINT

THERE ARE THOUGHT to be at least thirty species of mint. Until the 17th century, all mints were used in much the same way, with little attempt to differentiate between varieties. Today, peppermint (*M. piperita*) is preferred medicinally in the West; the Chinese use field mint (*M. arvensis*), known as *bo he*. Garden mint is usually spearmint (*M. spicata*). Not as strong as peppermint, this can be used in similar ways, and is good for children.

"If any man can name... all the properties of mint, he must know how many fish swim in the Indian ocean." Wilafried of Strabo, 12th century.

Character Pungent, dry, generally cooling.
Constituents Volatile oil (mainly menthol), tannins, flavonoids, tocopherols, choline, bitter principle.
Actions Antispasmodic, digestive tonic, prevents vomiting, carminative, relaxes peripheral blood vessels, promotes sweating but also cooling internally, promotes bile flow, analgesic.

Parts used

AERIAL PARTS
M. PIPERITA
These relax the muscles of the digestive tract and stimulate bile flow, so are useful for indigestion, flatulence, colic and similar conditions. They reduce nausea and can be helpful for travel sickness; they also promote sweating in fevers and influenza. Harvest just before flowering.

Fresh aerial parts

Dried aerial parts

ESSENTIAL OIL
M. PIPERITA
Peppermint oil contains large amounts of menthol. In fairly high doses, it is analgesic and calming. It is also cooling, so is good for skin complaints, fevers, or headaches and migraines linked to over-heating. Antibacterial, it can help combat infections. Used as an inhalant, it clears nasal congestion.

AERIAL PARTS
M. ARVENSIS
The Chinese use *bo he* as a cooling remedy for head colds and influenza, and also for some types of headache, sore throats and eye inflammations. As a liver stimulant, it is added to remedies for digestive disorders or liver *qi* (energy) stagnation.

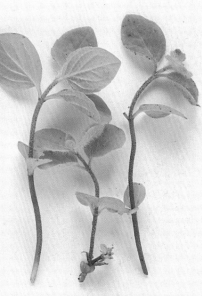

Fresh aerial parts

Applications

AERIAL PARTS
M. PIPERITA /M. ARVENSIS

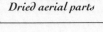 INFUSION Take for nausea, travel sickness, indigestion, flatulence, colic, feverish conditions and migraines.

 TINCTURE Use for the same conditions as the infusion.

 COMPRESS Soak a pad in the infusion to cool inflamed joints or for rheumatism or neuralgia.

 INHALATION Put a few fresh leaves in boiling water, and inhale to ease nasal congestion.

ESSENTIAL OIL
M. PIPERITA

WASH Use 2-3 drops of oil in 10 ml water for skin irritations, itching, burns, inflammations, scabies and ringworm, or to repel mosquitos.

INHALATION 2-3 drops of oil in a saucer of water left in the room at night will reduce nasal congestion.

MASSAGE OIL Dilute 5-10 drops peppermint oil in 25 ml almond or sunflower oil for headaches, fever or period pain, or to relieve milk congestion when breastfeeding.

CAUTIONS
• Avoid prolonged use of the essential oil as an inhalant.
• Mint can irritate the mucous membranes and should not be given to children for more than a week without a break. Do not give any form of mint directly to young babies.
• Peppermint can reduce milk flow, so take with caution internally while breastfeeding.

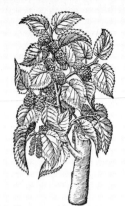

Morus nigra & M. alba
MULBERRY

"Mulberries taken in meate... do very speedily passe thorow the belly... and make a passage for other meates, as Galen saith."
John Gerard, 1597.

IN THE 16TH CENTURY, the berries, bark and leaves of the black mulberry (*M. nigra*) were all used medicinally: the berries for inflammations and to stop bleeding; the bark for toothache; and the leaves for "the bitings of serpents" and as an antidote to aconite poisoning. While mulberry has faded from the European *materia medica*, white mulberry (*M. alba*) is still widely used in China as a remedy for coughs, colds and high blood pressure, and as a *yin* tonic.

Character
Mainly sweet, cold; leaves also bitter; branch bitter and neutral.
Constituents
Flavonoids, coumarin, tannins, sugars; berries also contain vitamins A, B$_1$, B$_2$, C.
Actions
Berries: tonic, laxative.
Leaves: antibacterial, promote sweating, expectorant.
Branch: antirheumatic, reduces high blood pressure, analgesic.
Root bark: sedative, diuretic, expectorant, reduces high blood pressure.

Parts used

BERRIES
M. NIGRA & M. ALBA
In China, white mulberries, or *sang shen*, are used as a *yin* tonic to nourish the blood and "vital essence", and as a gentle laxative in constipation. In European tradition, black mulberries are also regarded as a tonic and taken for weakness. Harvest when ripe.

Fresh white mulberry

Dried white mulberry

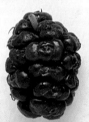

Fresh black mulberry

Crushed black mulberry

LEAVES
M. NIGRA & M. ALBA
In China, white mulberry leaves, *sang ye*, are generally used for colds with fevers, headaches and sore throats, to cool heat in the liver channel, which can lead to sore eyes and irritability, and to cool the blood. In Europe, black mulberry leaves have recently been used to stimulate insulin production in diabetes. Harvest in summer.

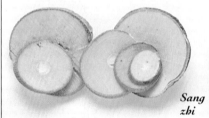

Sang zhi

BRANCH & TWIGS
M. ALBA
Sang zhi have been shown to be analgesic and to reduce high blood pressure, although traditionally they have been used for rheumatic disorders. The Chinese consider them more suitable for upper body pain.

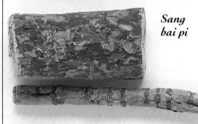

Fresh black mulberry leaves

Sang bai pi

ROOT BARK
M. ALBA
Sang bai pi is a good expectorant for coughs associated with "hot" conditions (usually typified by thick, sticky yellow phlegm). It can help asthma and is sedative and soothing.

Applications

BERRIES (*M. ALBA/M. NIGRA*)
TINCTURE Take as a tonic to nourish the blood and *yin*: combine with *wu wei zi* or *he shou wu*, or just eat the fresh fruits.

MOUTHWASH/GARGLE Crush the fresh berries, and use the juice for mouth ulcers and sore throats.

LEAVES (*M. ALBA/M. NIGRA*)
INFUSION Take for colds and chills: combines well with elderflower and mint.

DECOCTION Take for colds.

SYRUP Take a syrup made from the decoction for coughs.

TWIGS
M. ALBA
DECOCTION Use for rheumatic pains in the upper body: combine with herbs such as *wei ling xian*, Siberian ginseng, *fang feng*, *gui zhi* or *qin jiao*.

ROOT BARK
M. ALBA
DECOCTION Use for "hot" conditions affecting the lungs, for asthma, or as a diuretic in oedema (use with *fu ling*, *chen pi* and buchu).

CAUTIONS
• Avoid excess fruits if suffering from diarrhoea.
• Avoid the leaves and bark if the lungs are weak or "cold"; if in doubt, seek professional advice.

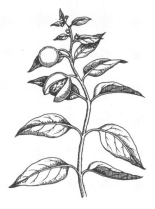

Myristica fragrans
NUTMEG

FIRST BROUGHT TO EUROPE from the Banda Islands by Portuguese sailors in around 1512, nutmeg gained the reputation of a cure-all, and was widely eaten as a tonic. Its hallucinogenic properties were soon discovered, with nutmeg eaters becoming "deliriously inebriated". It was also erroneously taken to procure abortions and acclaimed as a cure for the plague. Known as *rou dou kou* in China, it has been used there since the 7th century for stomach problems.

"...in large quantities it is apt to affect the head, and even to manifest an hypnotic power..."
Dr. E. Sibley, 1821.

Character
Pungent, warm.
Constituents
Volatile oil (inc. borneol, eugenol).
Actions
Carminative, digestive stimulant, antispasmodic, prevents vomiting, appetite stimulant, anti-inflammatory.

Parts used

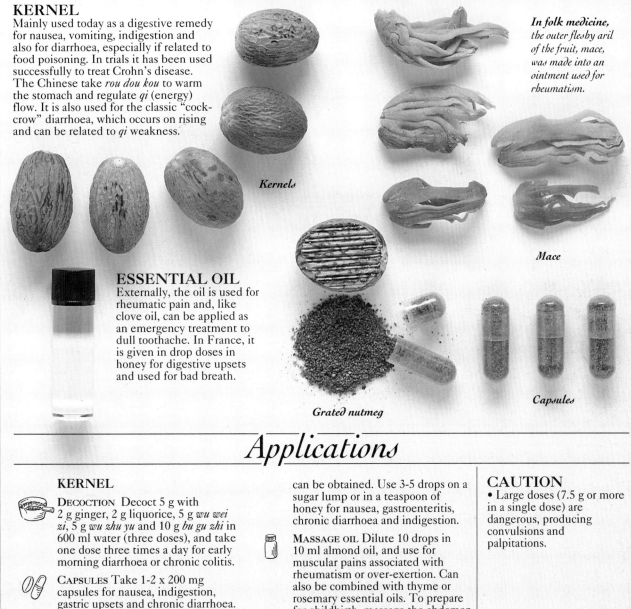

KERNEL
Mainly used today as a digestive remedy for nausea, vomiting, indigestion and also for diarrhoea, especially if related to food poisoning. In trials it has been used successfully to treat Crohn's disease. The Chinese take *rou dou kou* to warm the stomach and regulate *qi* (energy) flow. It is also used for the classic "cockcrow" diarrhoea, which occurs on rising and can be related to *qi* weakness.

Kernels

In folk medicine, the outer fleshy aril of the fruit, mace, was made into an ointment used for rheumatism.

Mace

ESSENTIAL OIL
Externally, the oil is used for rheumatic pain and, like clove oil, can be applied as an emergency treatment to dull toothache. In France, it is given in drop doses in honey for digestive upsets and used for bad breath.

Grated nutmeg

Capsules

Applications

KERNEL

DECOCTION Decoct 5 g with 2 g ginger, 2 g liquorice, 5 g *wu wei zi*, 5 g *wu zhu yu* and 10 g *bu gu zhi* in 600 ml water (three doses), and take one dose three times a day for early morning diarrhoea or chronic colitis.

CAPSULES Take 1-2 x 200 mg capsules for nausea, indigestion, gastric upsets and chronic diarrhoea.

ESSENTIAL OIL

OIL Put 1-2 drops on a cotton swab, and apply to the gums around an aching tooth until dental treatment can be obtained. Use 3-5 drops on a sugar lump or in a teaspoon of honey for nausea, gastroenteritis, chronic diarrhoea and indigestion.

MASSAGE OIL Dilute 10 drops in 10 ml almond oil, and use for muscular pains associated with rheumatism or over-exertion. Can also be combined with thyme or rosemary essential oils. To prepare for childbirth, massage the abdomen daily in the three weeks before the baby is due with a mixture of 5 drops nutmeg oil and no more than 5 drops sage oil in 25 ml almond oil.

CAUTION
• Large doses (7.5 g or more in a single dose) are dangerous, producing convulsions and palpitations.

Ocimum basilicum
BASIL

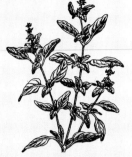

"This herb and rue will not grow together... and we know rue is as great an enemy of poison as any that grows."
Nicholas Culpeper, 1653.

FROM ITS NATIVE INDIA, basil was introduced into Europe in ancient times. Views and traditions associated with the herb have been mixed. Some cultures associated basil with hatred and misfortune; others regarded it as a love token. Dioscorides said that it should never be taken internally, while Pliny recommended smelling it in vinegar for fainting fits. In Ayurvedic medicine, basil is known as *tulsi* and the juice is widely used.

Character
Sweet, pungent, slightly bitter, very warm, dry.
Constituents
Volatile oil (including estragol), tannins, basil camphor.
Actions
Antidepressant, antiseptic, stimulates the adrenal cortex, prevents vomiting, tonic, carminative, febrifuge, expectorant, soothes itching.

Parts used

LEAVES
Good for rubbing on insect bites, the leaves can also be taken as a warming and uplifting tonic for nervous exhaustion or any cold condition. Harvest before flowering.

Fresh aerial parts

Dried aerial parts

ESSENTIAL OIL
In aromatherapy, the oil, extracted from the leaves, is often combined with hyssop, bergamot or geranium oils as a stimulating massage for depression.

In Ayurvedic medicine, the juice is recommended for snakebites, as a general tonic, for chills, coughs, skin problems and earache.

Applications

LEAVES

FRESH Rub on insect bites to reduce itching and inflammation.

INFUSION Combine with motherwort and drink immediately after childbirth to prevent a retained placenta.

TINCTURE Combine with wood betony and skullcap for nervous conditions, or with elecampane and hyssop for coughs and bronchitis.

WASH Combine the juice with an equal quantity of honey and use for ringworm and itching skin.

JUICE Mix with a decoction of cinnamon and cloves for chills.

SYRUP Combine the juice with an equal quantity of honey for coughs.

INHALATION Pour boiling water on to the leaves and inhale the steam for head colds.

ESSENTIAL OIL

OIL Add 5-10 drops to a bath for nervous exhaustion, mental fatigue, melancholy or fear.

CHEST RUB Dilute 5 drops basil oil in 10 ml almond or sunflower oil for asthma and bronchitis.

MASSAGE OIL Use the diluted oil for nervous weakness; can also be applied as an insect repellent.

CAUTION
• Do not use the essential oil externally (or internally) in pregnancy.

Paeonia spp.
PAEONY

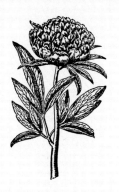

"This plant also prevents the mocking delusions that the Fauns bring on us in our sleep." Pliny, AD 77.

ALTHOUGH NOW REGARDED in the West as no more than a decorative garden flower, the paeony has a long tradition as a medicinal herb, and was used in the past to treat nervous conditions that included epilepsy. Today, the root is still valued in Chinese medicine, where two species are used: both the red- and white-flowered *P. lactiflora*, and *P. suffruticosa*, the tree paeony. The name is reputedly derived from Paeos, a physician during the Trojan Wars.

Character
P. LACTIFLORA: sour, bitter, cold.
P. SUFFRUTICOSA: more pungent.
Constituents
Alkaloids, volatile oil, benzoic acid, asparagin.
Actions
P. LACTIFLORA: antibacterial, anti-spasmodic, anti-inflammatory, analgesic, tranquillizing, reduces blood pressure.
P. SUFFRUTICOSA: antibacterial, circulatory stimulant, reduces blood pressure, anti-inflammatory, analgesic, sedative.

Parts used

ROOT
P. LACTIFLORA (RED)
Known as *chi shao yao* in China, the root of the red paeony is thought to cool the blood, move stagnating blood, and relieve pain. It has recently been used successfully in combination with other Chinese herbs to treat childhood eczema at Great Ormond Street Hospital in London.

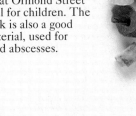

Chi shao yao

ROOT
P. LACTIFLORA (WHITE)
White paeony root has a much more specific action on the liver than red paeony, soothing liver energy and improving function. In Chinese medicine, *bai shao yao* is seen as nourishing the blood rather than cooling it, and is considered one of the great women's tonics, often used for menstrual disorders.

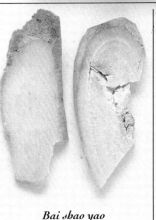

Bai shao yao

ROOT BARK
P. SUFFRUTICOSA
In China, tree paeony root bark, *mu dan pi*, is considered to cool the blood, and has been used in the eczema project at the Great Ormond Street Hospital for children. The root bark is also a good antibacterial, used for boils and abscesses.

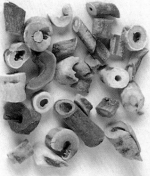

Mu dan pi

Applications

ROOT
P. LACTIFLORA (RED)

 DECOCTION Use up to 45 g herb in 600 ml water (enough for three doses) for any condition involving over-heated blood, including certain types of eczema, skin inflammations, nosebleeds, and pain associated with injury. Best in combination with herbs such as *mu dan pi* (*P. suffruticosa*) and *fang feng*.

ROOT
P. LACTIFLORA (WHITE)

DECOCTION Take for liver-associated problems and some menstrual disorders. As a regular tonic, ideal for women and reputed to beautify the skin, decoct 20 g *bai shao yao* and 5 g liquorice root for 15 minutes with 500 ml water, and drink two wine-glass doses a day.

ROOT BARK
P. SUFFRUTICOSA

DECOCTION Use 30 g herb in 600 ml water (enough for three doses) in combination with other herbs such as *sheng di huang* for feverish conditions involving nosebleeds, or add to remedies for hot, dry eczema. Combine with *shu di huang, shan zhu yu, fu ling, ze xie* and *shan yao* for liver disharmonies.

Panax spp.
GINSENG

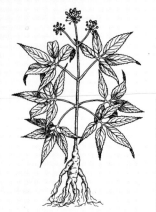

USED IN CHINA FOR over 5,000 years, ginseng (*P. ginseng*) was known to 9th-century Arab physicians. Marco Polo wrote of this prized wonder drug and, when a delegation from the King of Siam visited Louis XIV, they presented him with a root of *gintz-aen*. From then on, ginseng was widely used by wealthy Europeans for exhaustion and debility. By the 18th century, it was also popular in America, especially when *P. quinquefolius* was found to be indigenous.

"This, with the Chinese, is the medicine par excellence, the last resort when all other drugs fail..."
G. Stuart, 1911.

Character
All species: Sweet, slightly bitter.
P. GINSENG /P. NOTOGINSENG: warm.
P. QUINQUEFOLIUS: cool.
Constituents
Steroidal glycosides, saponins, volatile oil, vitamin D, acetyleneic compounds, sterols.
Actions
Tonic, stimulant, reduces blood sugar and cholesterol levels, stimulates the immune system.

Parts used

ROOT
P. GINSENG
Korean or Chinese ginseng, *ren shen*, is one of the most prized and expensive herbs. It is a *yang* tonic, replenishing *qi* (energy), especially in the spleen and lungs. Modern research has identified steroidal components similar to human sex hormones. *Ren shen* also strengthens the immune system and decreases fatigue.

Ren shen

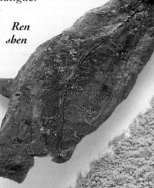

Powder

ROOT
P. QUINQUEFOLIUS
American ginseng, *xi yang shen*, is a *yin* tonic, taken in China for fevers and for exhaustion due to a chronic, wasting disease such as tuberculosis. It can help coughs related to lung weakness.

Xi yang shen

Powder

ROOT
P. NOTOGINSENG
Pseudoginseng, known as *san qi* in China, is used as an analgesic and to stop internal and external bleeding. It is also added to treatments for coronary heart disease and angina. *San qi* was used extensively by the Vietcong during the Vietnam war to increase recovery rates from gun-shot wounds.

San qi

Sliced root

Applications

ROOT
P. GINSENG

NOTE: It is often best to take P. ginseng for one month in autumn to strengthen the body for winter. If taking P. ginseng regularly, have a break of at least 2-3 weeks every two months.

 DECOCTION Take 3-10 g in 500 ml water as a general *yang* tonic.

 TINCTURE Use for diarrhoea related to weak digestive function. For asthma and chronic coughs, combine with walnut and ginger.

 POWDER Use in capsules or tablets in 500 mg -4 g doses as a tonic.

ROOT
P. QUINQUEFOLIUS

 TINCTURE Take as a tonic or combine with herbs such as elecampane and mulberry bark for chronic coughs and weak lungs.

 POWDER Use in capsules or tablets in 1-2 g doses for *yin* deficiency.

ROOT
P. NOTOGINSENG

 POWDER Use in capsules or tablets in 1-2 g doses for wounds, bleeding or pain. Combine with slippery elm for the pain of gastric ulceration.

CAUTIONS
• Avoid *P. notoginseng* in pregnancy; it may adversely affect the foetus.
• Although *P. ginseng* is generally safe, side effects have been reported: avoid high doses or prolonged use in pregnancy and hypertension.
• Avoid other stimulants such as tea, coffee and cola drinks when taking *P. ginseng*.

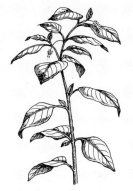

Phytolacca americana
POKEROOT

CALLED *POCON* BY NATIVE AMERICANS, pokeroot was mainly used in two ways: as an emetic, and externally for skin diseases. The Delaware Indians took it as a heart stimulant and in Virginia it was regarded as a strong purgative. Even today Appalachian backwoodsmen chew the seeds and berries for arthritis – all the more remarkable because the fresh plant is very toxic. It arrived in Europe in the 19th century and is used as an important lymphatic cleanser.

Character
Pungent, drying, slightly cold.
Constituents
Saponins, tannins, alkaloids, bitter principle, sugars.
Actions
Antirheumatic, stimulant, anticatarrhal, purgative, causes vomiting, antiparasitic, anti-inflammatory, immune stimulant, lymphatic stimulant, mild analgesic.

Parts used

DRIED ROOT
Used today as a lymphatic cleanser, particularly for glandular fever and tonsillitis, the dried root can also be helpful for mastitis, and is added to rheumatic remedies. Externally, it is used occasionally for skin infections such as scabies and ringworm; it can also be applied in poultices to soothe ulcers, haemorrhoids and inflamed joints.

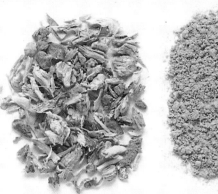

Dried root   *Powdered root*

BERRIES
Generally described as "milder" in action than the root, the fresh and dried berries are toxic, so the Appalachian practice of chewing them is not recommended. In the past, they were used externally for skin complaints and in poultices for rheumatism. The juice was applied for ulcers and tumours, but is not particularly effective.

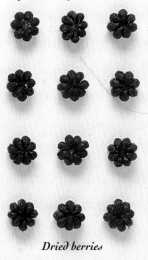

Tablets   *Capsules*

Tincture

Dried berries

Applications

DRIED ROOT

TINCTURE Use a maximum dose of 1 ml (20 drops) for acute lymphatic congestion and infection, including mastitis, tonsillitis, scrofula and glandular fever. Combine with wild indigo, purple coneflower or cleavers. Add to herbal remedies for rheumatism and rheumatoid arthritis. Can also be added to remedies used to stimulate the liver, or in prescriptions for gastric ulceration.

POULTICE Apply to inflamed joints, varicose ulcers and haemorrhoids.

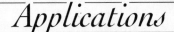

LOTION Use the diluted tincture or powder dispersed in water for lymphatic swellings.

POWDER Take internally in small doses (50-250 mg) for lymphatic disorders including mastitis and tonsillitis, or for rheumatism. Use a little powder as a dust for skin fungal infections, dry eczema, psoriasis and scabies.

CAUTIONS
• All parts of the fresh plant are toxic and can cause vomiting. Avoid growing pokeroot in the garden if you have young children, as fatalities have been reported.
• The dried berries are toxic.
• In large doses, the dried root is an extremely violent emetic (causes vomiting) and purgative. Do not exceed stated doses.
• Avoid pokeroot in pregnancy, as it can cause foetal abnormalities.

Plantago spp.
PLANTAIN

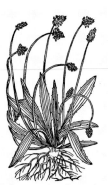

"And thou, waybread, Mother of worts, Open from Eastward, Mighty within."
The Lacnunga, 9th century.

CALLED WAYBREAD by the Anglo-Saxons, common plantain (*P. major*) was considered an important healing herb: Pliny even suggests that if several pieces of flesh are put in a pot with plantain it will join them back together again. Today, ribwort plantain (*P. lanceolata*) is mostly used in herbal medicine, although waybread still has a first-aid role in treating bee stings. The seeds of related species are used in patent laxatives.

Character
Slightly sweet, salty and bitter; cool, mainly drying.
Constituents
Leaves: mucilage, glycosides, tannins, minerals.
Seeds: mucilage, oils, protein, starch.
Actions
Leaves: relaxing expectorant, tonify mucous membranes, anti-catarrhal, antispasmodic, topically healing.
Seeds: demulcent, laxative.

Parts used

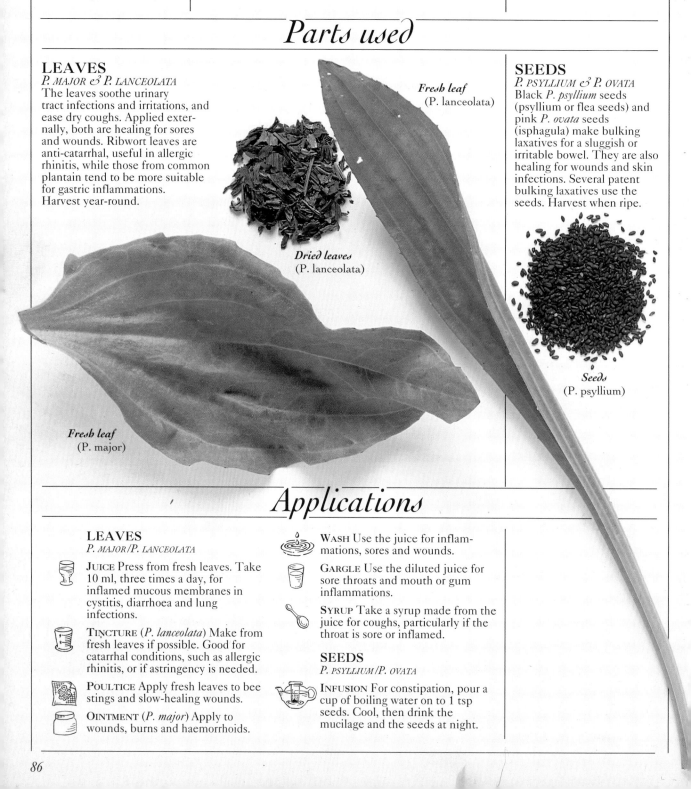

LEAVES
P. MAJOR & P. LANCEOLATA
The leaves soothe urinary tract infections and irritations, and ease dry coughs. Applied externally, both are healing for sores and wounds. Ribwort leaves are anti-catarrhal, useful in allergic rhinitis, while those from common plantain tend to be more suitable for gastric inflammations. Harvest year-round.

Dried leaves
(P. lanceolata)

Fresh leaf
(P. lanceolata)

SEEDS
P. PSYLLIUM & P. OVATA
Black *P. psyllium* seeds (psyllium or flea seeds) and pink *P. ovata* seeds (isphagula) make bulking laxatives for a sluggish or irritable bowel. They are also healing for wounds and skin infections. Several patent bulking laxatives use the seeds. Harvest when ripe.

Seeds
(P. psyllium)

Fresh leaf
(P. major)

Applications

LEAVES
P. MAJOR/P. LANCEOLATA

JUICE Press from fresh leaves. Take 10 ml, three times a day, for inflamed mucous membranes in cystitis, diarrhoea and lung infections.

TINCTURE (*P. lanceolata*) Make from fresh leaves if possible. Good for catarrhal conditions, such as allergic rhinitis, or if astringency is needed.

POULTICE Apply fresh leaves to bee stings and slow-healing wounds.

OINTMENT (*P. major*) Apply to wounds, burns and haemorrhoids.

WASH Use the juice for inflammations, sores and wounds.

GARGLE Use the diluted juice for sore throats and mouth or gum inflammations.

SYRUP Take a syrup made from the juice for coughs, particularly if the throat is sore or inflamed.

SEEDS
P. PSYLLIUM/P. OVATA

INFUSION For constipation, pour a cup of boiling water on to 1 tsp seeds. Cool, then drink the mucilage and the seeds at night.

Primula spp.
COWSLIP & PRIMROSE

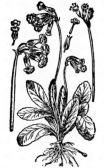

"...our city dames know well enough the ointment or distilled water of it aids beauty."
Nicholas Culpeper, 1653.

COWSLIPS (*P. VERIS*) TAKE THEIR NAME from the Anglo-Saxon *cu-sloppe*, a reminder of the days when they bloomed in meadows among dairy herds. Given their current rarity, primroses (*P. vulgaris*) have long been regarded as a good second-best, and the two plants are used almost interchangeably. The roots are high in saponins, irritant chemicals with expectorant properties. They are also a rich source of salicylates, which have similar actions to aspirin.

Character
Sweet, dry, slightly warm.
Constituents
Flowers: Volatile oil, glycosides, bitters.
Root: Saponins, glycosides, salicylates, volatile oil, tannin, flavonoids, sugars, silicic acid.
Actions
Flowers: sedating nervine, calming, astringent, promote sweating.
Root: stimulating expectorant, antispasmodic, anti-inflammatory, astringent.

Parts used

FLOWERS
Containing neither salicylates nor saponins, the flowers have markedly different properties from the root. The petals are very sedating, ideal for over-excited states or what Gerard described as "the frensies". They are also astringent and promote sweating, and can be used for feverish colds with headaches and nasal congestion. Harvest in spring.

Fresh primrose petals

Dried primrose flowers

Fresh primrose flowers

ROOT
Once a popular European standby for arthritis, the root is mainly used today for chesty coughs, as in chronic bronchitis. It helps to stimulate and warm the lungs, and can be very effective where there is a lot of sticky, white phlegm suggesting a "cold" condition. Harvest roots of established plants in autumn.

Dried cowslip flowers

Fresh cowslip flowers

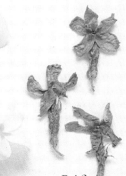

Tincture

Applications

FLOWERS

INFUSION Sip for headaches, feverish chills or head colds and catarrh.

TINCTURE Take 5-10 drops for insomnia, anxiety or over-excitement.

COMPRESS Soak a pad in the hot infusion and apply to facial or trigeminal neuralgia.

OINTMENT Use for sunburn and skin blemishes.

ESSENTIAL OIL For insomnia, use 5-10 drops in bath water at night.

MASSAGE OIL Dilute 5-10 drops oil in 25 ml almond or sunflower oil. Use for nerve pains, or apply to the temples for migraine.

ROOT

DECOCTION Take to clear the phlegm of stubborn coughs, especially chronic bronchitis. Can also relieve arthritis and rheumatism.

TINCTURE Take a standard dose for the same ailments as the decoction.

COMPRESS Soak a pad in the decoction for painful arthritic joints.

CAUTIONS
• Avoid the root if sensitive to aspirin.
• Do not take high doses of either herb during pregnancy, as they are uterine stimulants.
• Neither herb should be used by patients taking warfarin or other blood-thinning drugs.

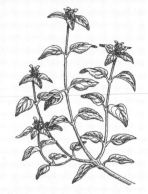

Prunella vulgaris
SELF-HEAL

A HIGHLY REGARDED EUROPEAN wound herb, self-heal is widely used to stop bleeding. In the past, the flower spikes were considered to resemble the throat, and under the Doctrine of Signatures theory, whereby plants cured those parts of the body that they most resembled, self-heal was also used for inflammations of the mouth and throat. In Chinese medicine, the flower spikes are used, and are known as *xia ku cao*, literally meaning "summer dry herb".

"...it serveth for the same that Bugle doth, and in the world, there are not two better wound herbes, as hath been often prooved."
John Gerard, 1597.

Character
Slightly bitter, pungent, cold, drying.
Constituents
Flavonoids (inc. rutin), vitamins A, B, C, K, fatty acids, volatile oil, bitter principle.
Actions
Aerial parts: antibacterial, reduce blood pressure, diuretic, astringent, heal wounds.
Flower spikes: liver stimulant, reduce blood pressure, antibacterial, cooling.

Parts used

AERIAL PARTS
The leaves and young shoots are used by Western herbalists to stop bleeding and applied fresh in poultices as emergency first aid on clean cuts. Culpeper recommended them for "green" (fresh) wounds, suggesting that they would be ideal to "close the lips of them" in the days before stitches. Harvest before flowering.

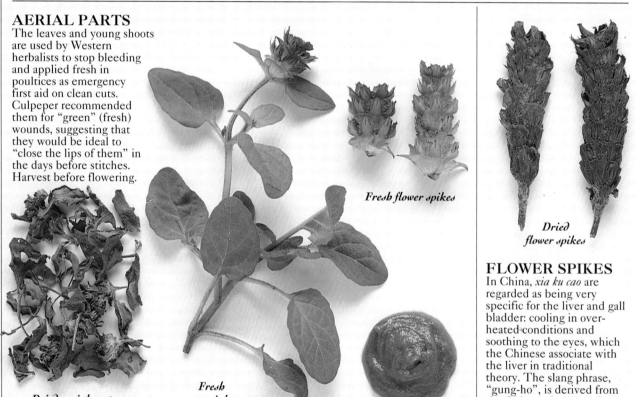

Fresh flower spikes

Dried flower spikes

Dried aerial parts

Fresh aerial parts

Ointment

FLOWER SPIKES
In China, *xia ku cao* are regarded as being very specific for the liver and gall bladder: cooling in over-heated conditions and soothing to the eyes, which the Chinese associate with the liver in traditional theory. The slang phrase, "gung-ho", is derived from the Chinese for "liver fire", *gan hao;* self-heal is ideal for cooling this over-exuberance.

Applications

AERIAL PARTS
TINCTURE Use for all sorts of bleeding, including heavy periods and blood in the urine.

INFUSION Use cool for the same ailments as the tincture. Can be helpful as an astringent, bitter herb in diarrhoea and as a spring tonic.

POULTICE Apply the fresh leaves to clean wounds.

OINTMENT Apply to bleeding haemorrhoids.

EYEWASH Use a very weak, well-strained infusion for hot, tired eyes or conjunctivitis.

MOUTHWASH/GARGLE Use a weak infusion or dilute tincture for bleeding gums, mouth inflammations and sore throats.

FLOWER SPIKES
DECOCTION In China, used to clear "liver fire" associated with irritability and anger, over-excitability, high blood pressure, headaches, hyperactivity in children, or eye problems. Often combined with *ju hua* (Chinese chrysanthemum flowers).

CAUTION
• Always seek professional advice for abnormal uterine bleeding or blood in the urine.

Rheum palmatum
RHUBARB

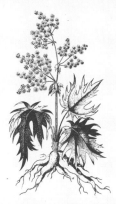

"...so effective for the liver that it is called the life, soul and treacle of the liver, purging... choler, phlegme and water humours."
William Cole, 1656.

ORIGINATING FROM NORTH-WEST China and Tibet, rhubarb has been used in medicine for more than 2,000 years. Its use gradually spread through India, reaching Europe during the Renaissance overland via Asia Minor – hence the common name, Turkey rhubarb. The plant was a favourite remedy with early Persian and Arabian physicians. The rhubarb grown for cooking and eating is usually *R. rhabarbarum*, an 18th-century cultivar.

Character
Bitter, cold, dry.
Constituents
Anthraquinones, tannins, calcium oxalate, resins, minerals.
Actions
Laxative, digestive remedy, astringent, antibacterial.

Parts used

ROOT
This is known as *da huang* in China, which translates as "big yellow" – the colour of rhubarb tinctures and decoctions. It is used very similarly in both East and West, as a purgative and liver cleanser. It is intrinsically "cold", and the Chinese use it to clear "heat" from the liver, stomach and blood; they also believe that it moves stagnant blood. Harvest in autumn.

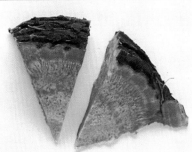

Fresh sliced root

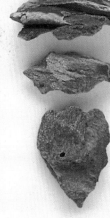

Tincture

Powdered root

Fresh root

Dried root

Applications

ROOT
 TINCTURE The action of the root varies considerably depending on dose. Low doses (5-10 drops) are astringent and can be used for diarrhoea. A slightly higher dose (1 ml) acts as a good liver stimulant and gentle laxative. Very high doses (up to 2.5 ml) have a strong cooling and purgative effect. Use increasing doses (0.5-2 ml) of carminatives such as fennel or mint with higher doses of rhubarb to prevent griping.

DECOCTION A weak decoction (up to 0.5 g root per dose) can be used for diarrhoea, while a strong decoction (3 g root per dose) is effective for chronic constipation or period cramps with delayed menstruation.

WASH The root is also antibacterial and astringent, and a strong decoction can be used on boils and suppurating skin diseases.

CAUTIONS
• Avoid the herb in pregnancy as it is a strong purgative.
• Rhubarb contains oxalates, and is best avoided in arthritic conditions and gout.
• Do not use the leaves, as they are potentially toxic and fatalities have been reported.

Rosa spp.
ROSE

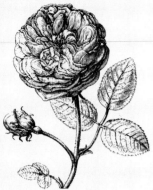

THERE IS A SAYING that roses are good for "the skin and the soul", and they have a long tradition of medicinal use. In Roman times, the wild rose, *R. canina*, was recommended for the bites of rabid dogs. Roses continued as an official medicine well into the 1930s, when tincture of apothecary's rose, *R. gallica*, was prescribed for sore throats. Today roses are still highly prized: the oil is extremely expensive, and is one of the most important oils in aromatherapy. In Ayurvedic medicine, roses are considered cooling and a tonic for the mind.

"...drye roses put to ye nose to smell do comforte the braine and the harte and quencheth sprite."
Askham's Herbal, 1550.

Character Sweet, astringent, generally either neutral or slightly cooling.
Constituents Volatile oil, vitamins C, B, E, K, tannins. Rose oil contains some 300 chemical constituents, of which only around 100 have been identified so far.
Actions Antidepressant, antispasmodic, aphrodisiac, astringent, sedative, digestive stimulant, increases bile production, cleansing, expectorant, antibacterial, antiviral, antiseptic, kidney tonic, blood tonic, menstrual regulator, anti-inflammatory.

Parts used

ROSEHIPS
R. CANINA
Valued as an important source of vitamin C, rosehips are still used in commercial teas, syrups and fruit drinks. The leaves were once used as a substitute for tea. Harvest in autumn.

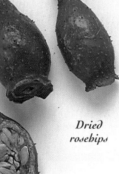

Dried rosehips

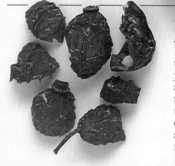

Jin ying zi

ROSEHIPS
R. LAEVIGATA
In China, the hips from this rose are known as *jin ying zi* and are mainly used as a kidney *qi* (energy) tonic, prescribed for urinary dysfunction. Like other rose remedies, they are astringent and taken for chronic diarrhoea. Harvest in autumn.

ESSENTIAL OIL
R. CENTIFOLIA
The cabbage rose is used to produce French rose oil, which differs significantly in its chemical composition from Bulgarian rose oil, and has a reputation as an aphrodisiac.

Fresh flower
(R. centifolia)

Applications

ROSEHIPS
R. CANINA

 TINCTURE Take as an astringent for diarrhoea, to relieve colic, or as a component in cough remedies.

 SYRUP Use to flavour other medicines, add to cough mixtures, or take as a source of vitamin C.

ROSEHIPS
R. LAEVIGATA

 DECOCTION Take with *dang shen, bai zhu* and *shan yao* for chronic diarrhoea with stomach weakness.

ESSENTIAL OIL
R. CENTIFOLIA/R. DAMASCENA

CREAM Add a few drops of oil to creams for dry or inflamed skin.

LOTION Apply 1 ml lady's mantle tincture in 10 ml rosewater for vaginal itching. The same combination can be made into a cream using a standard base. Combine rosewater with an equal amount of distilled witch hazel, and use as a cooling, moisturizing lotion for skin prone to spots or acne.

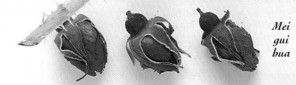

Fresh flower
(R. rugosa)

FLOWERS
R. RUGOSA
The Chinese use the flowers
(*mei gui hua*) as a *qi* (energy)
stimulant and blood tonic to
relieve stagnant liver energies.
They are used for digestive
irregularities, or with motherwort
for heavy periods. Harvest
during flowering.

PETALS
R. GALLICA
Red rose petals were listed
in the British Pharma-
copoeia until the 1930s, and
were used widely as mild
astringents and to flavour
other medicines. Harvest
in summer.

*Mei
gui
hua*

Fresh petals
(R. gallica)

ESSENTIAL OIL
R. DAMASCENA
The damask rose blooms for only a couple
of weeks. The petals are collected and
steam-distilled to produce true Bulgarian
rose oil, used in around 96% of all women's
perfumes. Medicinally, it is an important
nervine, used for depression and anxiety,
and is thought to help those who lack love
in their lives. It can also be added to skin
remedies or taken for digestive problems.

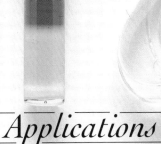

*Rosewater is a by-
product of the
steam distillation
of Bulgarian rose
oil, and makes a
good skin remedy.*

Applications

 OIL Add 2 drops of oil to bath water
for depression, grief or insomnia.

MASSAGE OIL Add up to 2 ml rose
oil to 20 ml almond or wheatgerm
oil, and use to relieve stress and
exhaustion, or for a sluggish
digestion.

FLOWERS
R. RUGOSA

 DECOCTION Take with motherwort
for heavy menstruation. Combine
with *bai shao yao* and *xiang fu* for
liver *qi* dysfunction.

PETALS
R. GALLICA

TINCTURE Take up to 3 ml three
times a day for diarrhoea or sluggish
digestion. Combine with lady's
mantle, white deadnettle or
shepherd's purse for irregular or
heavy menstruation.

GARGLE Use the infusion as a gargle
for sore throats. Can also be
combined with sage.

CAUTIONS
• Because of the high price
of rose oil, adulteration is
commonplace. Only use the
best quality, genuine oil
medicinally.
• Rose oil is non-toxic and
can be taken internally, but
seek professional advice first
if you are new to herbs.
• Use only the rose species
listed here, and not garden
hybrids.

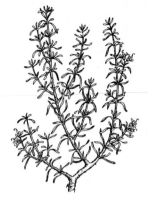

Rosmarinus officinalis
ROSEMARY

A FAVOURITE HERB both medicinally and as a symbol for remembrance, rosemary is a Mediterranean shrub which gradually spread north, and was reputedly first grown in England by Philippa of Hainault, wife of Edward III, in the 14th century. The plant is an excellent tonic and all-round stimulant, and has always been regarded as uplifting and energizing: Gerard said that it "comforteth the harte and maketh it merie".

"If thou be feeble boyle the leaves in cleane water and washe thyself and thou shalt be shiny... smell it oft and it shall keep thee youngly."
Banckes' Herbal, 1525.

Character
Warming, dry, pungent, bitter.
Constituents
Volatile oil, bitter, tannin.
Actions
Aerial parts: astringent, digestive remedy, nervine, carminative, antiseptic, diuretic, promote sweating, promote bile flow, antidepressant, circulatory stimulant, antispasmodic, restorative tonic for nervous system, cardiac tonic.
Essential oil: Topical: increases blood flow to an area, analgesic, antirheumatic, stimulant.

Parts used

AERIAL PARTS
Ideal in exhaustion, weakness and depression, the aerial parts invigorate the circulation, stimulate the digestion, and are good for "cold" conditions, including chills and rheumatism. They are useful for headaches that are eased by warm towels rather than ice packs. Harvest fresh year-round.

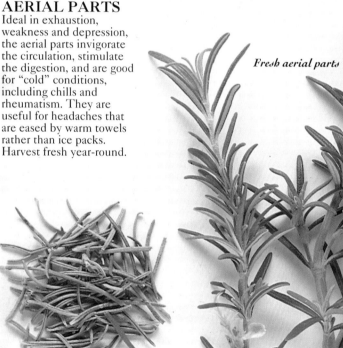

Fresh aerial parts

Tincture

Dried aerial parts

ESSENTIAL OIL
The oil makes a stimulating rub for arthritic conditions and is also used as a hair tonic, encouraging growth and restoring colour. Extracts are commonly found in commercial shampoos.

Applications

AERIAL PARTS

INFUSION Take the hot infusion for colds, influenza, rheumatic pains and indigestion; also as a stimulating drink for fatigue or headaches.

TINCTURE Take as a stimulant tonic. Combine with oats, skullcap or vervain for depression.

COMPRESS Soak a pad in the hot infusion and use for sprains. Alternate two to three minutes of the hot compress with two to three minutes of applying an ice pack to the injury.

HAIR RINSE Use the infusion as the final rinse for dandruff.

ESSENTIAL OIL

OIL Add 10 drops to the bath to soothe aching limbs or to act as a stimulant in nervous exhaustion.

MASSAGE OIL Dilute 1 ml rosemary oil in 25 ml sunflower or almond oil and massage into aching joints and muscles, into the scalp to stimulate hair growth, or use on the temples for headaches.

Rubus idaeus
RASPBERRY

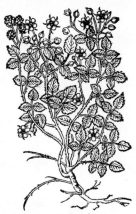

"The fruit is good to be given to those that have weake and queasie stomackes."
John Gerard, 1597.

THE RASPBERRY PLANT was a favourite household remedy. Raspberry vinegars were used for sore throats and coughs; the leaves in infusions for diarrhoea or as poultices for haemorrhoids; and raspberry syrup to prevent a build-up of tartar on teeth. Gerard considered the fruit "of a temperate heat", so it was easier on the stomach than strawberries, which could cause excess phlegm and chilling. Today, raspberry leaf tea is still taken to prepare for childbirth.

Character
Dry, astringent, generally cooling.
Constituents
Leaves: fragarine (uterine tonic), tannins, polypeptides.
Fruit: vitamins A, B, C, E, sugars, minerals, volatile oil.
Actions
Leaves: astringent, preparative for childbirth, stimulant, digestive remedy, tonic.
Fruit: diuretic, laxative, diaphoretic, cleansing.

Parts used

LEAVES
Taken during late pregnancy and childbirth, the leaves are an effective uterine stimulant. They are also astringent, so are useful for diarrhoea, wounds, sore throats and mouth ulcers. They have been included in rheumatic remedies as a cleansing diuretic, and in France they are regarded as a tonic for the prostate gland. Harvest during summer before the fruit ripens.

BERRIES
Traditionally taken for indigestion and rheumatism, the berries are rich in vitamins and minerals and highly nutritious. Harvest when ripe in late summer.

Fresh berries

The juice has been used in folk medicine as a cooling remedy for fevers, childhood illnesses and cystitis.

Fresh leaves

Dried leaves

Applications

LEAVES
INFUSION To ease childbirth, take one cup daily in the last six to eight weeks of pregnancy, and drink plenty of the warm tea during labour. Can also be used for mild diarrhoea, or as a gargle for mouth ulcers and sore throats.

TINCTURE More astringent than the infusion, the diluted tincture is used on wounds and inflammations, or as a mouthwash for ulcers and gum inflammations.

WASH Use the infusion for bathing wounds, and apply regularly to varicose ulcers and sores. It also makes a soothing eyewash.

BERRIES
VINEGAR Steep 500 g fruit in 1 litre wine vinegar for two weeks, then strain. This thick red liquid can be added to cough mixtures or used in gargles for sore throats. Its pleasant taste can help disguise the flavour of other herbal expectorants.

CAUTION
• Avoid high doses of the leaves during early pregnancy, as they can stimulate the uterus.

Salix alba
WILLOW

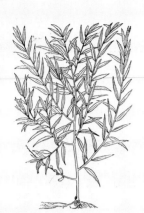

"The leaves... stay the heat of lust in man or woman, and quite extinguishes it, if it be long used; the seed also has the same effect."
Nicholas Culpeper, 1653.

IN TRADITIONAL HERBAL MEDICINE, white willow was widely used for fevers and other "hot" conditions. It was one of the first herbs to be scientifically investigated, and in the 19th century, a French chemist, Leroux, extracted the active constituent and named it "salicine". By 1852 this chemical was being produced synthetically, and by 1899 a less irritant and unpleasant-tasting variant of the substance (acetylsalicylic acid) was manufactured and marketed as aspirin, the first of the modern generation of plant-derived drugs.

Character
Cool, dry, slightly bitter.
Constituents
Salicin, tannins, flavonoids, glycosides.
Actions
Antirheumatic, anti-inflammatory, reduces heat, antihydrotic, analgesic, antiseptic, astringent, bitter digestive tonic.

Parts used

BARK
In modern herbalism only the bark is generally used. It is prescribed for many inflammatory conditions, including rheumatism and arthritis; it helps control fevers, and relieves neuralgia, headaches and pain in general. As a gentle bitter, it also acts as a mild digestive stimulant and is used for gastroenteritis and diarrhoea related to heat and inflammation. Harvest in summer.

Dried bark

Fresh bark

Powdered bark

Tincture

LEAVES
In the past, the leaves were a popular home remedy, used much as the bark today. Willow leaf tea was taken for fevers or colicky pains, and the infusion was recommended for dandruff.

Fresh leaves

Applications

BARK

 FLUID EXTRACT Stronger than the tincture; take for rheumatic conditions, headaches and neuralgia.

 TINCTURE Take up to 15 ml per dose for fever, or combine with boneset, elder, and bitter remedies like gentian. Use with soothing herbs such as plantain for infections and gastric inflammations (take non-alcoholic tincture, see p. 125).

 POWDER Take in doses of up to 10 g for fevers and headaches; mix with a teaspoon of honey.

DECOCTION Take for feverish chills and headaches, or as part of arthritic treatments.

LEAVES

 INFUSION Drink after meals for digestive problems.

Salvia spp.
SAGE

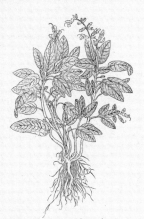

"Why of seknesse deyeth man
Whill sawge in gardeyn he may
han?"
Macer's herbal, 10th century.

TRADITIONALLY ASSOCIATED with longevity, sage has a reputation for restoring failing memory in the elderly. Like other memory-enhancing herbs, it was also planted on graves. It is said that when the British started importing tea from China, the Chinese so valued the herb they would trade two cases of tea for one of dried English sage. The purple variety of *S. officinalis* is generally used in medicine, and is more effective than the common green plant. In China, the root of a related plant, *S. miltiorrhiza* (*dan shen*), is used as a tonic herb.

Character
Pungent, bitter, cool, drying.
Constituents
S. OFFICINALIS: volatile oil, diterpene bitters, tannins, triterpenoids, resin, flavonoids, oestrogenic substances, saponins.
S. MILTIORRHIZA: vitamin E.
Actions
S. OFFICINALIS: carminative, anti-spasmodic, astringent, antiseptic, relaxes peripheral blood vessels, reduces perspiration, salivation and lactation, uterine stimulant, antibiotic, reduces blood sugar levels, promotes bile flow.
S. MILTIORRHIZA: circulatory stimulant, sedative, clears heat.

Parts used

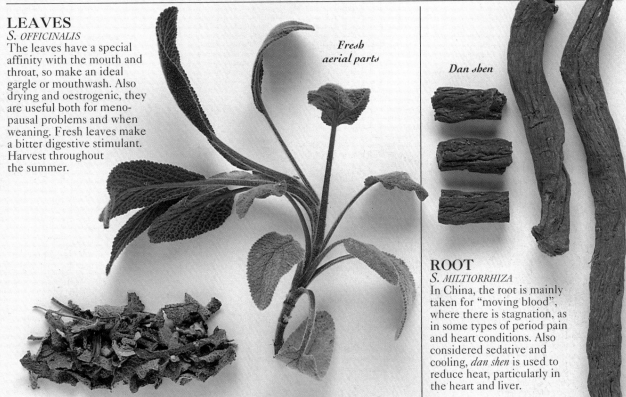

LEAVES
S. OFFICINALIS
The leaves have a special affinity with the mouth and throat, so make an ideal gargle or mouthwash. Also drying and oestrogenic, they are useful both for menopausal problems and when weaning. Fresh leaves make a bitter digestive stimulant. Harvest throughout the summer.

Fresh aerial parts

Dan shen

ROOT
S. MILTIORRHIZA
In China, the root is mainly taken for "moving blood", where there is stagnation, as in some types of period pain and heart conditions. Also considered sedative and cooling, *dan shen* is used to reduce heat, particularly in the heart and liver.

Dried aerial parts

Applications

LEAVES
S. OFFICINALIS

 INFUSION Use 20 g leaves to 50 ml water as a tonic and liver stimulant, or to improve digestive function and circulation in debility. Can reduce lactation when weaning and relieve night sweats at the menopause.

TINCTURE Use for menopausal problems. Prescribed to reduce salivation in Parkinson's disease.

COMPRESS Apply a pad soaked in the infusion to slow-to-heal wounds.

 GARGLE/MOUTHWASH Use a weak infusion for sore throats, tonsillitis, mouth ulcers or gum disease.

 HAIR RINSE Use the infusion as a rinse for dandruff or to restore colour to greying hair.

ROOT
S. MILTIORRHIZA

DECOCTION Prescribed for period pain caused by blood stagnation; also prescribed in Chinese medicine for angina and coronary heart disease.

CAUTIONS
• Avoid therapeutic doses in pregnancy. Small amounts of sage used in cooking are quite safe.
• Only take *dan shen* where the condition is caused by blood stagnation.
• Sage contains thujone, which can trigger fits in epileptics, who should avoid the herb.

Sambucus nigra
ELDER

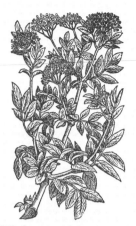

"The decoction of the root... cureth the biting of an adder."
Nicholas Culpeper, 1653.

A WEALTH OF FOLKLORE attaches to this plant, often described as a "complete medical chest", because of its countless therapeutic and prophylactic qualities. Classed as "hot and dry" by Galen, the herb was used for cold, damp conditions, such as catarrh or excessive mucus. In the 17th century, it was a favourite remedy for "clearing phlegm", both as an expectorant for coughs, and as a diuretic and violent purgative. Elderflower water was much praised in the 18th century for whitening the skin and removing freckles.

Character
Flowers/Berries: bitter, drying, cool, slightly sweet.
Bark: hot, bitter, drying.
Constituents
Volatile oil, flavonoids, mucilage, tannins, vitamins A, C, cyanogenic glycoside, viburnic acid, alkaloid.
Actions
Flowers: expectorant, anti-catarrhal, circulatory stimulant, promote sweating, diuretic, topically anti-inflammatory.
Berries: promote sweating, diuretic, laxative.
Bark: purgative, promotes vomiting (in large doses), diuretic. Topical: emollient.

Parts used

Fresh flower heads

BERRIES
The ripe berries are rich in vitamins A and C. In the days before imported winter fruits, they were made into wines and syrups, taken to prevent winter colds. Harvest in autumn.

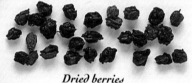

Dried berries

BARK
Warming in character, the bark is an effective liver stimulant, taken in the past for stubborn constipation and arthritic conditions. It is rarely used today.

FLOWERS
These are anticatarrhal and encourage sweating, so are ideal for feverish colds and influenza. They are also helpful for hay fever, taken as a prophylactic early in the year to strengthen the upper respiratory tract before the pollen count rises. Topically anti-inflammatory, they are used in skin creams and for chilblains. Harvest in early summer.

The leaves were once popular in green elder ointment, used for bruises, sprains, wounds and haemorrhoids.

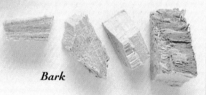

Bark

Applications

FLOWERS

INFUSION Drink hot for feverish and catarrhal conditions of the lungs or upper respiratory tract, including hay fever. Can be combined with yarrow, boneset and peppermint.

TINCTURE Take for colds and influenza, or in early spring to help reduce later hay fever symptoms.

CREAM Apply to chapped skin and sores on the hands or to chilblains.

EYEWASH Use the cold, strained infusion for inflamed or sore eyes.

MOUTHWASH/GARGLE Use the infusion for mouth ulcers, sore throats and tonsillitis.

BERRIES

SYRUP Make from the decoction and take as a prophylactic for winter colds or in combination with other expectorant herbs, such as thyme, for coughs.

TINCTURE Use in combination with other herbs, such as bogbean or willow, for rheumatic conditions.

CAUTIONS
• Do not take any parts of elder if the condition would be worsened by further drying or fluid depletion.
• Do not use the bark in pregnancy as it is very strongly purgative.

Scrophularia spp.
FIGWORT

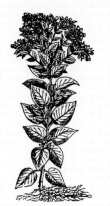

"...it taketh away all redness, spots and freckles in the face, as also the scurf, and any foul deformity therein..."
Nicholas Culpeper, 1653.

IN BOTH EASTERN AND WESTERN traditions, figwort (*S. nodosa*) is a very cleansing herb. In the past, it was known as the scrofula plant (hence the botanical name) as it was used to treat abscesses, purulent wounds and the "King's Evil" or scrofula (tuberculosis of the lymph glands in the neck). Culpeper calls the herb throatwort because of its use in treating this disease. The Chinese use *xuan shen*, the root of a related species, *S. ningpoensis*, as a prime remedy for "fire poisons", the kind of purulent conditions associated with the herb in the West.

Character
Bitter, cold, drying; salty (*S. ningpoensis*).

Constituents
S. NODOSA: saponins, cardioactive glycosides, alkaloids, flavonoids, iridoids.
S. NINGPOENSIS: saponins, phytosterol, essential fatty acids, asparagine.

Actions
S. NODOSA: diuretic, laxative, heart stimulant, circulatory stimulant, anti-inflammatory.
S. NINGPOENSIS: tonic, cooling, anti-inflammatory, antibacterial, heart tonic, reduces high blood pressure, sedative.

Parts used

AERIAL PARTS
S. NODOSA
Best known for treating skin problems, the aerial parts are suitable for any sort of cleansing – for example, in rheumatic disorders and gout, when there is stagnation in the lymphatic system, or for a sluggish digestion with constipation. Harvest after flowering in summer.

ROOT
S. NINGPOENSIS
Unlike *S. nodosa*, the Chinese variety relaxes the heart, reducing blood pressure, and sedating slightly. It also replenishes *jing* (vital essence).

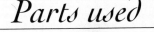

Flowers

Fresh aerial parts

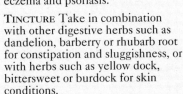

Dried aerial parts

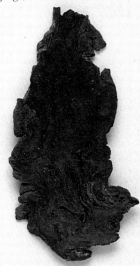

Xuan shen

Applications

AERIAL PARTS
S. NODOSA

 INFUSION Use whenever there is a build-up of toxins to cleanse: for rheumatic conditions, lymphatic disorders or skin conditions such as eczema and psoriasis.

TINCTURE Take in combination with other digestive herbs such as dandelion, barberry or rhubarb root for constipation and sluggishness, or with herbs such as yellow dock, bittersweet or burdock for skin conditions.

 COMPRESS Soak a pad in the infusion and apply to painful swellings, wounds and ulcers.

WASH Use the infusion for eczema, skin inflammations and fungal infections.

ROOT
S. NINGPOENSIS

 DECOCTION Use for throat problems, including swollen glands and tonsillitis. Prescribed for deep-seated abscesses and lymphatic swellings. As a *yin* tonic, it is taken with salt in China.

CAUTION
• *S. nodosa* stimulates the heart, so avoid in cases of abnormally rapid heartbeat.

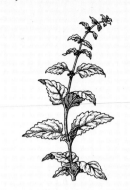

Scutellaria spp.
SKULLCAP

"Skullcap is perhaps the most widely relevant nervine available to us in the materia medica.*"*
David Hoffman, *The Holistic Herbal*, 1983.

A COMPARATIVE NEWCOMER to the European herbal repertoire, Virginian skullcap was used by Native Americans for rabies and to promote menstruation. It is characterized by dish-shaped seed pods and flowers that grow on only one side of the stem; hence its botanical name, *S. lateriflora*. Today, it is one of the best herbs for treating nervous disorders. The Chinese use a related plant, *S. baicalensis* or *huang qin*.

Character
Bitter, cold, drying.
Constituents
S. LATERIFLORA: flavonoids, tannins, bitter, volatile oil, minerals.
S. BAICALENSIS: flavonoids, sitosterols.
Actions
S. LATERIFLORA: relaxing nervine, antispasmodic.
S. BAICALENSIS: antibacterial, cooling, diuretic, antispasmodic, promotes bile flow.

Parts used

Fresh aerial parts

Dried aerial parts

ROOT
S. BAICALENSIS
In China, *huang qin* is mainly used to clear heat from the respiratory and digestive systems. It can be helpful for infections of the urinary tract and skin, and is also used where high blood pressure is related to over-heated conditions.

AERIAL PARTS
S. LATERIFLORA
Calming for many nervous conditions, the aerial parts also have a tonic effect on the central nervous system, so are ideal for nervous exhaustion. They can be helpful in pre-menstrual tension and have been used for epilepsy. Harvest late in the flowering period, when the characteristic skullcap-shaped seed pods have appeared on the plant.

Tincture

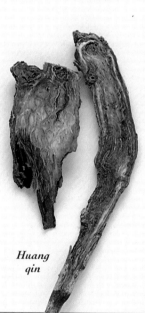

Huang qin

Applications

AERIAL PARTS
S. LATERIFLORA

INFUSION Use the herb fresh, if possible, to make a soothing tea for nervous exhaustion, excitability, over-anxiety and pre-menstrual tension. For insomnia, combine skullcap with wild lettuce or passionflower and take at night.

TINCTURE Best made from the fresh herb, this is a potent remedy for calming the nerves. Take 5 ml or combine with 10 drops lemon balm for nervous stress or depression.

ROOT
S. BAICALENSIS

DECOCTION Use in combination with other cold, bitter herbs such as *huang lian* or goldenseal to purge heat from the system in gastric, chest and urinary infections, including diarrhoea, jaundice, gastroenteritis, bronchitis and cystitis. Combine with herbs such as *ju hua* to reduce high blood pressure.

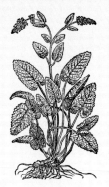

Stachys officinalis
WOOD BETONY

THE MOST IMPORTANT Anglo-Saxon herb, wood betony had no fewer than 29 uses in treating physical diseases, and was also possibly the most popular amulet herb, used well into the Middle Ages to ward off evil or ill humours. Gerard, in 1597, gives a long list of applications, adding that "it maketh a man to pisse well". Today, wood betony is neglected by many herbalists: it is, however, worth rediscovering.

"...it is good whether for a man's soul or his body; it shields him against visions and dreams."
Herbarium Apuleii, Saxon translation, *c.* 9th century.

Character
Cool, drying, bitter-sweet.
Constituents
Alkaloids (including stachydrine and trigonelline), tannins, saponins.
Actions
Sedative, bitter digestive remedy, nervine, mild diuretic, circulatory tonic particularly for the cerebral circulation, astringent.

Parts used

AERIAL PARTS
Mainly used for headaches and nervous disorders, the aerial parts are also a good digestive remedy, stimulating and cleansing for the system, with a mild diuretic action. Harvest in summer while flowering.

ROOT
Although not commonly used today, the root is regarded as more bitter and specific for the liver with a gentle laxative action.

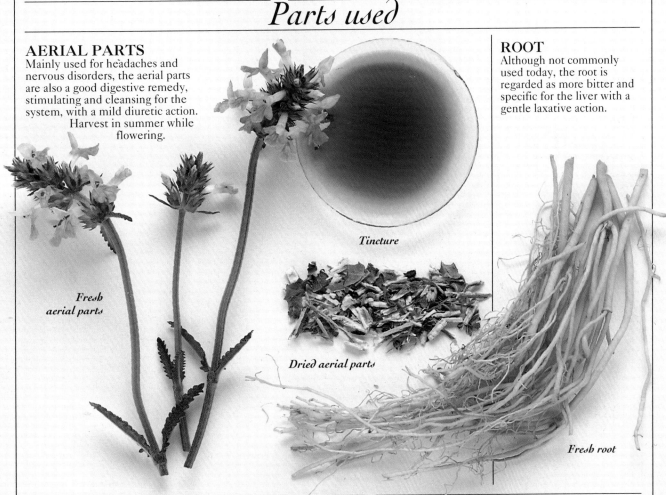

Tincture

Fresh aerial parts

Dried aerial parts

Fresh root

Applications

AERIAL PARTS

INFUSION Take low doses (1 tsp per cup) as a relaxing and tonic herb for general use. Take in therapeutic doses for period pain, migraines and other headaches, nervous tension, or as a digestive stimulant and cleanser. During difficult or painful labour, drink a hot infusion.

TINCTURE Use as the infusion. It is especially helpful for nervous headaches; combines well with lavender. Also useful as a cleansing herb in toxic and arthritic conditions.

POULTICE Apply pounded fresh herb to wounds and bruises.

WASH Bathe leg ulcers and infected wounds in the infusion.

MOUTHWASH/GARGLE Use the infusion for mouth ulcers, gum inflammations and sore throats.

TONIC WINE Macerate 50 g betony with 25 g each of vervain and hyssop in 75 cl white wine for two weeks. Take liqueur-glass doses for nervous headaches and tension.

CAUTION
• The herb is a uterine stimulant, so avoid high doses in pregnancy; may be taken during labour.

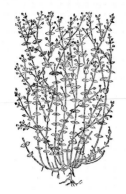

Stellaria spp.
CHICKWEED

IN GERARD'S DAY, chickweed (*S. media*) was given as a tonic to caged linnets. It is probably the most common of weeds, growing in virtually all corners of the world. Instead of rooting it out, it is worth remembering that chickweed was traditionally harvested as a vegetable. It was also used to heal wounds and in poultices for drawing boils. In China, the root of *S. dichotoma*, or *yin chai hu*, is used.

"...in a word, it comforteth, digesteth, defendeth and suppurateth very notably."
John Gerard, 1597.

Character
Sweet, moist, cool.
Constituents
Mucilage, saponins, silica, minerals, vitamins A, B, C, fatty acids.
Actions
Astringent, antirheumatic, heals wounds, demulcent.

Parts used

AERIAL PARTS
S. MEDIA
Made into creams, the aerial parts are still used today for eczema and skin irritations. In mainland Europe, they are a traditional folk remedy, mainly taken internally as a cleansing diuretic and tonic for rheumatic pains and weak conditions. Harvest throughout the growing period.

ROOT
S. DICHOTOMA
In China, *yin chai hu* is used as a cooling herb in fevers, and to stop nosebleeds and heavy menstrual bleeding. It is also given as a tonic for malnourished children, reflecting its use in poor European rural areas as a "free food" in hard times.

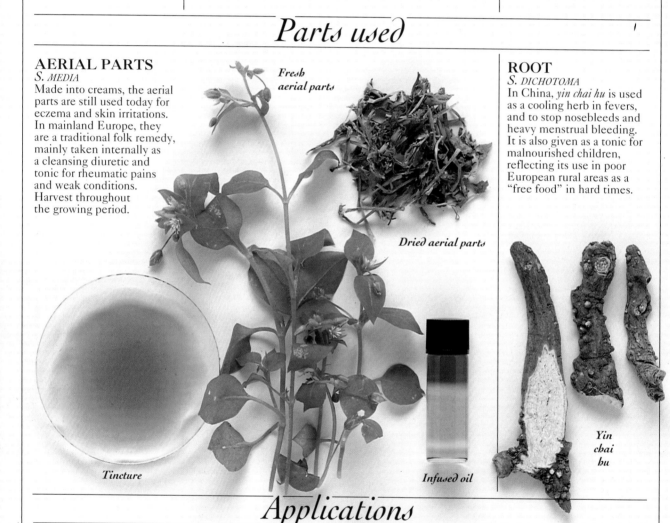

Fresh aerial parts

Dried aerial parts

Tincture

Infused oil

Yin chai hu

Applications

AERIAL PARTS
S. MEDIA

 DECOCTION Use the herb fresh if possible for a cleansing, tonic mixture to relieve tiredness and debility. Also helpful for urinary tract inflammations, such as cystitis.

 TINCTURE Add to remedies for rheumatism.

 POULTICE Apply the fresh plant to boils and abscesses; also to painful rheumatic joints.

 COMPRESS Soak a pad in the hot decoction, or tincture diluted in hot water, for painful rheumatic joints.

 CREAM Apply to eczema, especially if it is itching. Use to draw insect stings or splinters, and on burns and scalds.

 INFUSED OIL Follow the hot infusion method (see p. 122), and apply the oil as an alternative to creams for irritant skin rashes, or add 1 tbsp to bath water for eczema.

ROOT
S. DICHOTOMA

DECOCTION Use for hot fevers related to weakness in chronic illness.

Symphytum officinale
COMFREY

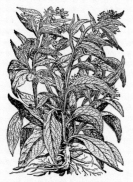

"...given to drinke against the paine of the backe, gotten by violent motion as wrastling or overmuch use of women...
John Gerard, 1597.

A COUNTRY NAME for comfrey was knitbone, a reminder of its traditional use in healing fractures. The herb contains allantoin, which encourages bone, cartilage and muscle cells to grow. When the crushed herb is applied to an injured limb, the allantoin is absorbed through the skin and speeds up healing. In the past, comfrey baths were popular before marriage to repair the hymen and thus "restore virginity".

Character
Cool, moist, sweet.
Constituents
Mucilage, steroidal saponins, allantoin (mainly flowering tops), tannins, pyrrolizidine alkaloids (mainly root), inulin, vitamin B$_{12}$, protein.
Actions
Cell proliferator, astringent, demulcent, heals wounds, expectorant.

Parts used

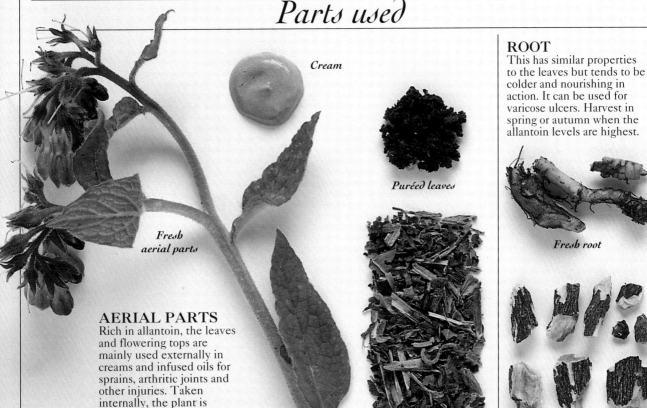

Cream

Puréed leaves

ROOT
This has similar properties to the leaves but tends to be colder and nourishing in action. It can be used for varicose ulcers. Harvest in spring or autumn when the allantoin levels are highest.

Fresh aerial parts

Fresh root

AERIAL PARTS
Rich in allantoin, the leaves and flowering tops are mainly used externally in creams and infused oils for sprains, arthritic joints and other injuries. Taken internally, the plant is equally healing and is used for digestive tract ulceration. Harvest during flowering in early summer.

Dried aerial parts

Dried root

Applications

AERIAL PARTS/ROOT

TINCTURE Prescribed for gastric ulceration or oesophageal damage.

POULTICE Purée the leaves only, and apply to minor fractures that would not normally be set in plaster, such as broken toes, ribs or hairline cracks in larger bones.

CREAM Use for bone or muscle damage, including osteoarthritis.

INFUSED OIL Make by the hot infusion method (see p. 122), and use for arthritic joints, bruises, sprains and other traumatic injuries; also for inflamed bunions.

ROOT

DECOCTION Prescribed for inflammations and ulceration of the digestive tract.

POULTICE Make a paste of powdered root with a little water and use on varicose ulcers and other stubborn wounds; also for bleeding haemorrhoids.

SYRUP Take a syrup made from the decoction for dry coughs or stubborn, thick phlegm.

CAUTIONS
• Avoid excessive internal consumption of the herb because of pyrrolizidine alkaloids, which have been linked by some research to liver cancer in rats.
• Topical application is safer and more effective for arthritis than internal use.
• Avoid using on dirty wounds, as rapid healing can trap dirt or pus.
• Restricted herb in Australia and New Zealand.

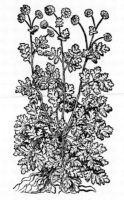

"... the herb bruised... and applied to the wrists before the coming of the ague-fits, does take them away."
Nicholas Culpeper, 1653.

Tanacetum parthenium
FEVERFEW

RECENTLY, FEVERFEW has been hailed as a "cure" and prophylactic for migraines. In the past, the herb was also used for headaches, but it was largely applied externally; feverfew was thought too bitter and potentially damaging to be taken internally. Nevertheless, it was popularly taken by women, to expel the placenta after birth, and for various womb disorders. The name feverfew is a corruption of featherfew, referring to the plant's fine petals.

Character
Bitter, warm, drying.
Constituents
Sesquiterpene lactones, volatile oil, pyrethrin, tannins.
Actions
Anti-inflammatory, relaxes blood vessels, relaxant, digestive stimulant, promotes menstruation, expels worms.

Parts used

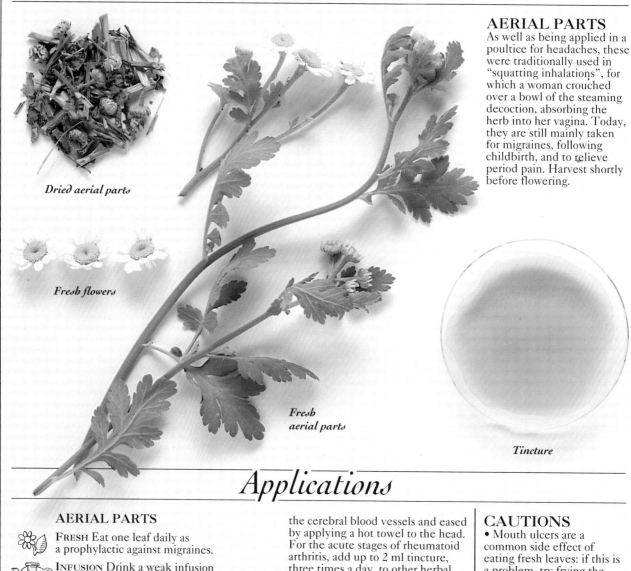

Dried aerial parts

Fresh flowers

Fresh aerial parts

Tincture

AERIAL PARTS
As well as being applied in a poultice for headaches, these were traditionally used in "squatting inhalations", for which a woman crouched over a bowl of the steaming decoction, absorbing the herb into her vagina. Today, they are still mainly taken for migraines, following childbirth, and to relieve period pain. Harvest shortly before flowering.

Applications

AERIAL PARTS

FRESH Eat one leaf daily as a prophylactic against migraines.

INFUSION Drink a weak infusion (15 g herb to 500 ml water) after childbirth to encourage cleansing and tonifying of the uterus; also for period pain associated with sluggish flow and congestion.

TINCTURE Take 5 -10 drops every 30 minutes at the onset of a migraine; it is best for "cold"-type migraines, involving tightening of the cerebral blood vessels and eased by applying a hot towel to the head. For the acute stages of rheumatoid arthritis, add up to 2 ml tincture, three times a day, to other herbal remedies.

POULTICE Fry the fresh herb in a little oil, and apply hot to the abdomen for colicky pains.

CAUTIONS
• Mouth ulcers are a common side effect of eating fresh leaves: if this is a problem, try frying the leaves first.
• The herb should be avoided by patients taking warfarin or other blood-thinning drugs, as it can affect clotting rates.

Taraxacum officinale
DANDELION

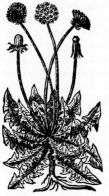

"It is colde, but drieth more and doth withall clense and open by reason of the bitternes which it hath joined with it…"
John Gerard, 1597.

A RELATIVELY RECENT ADDITION to the medicinal repertoire, dandelion was not mentioned in Chinese herbals until the 7th century, while in Europe it first appears in the *Ortus Sanitatis* of 1485. The name dandelion was apparently invented by a 15th-century surgeon, who compared the shape of the leaves to a lion's tooth, or *dens leonis*. In the West, we separate the leaves and root; the Chinese use the whole plant, which they call *pu gong ying*.

Character
Cold, bitter, sweet.
Constituents
Leaves: bitter glycosides, carotenoids, terpenoids, choline, potassium salts, iron and other minerals, vitamins A, B, C, D.
Root: bitter glycosides, tannins, triterpenes, sterols, volatile oil, choline, asparagin, inulin.
Actions
Leaves: diuretic, liver and digestive tonic.
Root: liver tonic, promotes bile flow, diuretic, mild laxative, antirheumatic.

Parts used

WHOLE HERB
In China, the flowers, leaves, root, and seed heads of either the common dandelion or an Oriental species, *T. mongolicum*, are used as a diuretic and liver stimulant. They are also considered to clear heat and toxins from the blood, so are used for boils and abscesses.

LEAVES
An effective diuretic, the leaves are rich in potassium, which is generally lost with frequent urination. They are used for fluid retention, especially with heart problems, and for other urinary disorders. The leaves are also an effective liver and digestive tonic. Harvest throughout the growing season.

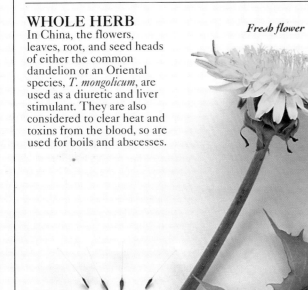

Fresh flower

Fresh leaf

Fresh seeds

The white sap from the stem and root can be used as a topical remedy for warts.

ROOT
A favourite liver stimulant with many herbalists, the root is used as a gentle cleansing tonic for a range of problems including gallstones and jaundice. It can be useful for constipation and in chronic toxic conditions such as joint inflammations, eczema and acne. Harvest in autumn.

Fresh root

Applications

LEAVES

 FRESH Add to spring salads as a cleansing remedy.

JUICE Liquidize the leaves when a diuretic action is needed. Take up to 20 ml juice, three times a day.

INFUSION A less effective diuretic than the juice, the infusion makes a cleansing remedy for toxic conditions including gout and eczema. Also use as a gentle liver and digestive stimulant. Make with freshly dried leaves.

TINCTURE Often added to remedies for a failing heart to ensure adequate potassium intake.

ROOT

TINCTURE Use the fresh root for toxic conditions such as gout, eczema or acne. Also prescribed as a liver stimulant in liver disorders and related constipation.

 DECOCTION Use for the same conditions as the tincture.

Thymus spp. THYME

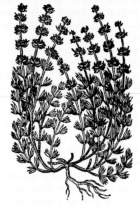

"For headaches a decoction in vinegar is applied to the temples…"
Pliny, AD 77.

GARDEN THYME (*T. vulgaris*) is the cultivated form of wild thyme (*T. serpyllum*). Known as "mother of thyme", probably because of its traditional use for menstrual disorders, wild thyme derives its Latin name from the plant's serpent-like growth. Pliny recommends it as an antidote for snake bites, "poison of marine creatures" and headaches. The Romans also burned the plant in the belief that the fumes would repel scorpions.

Character
Pungent, slightly bitter, warm, drying.
Constituents
Volatile oil, bitter principle, saponins, triterpenes, flavonoids, tannins.
Actions
Antiseptic expectorant, antispasmodic, antiseptic, astringent, antimicrobial, diuretic, soothes coughs, antibiotic, heals wounds.
Topical: increases blood flow to an area.

Parts used

AERIAL PARTS
T. VULGARIS
An antiseptic expectorant, the aerial parts are ideal for deep-seated chest infections marked by thick yellow phlegm. They are also a useful digestive remedy, warming for stomach chills and associated diarrhoea. Harvest before and during flowering in summer; discard the woody stems.

Fresh aerial parts

Dried aerial parts

ESSENTIAL OIL
T. VULGARIS
Extremely antibacterial and antifungal, the oil also stimulates the immune system. A concentrated form of the herb, it is good for respiratory and digestive problems. Several qualities of thyme oil are available commercially: all have similar actions.

AERIAL PARTS
T. SERPYLLUM
The leaves and flowers have similar actions to the cultivated garden variety, but are slightly more stimulating and effective at preventing spasms. They can also be taken for period pain. Harvest before and during flowering.

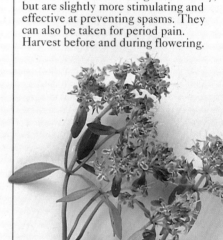

Fresh aerial parts

Applications

AERIAL PARTS
T. VULGARIS/T. SERPYLLUM

INFUSION Use for chest infections, stomach chills or irritable bowel.

TINCTURE Use for diarrhoea associated with stomach chills or as an expectorant in chest infections.

GARGLE Use the infusion or diluted tincture for sore throats.

SYRUP Take a syrup made from the infusion for coughs and lung infections.

ESSENTIAL OIL

CHEST RUB Dissolve 10 drops thyme oil in 20 ml almond or sunflower oil for chest infections.

OIL Dissolve 10 drops in 20 ml water, and apply to insect bites and infected wounds. Add 5 drops to bath water for weakness and arthritic conditions.

MASSAGE OIL Dissolve 10 drops each of thyme and lavender oil in 25 ml almond or sunflower oil for rheumatic pains or strained muscles.

CAUTIONS
• Avoid therapeutic doses of thyme and thyme oil in any form in pregnancy, as the herb is a uterine stimulant.
• Thyme oil can irritate the mucous membranes, so always dilute well.

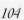

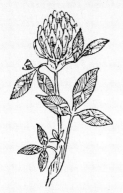

Trifolium pratense
RED CLOVER

THE RED CLOVER we now use medicinally was mainly used in the past as a fodder crop for cattle. Gerard knew it as meadow trefoil or "three-leaved grasse", and its familiar three-lobed leaves were associated by medieval Christians with the Trinity. The Romans used strawberry-leaved clover (*T. fragiferum*), a Mediterranean plant which Pliny suggested taking in wine for urinary stones, while recommending the root for dropsy.

"Plinie writeth and setteth it downe for certaine, that the leaves hereof do tremble and stande right up against the comming of a storme or tempest."
John Gerard, 1597.

Character
Slightly sweet, cool.
Constituents
Phenolic glycosides, flavonoids, salicylates, coumarins, cyanogenic glycosides, mineral acids.
Actions
Alterative, antispasmodic, diuretic, anti-inflammatory, possible oestrogenic activity.

Parts used

FLOWERS
Mainly used as a cleansing herb for skin complaints, the flowers are also useful for coughs, and have been widely used for bronchitis and whooping cough. In the 1930s, they became popular as an anti-cancer remedy, and may still be prescribed to breast, ovarian and lymphatic cancer sufferers. Harvest during flowering.

Fresh flowers

Tincture

Crushed fresh flower

Ointment

Dried flowers

Applications

FLOWERS

 FRESH Crush the flowers, and apply to insect bites and stings.

 TINCTURE Take internally for eczema and psoriasis.

COMPRESS Use for arthritic pains and gout.

 OINTMENT For lymphatic swellings, cover fresh flowers with water, and simmer in a slow cooker for 48 hours. Strain, evaporate the residue to semi-dryness and combine with an equal amount of ointment base.

EYEWASH Use 5-10 drops tincture in 20 ml water (a full eyebath) or a well-strained infusion for conjunctivitis.

DOUCHE Use the infusion for vaginal itching.

SYRUP Take a syrup made from the infusion for stubborn, dry coughs.

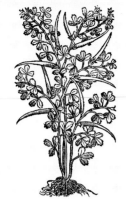

Trigonella foenum-graecum
FENUGREEK

"When the body is rubbed with it, the skin is left beautiful without any blemishes."
Ancient Egyptian recipe for fenugreek ointment, *c.* 1500 BC.

HIGHLY REGARDED BY HIPPOCRATES, fenugreek is one of the oldest medicinal herbs. In Ancient Egypt, it was used to ease childbirth and to increase milk flow; today, it is still taken by Egyptian women for period pain, and as *hilba* tea it is a popular standby to ease stomach cramps for tourists afflicted by "gippy tummy". In China, fenugreek or *hu lu ba* is also used for abdominal pain. Western research has recently highlighted hypoglycaemic properties.

Character
Very warming, pungent, bitter.
Constituents
Steroidal saponins, alkaloids (inc. trigonelline and gentianine), mucilage, protein, vitamins A, B, C, minerals.
Actions
Seeds: anti-inflammatory, digestive tonic, promote milk flow, locally demulcent, uterine stimulant, reduce blood sugar levels, aphrodisiac.
Aerial parts: antispasmodic.

Parts used
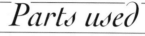

SEEDS
Traditionally used as an aphrodisiac, the seeds are warming for the kidneys and reproductive organs, and are used in China to treat male impotence. They can be taken for period pain and menopausal problems related to kidney *qi* (energy) weakness. They are also a bitter digestive remedy, and can be used in diabetes and, externally, for skin inflammations. Harvest when ripe.

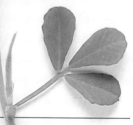

Fresh aerial parts

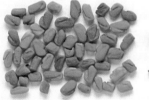

Seeds

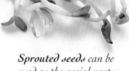

Sprouted seeds can be used as the aerial parts.

Tincture

Dried aerial parts

Capsules

AERIAL PARTS
In the Middle East and the Balkans, the aerial parts are a folk remedy for abdominal cramps associated with both period pain and diarrhoea or gastroenteritis. They are also used to ease labour pains. Harvest in late summer.

Applications

SEEDS

DECOCTION Take as a warming drink for period pain, stomach upsets and, if a nursing mother, to increase milk flow. Disguise the bitter taste with a little fennel.

TINCTURE Take for reproductive disorders and conditions involving kidney *qi* (energy) weakness. Prescribed with other hypo-glycaemic herbs in diabetes.

CAPSULES Prescribed to help control glucose metabolism in late-onset diabetes.

POULTICE Make the powdered herb into a paste and apply to boils and cellulitis.

AERIAL PARTS

INFUSION Take for abdominal cramps, labour and period pain. May also be made from sprouted seeds.

CAUTIONS
• Fenugreek is a uterine stimulant, so avoid in pregnancy. The aerial parts may be used in labour.
• Insulin-dependent diabetics should seek professional advice before using fenugreek as a hypoglycaemic.

Tussilago farfara
COLTSFOOT

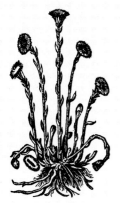

SMOKING COLTSFOOT for coughs and asthma was recommended by the Greek physician Dioscorides. The plant's Latin name means "cough dispeller" and even now, herbal cigarettes often contain coltsfoot. The plant flowers in early spring and the leaves only appear when the flowers have died down; hence the plant's old name, *filius ante patrem* ("the son before the father"). In China, only the flowers, known as *kuan dong hua*, are used.

"The smoke of this plant, dried with the root and burnt, is said to cure, if inhaled deeply through a reed, an inveterate cough."
Pliny, AD 77.

Character
Warm, pungent, slightly sweet.
Constituents
Mucilage, tannins, pyrrolizidine alkaloids, inulin, zinc, bitter principle, sterols, flavonoids (inc. rutin), potassium, calcium.
Actions
Relaxing expectorant, anticatarrhal, antispasmodic, demulcent. Topical: tissue healer, emollient.

Parts used

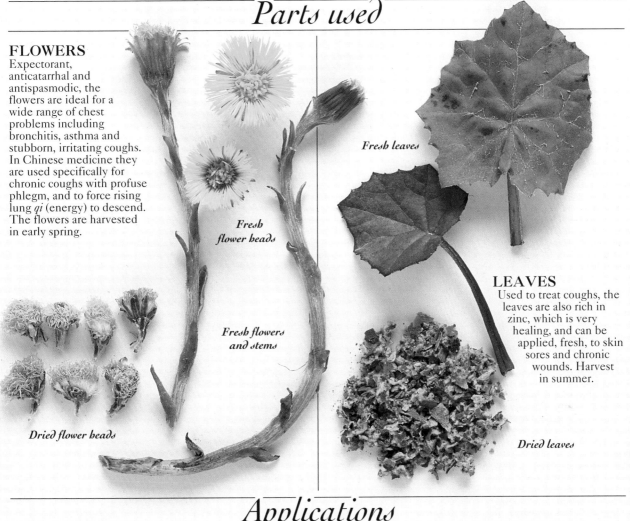

FLOWERS
Expectorant, anticatarrhal and antispasmodic, the flowers are ideal for a wide range of chest problems including bronchitis, asthma and stubborn, irritating coughs. In Chinese medicine they are used specifically for chronic coughs with profuse phlegm, and to force rising lung *qi* (energy) to descend. The flowers are harvested in early spring.

Fresh leaves

Fresh flower heads

Fresh flowers and stems

LEAVES
Used to treat coughs, the leaves are also rich in zinc, which is very healing, and can be applied, fresh, to skin sores and chronic wounds. Harvest in summer.

Dried flower heads

Dried leaves

Applications

FLOWERS

 DECOCTION Prescribed for irritable coughs and catarrh; also for coughs associated with colds or influenza.

TINCTURE Prescribed for chronic or persistent coughs; combines well with thyme and elecampane.

SYRUP Prescribed for coughs; a syrup made from the decoction is more moistening for dry, stubborn coughs than the infusion.

LEAVES

DECOCTION Prescribed for coughs and catarrh.

TINCTURE Prescribed for chronic or persistent coughs.

POULTICE Apply the fresh leaf externally to ulcers, sores and other slow-to-heal wounds.

CAUTION
• Restricted herb in Australia and New Zealand. In the UK, it may be used internally only under professional guidance. (The herb contains pyrrolizidine alkaloids, which have caused liver damage in rats. The quantities in the plant are, however, minute, and Swedish research also suggests that in coltsfoot they are destroyed when making a decoction.)

Urtica dioica
STINGING NETTLE

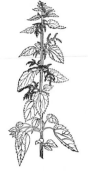

"...they consume the phlegmatic superfluities which Winter has left behind."
Nicholas Culpeper, 1653.

ACCORDING TO TRADITION, Caesar's troops introduced the Roman nettle (*U. pilulifera*) into Britain because they thought that they would need to flail themselves with nettles to keep warm, and until recently "urtication", or beating with nettles, was a standard folk remedy for arthritis and rheumatism. Nettles are still used medicinally and make a cleansing spring tonic and a nourishing vegetable if gathered when the leaves are young.

Character
Cool, dry; astringent, slightly bitter taste.
Constituents
Histamine, formic acid, acetylcholine, serotonin, glucoquinones, many minerals (inc. silica), vitamins A, B, C, tannins.
Actions
Astringent, diuretic, tonic, nutritive, stops bleeding, circulatory stimulant, promotes milk flow, lowers blood sugar levels, prevents scurvy.

Parts used

AERIAL PARTS
Nettles take minerals, including iron, from the soil and the aerial parts are a good tonic for anaemia; the high vitamin C content in the plant helps ensure that the iron is properly absorbed by the body. They clear uric acid from the system so relieve gout and arthritis, and their astringency stops bleeding. Nettles "sting" because of histamine and formic acid in the hairs which trigger the familiar allergic response. Harvest while flowering.

ROOT
Traditionally used as a conditioner for falling hair and dandruff. Harvest in autumn.

The hairs are the stinging part of the plant.

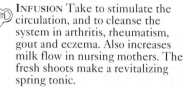

Dried leaves and stalks

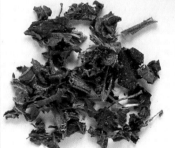

Ointment

Fresh aerial parts

Fresh root

Applications

AERIAL PARTS

 INFUSION Take to stimulate the circulation, and to cleanse the system in arthritis, rheumatism, gout and eczema. Also increases milk flow in nursing mothers. The fresh shoots make a revitalizing spring tonic.

 TINCTURE Used in combinations for arthritic disorders, skin problems and heavy uterine bleeding.

 COMPRESS Soak a pad in the tincture, and apply to painful arthritic joints, gout, neuralgia, sprains, tendinitis and sciatica.

 OINTMENT Apply to haemorrhoids.

WASH Apply to burns, insect bites and wounds.

JUICE Liquidize the whole fresh plant to make a good tonic for debilitated conditions and anaemia, and to soothe nettle stings. Prescribed for cardiac insufficiency with oedema.

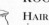 **POWDER** Inhale the powdered leaves as snuff for nosebleeds.

ROOT

HAIR RINSE Use the decoction as a rinse for dandruff, falling hair and as a general conditioner.

Vaccinium myrtillus & V. vitisidaea
BILBERRY & COWBERRY

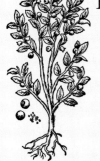

ONCE HIGHLY REGARDED medicinal herbs, the bilberry and cowberry plants are near relatives of bearberry (*Arctostaphylos uva-ursi*), an important urinary antiseptic, and their leaves have been used in very similar ways in folk medicine. Elizabethan apothecaries made a syrup of the berries with honey, called *rob*, as a remedy for diarrhoea. The berries were also believed to be cooling, so were used where there was excess choleric humour to be purged.

"...they cure the bloody flixe proceeding of choler..."
John Gerard, 1597.

Character
Sour, astringent, cold, drying.
Constituents
Tannins, sugars, fruit acids, glucoquinone, glycosides. Cowberry leaves contain arbutin.
Actions
Astringent, reduce blood sugar levels, tonic, antiseptic, prevent vomiting, urinary antiseptic.

Parts used

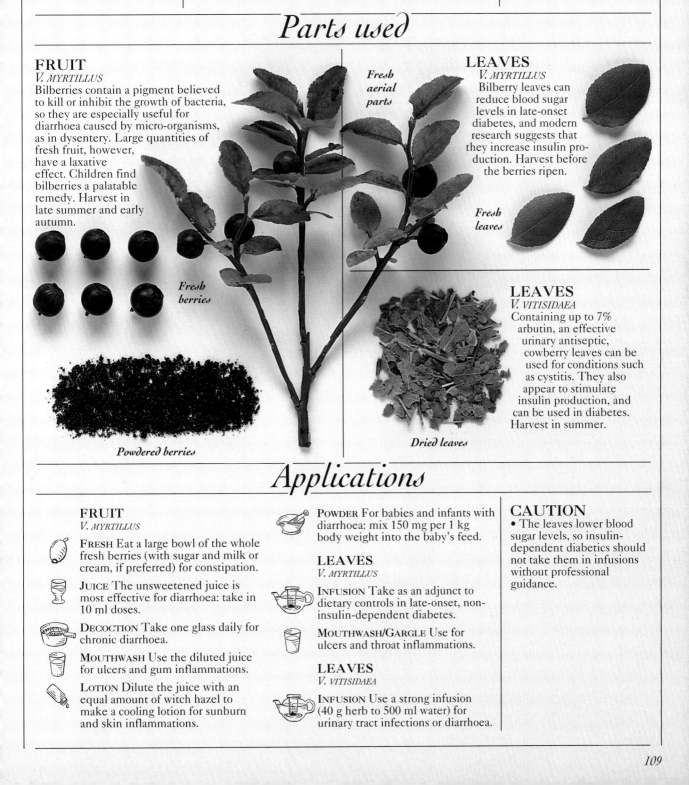

FRUIT
V. MYRTILLUS
Bilberries contain a pigment believed to kill or inhibit the growth of bacteria, so they are especially useful for diarrhoea caused by micro-organisms, as in dysentery. Large quantities of fresh fruit, however, have a laxative effect. Children find bilberries a palatable remedy. Harvest in late summer and early autumn.

Fresh berries

Powdered berries

Fresh aerial parts

LEAVES
V. MYRTILLUS
Bilberry leaves can reduce blood sugar levels in late-onset diabetes, and modern research suggests that they increase insulin production. Harvest before the berries ripen.

Fresh leaves

LEAVES
V. VITISIDAEA
Containing up to 7% arbutin, an effective urinary antiseptic, cowberry leaves can be used for conditions such as cystitis. They also appear to stimulate insulin production, and can be used in diabetes. Harvest in summer.

Dried leaves

Applications

FRUIT
V. MYRTILLUS

FRESH Eat a large bowl of the whole fresh berries (with sugar and milk or cream, if preferred) for constipation.

JUICE The unsweetened juice is most effective for diarrhoea: take in 10 ml doses.

DECOCTION Take one glass daily for chronic diarrhoea.

MOUTHWASH Use the diluted juice for ulcers and gum inflammations.

LOTION Dilute the juice with an equal amount of witch hazel to make a cooling lotion for sunburn and skin inflammations.

POWDER For babies and infants with diarrhoea: mix 150 mg per 1 kg body weight into the baby's feed.

LEAVES
V. MYRTILLUS

INFUSION Take as an adjunct to dietary controls in late-onset, non-insulin-dependent diabetes.

MOUTHWASH/GARGLE Use for ulcers and throat inflammations.

LEAVES
V. VITISIDAEA

INFUSION Use a strong infusion (40 g herb to 500 ml water) for urinary tract infections or diarrhoea.

CAUTION
• The leaves lower blood sugar levels, so insulin-dependent diabetics should not take them in infusions without professional guidance.

Valeriana officinalis
VALERIAN

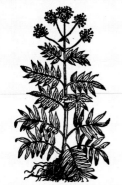

"...for such as be troubled with the crampe and other convulsions, and for all those that are brused with falles."
John Gerard, 1597.

NATURE'S TRANQUILLIZER, valerian calms the nerves without the side effects of comparable orthodox drugs. It has a distinctive, rather unpleasant smell, and was aptly called *phu* by the Greek physician Galen. In recent years, it has been well researched, with chemicals called valepotriates developing in valerian extracts. These seem to depress the nervous system, while the fresh plant is more sedating.

Character
Pungent, slightly bitter, cool, dry.
Constituents
Volatile oil (inc. isovalerianic acid, borneol), valepotriates, alkaloids, iridoids.
Actions
Tranquillizer, antispasmodic, expectorant, diuretic, reduces blood pressure, carminative, mild anodyne.

Parts used

ROOT
Good for nervous tension, especially anxiety and insomnia, the root also strengthens the heart and can sometimes reduce high blood pressure. It encourages healing in wounds and ulcers, and is effective, topically, for muscle cramps. It may also be used as an expectorant, and can help tickling, nervous coughs. Harvest in autumn.

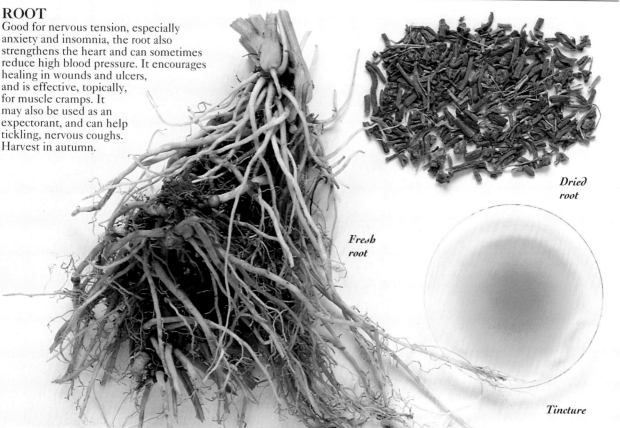

Fresh root

Dried root

Tincture

Applications

ROOT

MACERATION Soak 2 tsp of the chopped, preferably fresh root for 8-10 hours in a cup of cold water. Use as a sedating brew for anxiety and insomnia. Add 2-3 drops of peppermint water (available from chemists) to disguise the flavour.

INFUSION Use for anxiety and insomnia.

TINCTURE Use as a sedative or for insomnia. The dosage can vary considerably with individuals: up to 5 ml may be required, but in some

people this can cause headaches, so start with low doses of 1-2 ml. Combine with liquorice and other expectorants such as hyssop for coughs. Can be added to mixtures for high blood pressure where tension or anxiety is a contributory factor.

COMPRESS Soak a pad in the tincture to ease muscle cramps.

WASH Use the infusion or maceration for chronic ulcers and wounds, and for drawing splinters.

CAUTIONS
• Do not take for more than 2-3 weeks without a break, as continual use or high doses may lead to headaches and palpitations.
• Valerian enhances the action of sleep-inducing drugs, so avoid if taking this type of medication.
• Do not confuse with the garden plant, red "American" valerian (*Centranthus ruber*), which has no medicinal properties.

Verbascum thapsus
MULLEIN

THE TALL STEMS OF MULLEIN, covered in fine down, were once burned as tapers in funeral processions. Dioscorides used the herb for scorpion stings, eye complaints, toothache, tonsillitis and coughs. It was also traditionally taken for wasting diseases such as tuberculosis. An infused oil made from the flowers was a standby in many parts of Europe for ailments as diverse as haemorrhoids and ear infections.

"...beasts of burden that are not only suffering from cough but also broken-winded, are relieved by a draught."
Pliny, AD 77.

Character
Slightly sweet, cool, moist.
Constituents
Mucilage, saponins, volatile oil, flavonoids, bitter glycosides (inc. aucubin).
Actions
Expectorant, demulcent, mild diuretic, sedative, heals wounds, astringent, anti-inflammatory.

Parts used

FLOWERS
A relaxing expectorant for dry, chronic, hard coughs such as in whooping cough, tuberculosis, asthma and bronchitis. The flowers are also effective for throat inflammations. Still made today, the infused oil is used to soothe inflammations, wounds and earache. Harvest flowers individually.

Fresh flower spike

Fresh flowers

Infused oil

LEAVES
Used mainly for respiratory disorders, the leaves were at one time made into herbal "tobacco" and smoked for asthma and tuberculosis. Traditionally, the plant was regarded as antiseptic and the large leaves produced in the second season were wrapped around fruits to preserve them. Harvest before flowering in the second year.

Fresh leaf

Flowers and leaves are not often separated in commercially dried mullein; leaves generally predominate.

Applications

FLOWERS

 TINCTURE Take up to 20 ml a day for chronic, dry coughs and throat inflammations.

GARGLE Use an infusion for throat inflammations.

SYRUP Take a syrup made from the infusion for chronic, hard coughs.

INFUSED OIL Make by the cold infusion method and use drops for earache (only if certain that the eardrum is not perforated). Use as a salve on wounds, haemorrhoids, eczema or inflamed eyelids.

LEAVES

 INFUSION Use a strong infusion of dried herb (50 g to 500 ml water) for chronic coughs and throat inflammations. Also promotes sweating, so can be useful for feverish chills with hard coughs.

TINCTURE Use for chronic respiratory disorders; combine with stimulating expectorants if required, such as mulberry bark, cowslip root, elecampane, sweet violet, anise or thyme.

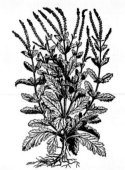

Verbena officinalis
VERVAIN

"...the Magi make the maddest statements about the plant: that people who have been rubbed with it will obtain their wishes, banish fever... and cure all diseases..."
Pliny, AD 77.

ONE OF THE DRUIDS' most sacred herbs, vervain was called *hiera botane* (sacred plant) by the Romans, who used it to purify homes and temples. Its association with magic and ritual was still popular in the 17th century, and Gerard warns against using it for "witchcraft and sorceries". The herb was traditionally used for dropsy; cardioactive glycosides have been identified in the plant to support this use.

Character
Pungent, bitter, cool.
Constituents
Volatile oil (inc. citral), bitter glycosides (inc. iridoids), tannins.
Actions
Relaxant tonic, promotes milk flow, promotes sweating, nervine, sedative, antispasmodic, liver restorative, laxative, uterine stimulant, bile stimulant.

Parts used

AERIAL PARTS
An effective nerve tonic, liver stimulant, urinary cleanser and fever remedy, the aerial parts also encourage milk flow, and can be taken during labour to stimulate contractions. They have a number of topical uses for sores, wounds and gum disorders. In China, the plant is known as *ma bian cao*, and the aerial parts are used mainly as a fever remedy for malaria and influenza. Gather while flowering in summer.

Fresh aerial parts

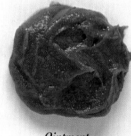

Vervain is one of Dr. Bach's original 12 flower remedies, used for mental stress and over-exertion, with related insomnia and inability to relax.

Dried aerial parts

Ointment

Applications

AERIAL PARTS

 INFUSION Take for insomnia and nervous tension, or to encourage sweating and stimulate the immune system in feverish conditions. Can also be used as a liver stimulant to improve poor appetite and digestive function. Sip during labour to encourage contractions, and during lactation to stimulate milk flow.

 TINCTURE Take for nervous exhaustion and depression (combines well with oats); as a liver stimulant for sluggish digestion, toxic conditions or jaundice; and

with other urinary herbs for stones and conditions related to excess uric acid, such as gout.

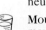 POULTICE Apply to insect bites, sprains and bruises.

OINTMENT Use on eczema, wounds and weeping sores. Also for painful neuralgia.

MOUTHWASH Use the infusion for mouth ulcers and soft, spongy gums.

CAUTIONS
• Avoid the herb in pregnancy, as it is a uterine stimulant; may be taken during labour.
• If taking the tincture for liver disorders, use the hot-water method (see p. 125) to reduce the alcohol.

Viburnum spp.
GUELDER ROSE & BLACK HAW

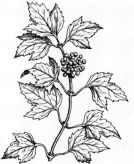

"...for sympathetic disturbances of the heart, stomach and nervous system, common to ladies..."
Finley Ellingwood, 1910.

AN ALTERNATIVE NAME for the guelder rose (*V. opulus*) is cramp bark, which neatly sums up its main medicinal action as a muscle relaxant. The plant was known in the 14th century, as Chaucer suggests eating the berries. It was also used by Native Americans for mumps and other swellings. A close relative, black haw (*V. prunifolium*), is an even more important American variety, known for its significant relaxing action on the uterus. Black haw was a favourite with the Eclectics of 19th-century America (see pp. 20-1).

Character
Astringent, bitter, cool, dry.
Constituents
Bitter substance (viburnin), valerianic acid, tannins, saponins. *V. prunifolium* also contains scopoletin (a coumarin).
Actions
Antispasmodic, sedative, astringent, muscle relaxant, cardiac tonic, uterine relaxant, anti-inflammatory.

Parts used

BARK
V. OPULUS
Guelder rose bark is a muscle relaxant. It also sedates the nervous system, and is useful when physical and emotional tensions combine: typical symptoms include tense, raised shoulders and tight breathing. It relaxes the cardiovascular system in high blood pressure and eases constipation associated with tension. Applied externally, it relieves muscle cramps. Strip from stems in spring before flowering.

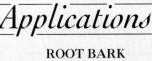
Dried bark

ROOT BARK
V. PRUNIFOLIUM
A potent muscle relaxant, black haw root bark has a very specific action on the uterus and is one of the best remedies for period pain. It can be helpful for pain and bleeding after childbirth and for heavy menstrual bleeding linked to menopausal syndrome. It can also help to reduce high blood pressure and relieve cramp. Dig up the root in autumn and strip off the bark.

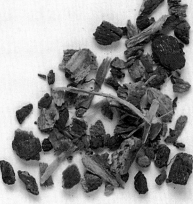

Tincture

Cream

Dried root bark

Applications

BARK
V. OPULUS

TINCTURE Take as a relaxant for nervous or muscular tension. Use for colicky conditions of the intestines, gall bladder or urinary system. Add to digestive remedies for an irritable bowel, or combine with butternut or rhubarb root for constipation caused by tension.

CREAM Mix the tincture with a standard base (such as emulsifying ointment) to make a cream, and apply for muscle cramps or shoulder tension.

ROOT BARK
V. PRUNIFOLIUM

TINCTURE Use for period pain or pain after childbirth, either in 1-1.5 ml doses every 15-20 minutes, or as a single 20 ml dose taken at the first hint of muscle cramps. Use in standard doses for other menstrual irregularities and menopausal syndrome. Can be added to remedies for high blood pressure.

DECOCTION Less effective than the tincture. Drink a cup of strong decoction for period pain.

Viola spp.
SWEET VIOLET & HEARTSEASE

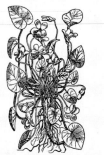

"The lytylnes... in substaunce is nobly rewarded in gretnesse of sauour and of vertue."
Bartholomaeus Anglicus, c. 1250.

SWEET VIOLET AND HEARTSEASE (*V. odorata* and *V. tricolor*) have been used medicinally since ancient times. Homer relates how the Athenians used violets to "moderate anger", while Pliny recommends wearing a garland of violets to prevent headaches and dizziness. Heartsease was once used in love potions, hence the name. The Chinese use a related species, *V. yedoensis*, in similar ways. This has also been used successfully, with other herbs, to treat severe childhood eczema at a London hospital.

Character
Moist, pungent, cold, slightly bitter.
Constituents
Saponins, salicylates, alkaloids, flavonoids, volatile oil.
Actions
V. ODORATA: anti-inflammatory, stimulating expectorant, diuretic, anti-tumour remedy.
V. TRICOLOR: expectorant, anti-inflammatory, diuretic, antirheumatic, laxative, stabilizes capillary membranes.
V. YEDOENSIS: antimicrobial, anti-inflammatory.

Parts used

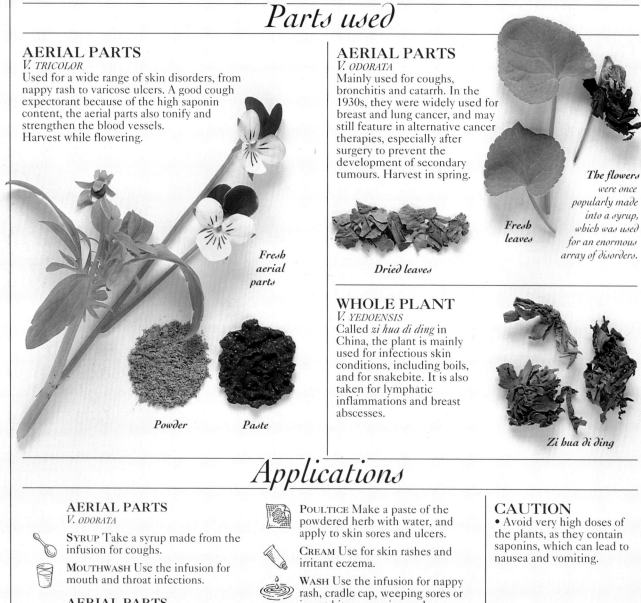

AERIAL PARTS
V. TRICOLOR
Used for a wide range of skin disorders, from nappy rash to varicose ulcers. A good cough expectorant because of the high saponin content, the aerial parts also tonify and strengthen the blood vessels.
Harvest while flowering.

Fresh aerial parts

Powder

Paste

AERIAL PARTS
V. ODORATA
Mainly used for coughs, bronchitis and catarrh. In the 1930s, they were widely used for breast and lung cancer, and may still feature in alternative cancer therapies, especially after surgery to prevent the development of secondary tumours. Harvest in spring.

Dried leaves

Fresh leaves

The flowers were once popularly made into a syrup, which was used for an enormous array of disorders.

WHOLE PLANT
V. YEDOENSIS
Called *zi hua di ding* in China, the plant is mainly used for infectious skin conditions, including boils, and for snakebite. It is also taken for lymphatic inflammations and breast abscesses.

Zi hua di ding

Applications

AERIAL PARTS
V. ODORATA

SYRUP Take a syrup made from the infusion for coughs.

MOUTHWASH Use the infusion for mouth and throat infections.

AERIAL PARTS
V. TRICOLOR

INFUSION Take for chronic skin disorders, and as a gentle circulatory and immune system stimulant.

TINCTURE Use for lung and digestive disorders, capillary fragility and urinary problems.

POULTICE Make a paste of the powdered herb with water, and apply to skin sores and ulcers.

CREAM Use for skin rashes and irritant eczema.

WASH Use the infusion for nappy rash, cradle cap, weeping sores or insect bites, or varicose ulcers.

WHOLE PLANT
V. YEDOENSIS

DECOCTION Use in combination with other cooling, cleansing herbs such as *chi shao yao* and *fang feng* for skin diseases and abscesses.

CAUTION
• Avoid very high doses of the plants, as they contain saponins, which can lead to nausea and vomiting.

Zingiber officinalis
GINGER

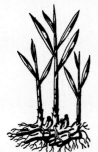

"...it is of an heating and digesting qualitie, and is profitable for the stomacke."
John Gerard, 1597.

ORIGINALLY FROM TROPICAL ASIA, ginger has been used as a medicinal herb in the West for at least 2,000 years. It was introduced into the Americas by the Spaniards, and is now cultivated extensively in the West Indies. As a hot, dry herb, ginger was traditionally used to warm the stomach and dispel chills. In the 18th century, it was added to remedies to modify their action and reduce the irritant effects on the stomach. Ginger is still used in this way in China to reduce the toxicity of some herbs.

Character
Pungent, hot, dry.
Constituents
Volatile oil (inc. borneol, citral), phenols, alkaloid, mucilage.
Actions
Circulatory stimulant, relaxes peripheral blood vessels, promotes sweating, expectorant, prevents vomiting, antispasmodic, carminative, antiseptic. Topical: increases blood flow to an area.

Parts used

FRESH ROOT
In China, the fresh root, *sheng jiang,* is mainly used to promote sweating and as an expectorant for colds and chills. It is also roasted in hot ashes and used for diarrhoea or to stop bleeding. As well as prescribing fresh root for chills, Western herbalists regard it as a good circulatory stimulant.

Sliced fresh root

Fresh root

DRIED ROOT
Called *gan jiang* in China, the dried root is mainly used to warm and stimulate the stomach and lungs, and is an effective *yang* restorative. In the West, it is used for travel sickness; in recent trials it has been used successfully for very severe sickness in pregnancy.

Gan jiang

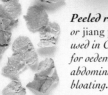

Peeled root skin or jiang pi *is used in China for oedema and abdominal bloating.*

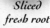
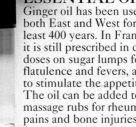

ESSENTIAL OIL
Ginger oil has been used in both East and West for at least 400 years. In France, it is still prescribed in drop doses on sugar lumps for flatulence and fevers, and to stimulate the appetite. The oil can be added to massage rubs for rheumatic pains and bone injuries.

Capsules

Applications

FRESH ROOT
DECOCTION For chills and catarrhal colds, use 1-2 slices to a mug of water and simmer for 10 minutes. A pinch of cinnamon can be added.

TINCTURE Use 2-10 drops per dose as a warming circulatory stimulant; also for flatulence, indigestion and nausea.

DRIED ROOT

CAPSULES Take 1-2 x 200 mg capsules before a journey for travel sickness. Use up to 1 g doses for morning sickness in pregnancy.

DECOCTION The Chinese use dried ginger in combination with other herbs as a restorative for *yang* or spleen energies, for abdominal fullness, nausea and excess phlegm.

ESSENTIAL OIL
MASSAGE OIL Add 5-10 drops ginger oil to 25 ml almond oil for rheumatism or lumbago. Combines well with juniper or eucalyptus oil.

OIL Use 1-2 drops on a sugar lump or in half a teaspoon of honey for flatulence, menstrual cramps, nausea or stomach upsets.

CAUTIONS
• Avoid excessive amounts of ginger if the stomach is already hot and over-stimulated, as in peptic ulceration.
• Use ginger with respect in early pregnancy, although it can be safely taken for morning sickness in the doses described.

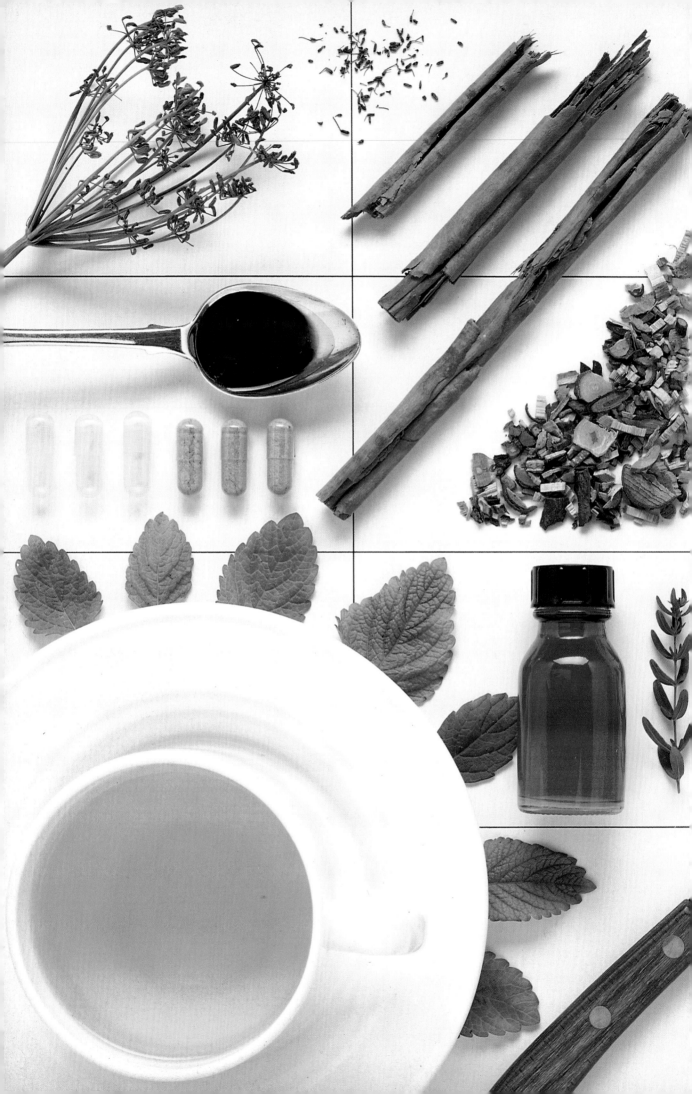

HERBAL REMEDIES

In many parts of the world, herbs are the only option
for all types of health problems. While professional
herbalists in the West may use herbs for severe health
disorders, there is also a wide range of gentler remedies
suitable for home treatment of common complaints.
This section includes instructions on preparing
remedies and an ailment-by-ailment guide.
The focus is on herbs that can be safely used at
home as an alternative to over-the-counter drugs.
Other herbs that are commonly prescribed
are included where appropriate.

HARVESTING & DRYING HERBS

THE CONSTITUENT CHEMICALS and thus the therapeutic properties of herbs can be affected by exactly when they are gathered. Harvest herbs on a dry day, when they are at the peak of maturity and the concentration of active ingredients is highest. Dry them quickly, away from bright sunlight, to preserve the aromatic ingredients and prevent oxidation of other chemicals. To ensure good air circulation, leave in a dry, airy, warm place. An airing cupboard with the door open is ideal, or a sunny room. A damp-free garden shed with a low-powered fan

running can also be effective. Avoid using a garage, as the herbs become contaminated with petrol fumes. It is possible to dry herbs completely within six days; the longer it takes the more likely the plant is to discolour and lose its flavour. Keep the drying room between 20-32°C/70-90°F. When the herbs are dry, store in clean, dry, dark glass or pottery containers, with an airtight lid, out of direct sunlight. If stored when damp, the herbs will go mouldy. Label dried herbs with the variety, source and date: most will keep for 12-18 months.

Flowers

Harvest after the morning dew has evaporated, when fully open: handle carefully, as they are easily damaged. Cut flower heads from the stems and dry whole on trays. Treat small flowers, such as lavender, like seeds; pick before the flowers wither completely. If the stem is large or fleshy, like mullein, remove the individual flowers and dry them separately.

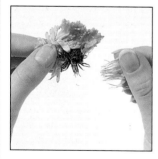

1 Remove obvious dirt, grit and insects. Spread the flowers on a paper-lined tray or newspaper to dry.

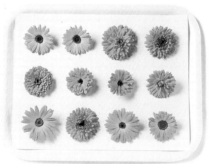

2 When dry, store whole in a dark, airtight container. If using marigolds, as shown here, remove the dried petals and store individually, discarding the central part of the flower.

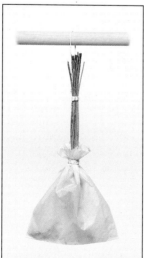

Lavender - dry on the stem in a paper bag or over a tray.

Aerial parts and leaves

Large leaves, such as burdock, can be harvested and dried individually; smaller leaves, such as lemon balm, are best left on the stem. Gather leaves of deciduous herbs just before flowering and evergreen herbs, such as rosemary, throughout the year. If using all the aerial parts, harvest in the midst of flowering, giving a mixture of leaves, stem, flowers and seed head.

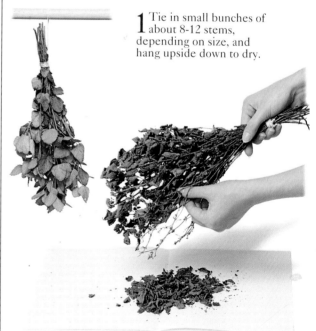

1 Tie in small bunches of about 8-12 stems, depending on size, and hang upside down to dry.

2 When the leaves are brittle to the touch, but not so dry that they turn to powder, rub them from the stem on to paper and discard the larger pieces. If all aerial parts are being used, crumble together.

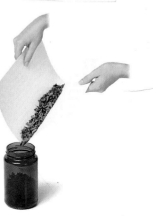

3 Pour or spoon the dried herbs from the paper into an airtight storage container.

Seeds

Harvest entire seed heads with about 15-25 cm of stalk when the seeds are almost ripe, before too many have been dispersed by the wind or eaten by birds. Hang upside down over a paper-lined tray or in a paper bag, away from direct sunlight; seeds will fall off when ripe.

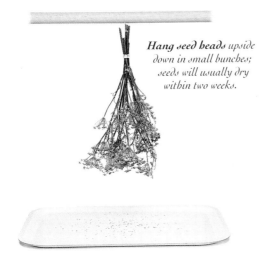

Hang seed heads upside down in small bunches; seeds will usually dry within two weeks.

Roots

Harvest most roots in autumn, when the aerial parts of the plant have died down and before the ground becomes too hard to make digging difficult. An exception is dandelion where the roots should be gathered in spring. Some roots reabsorb moisture from the air so discard if they become soft.

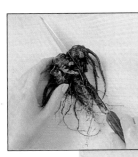

1 Wash thoroughly to remove soil and dirt. Chop large roots into small pieces while still fresh, as they can be difficult to cut when dry.

2 Spread the pieces of root on a tray lined with paper and dry for 2-3 hours in a cooling oven (or 4-6 hours for larger roots). Transfer to an airing cupboard or warm, sunny room to complete drying.

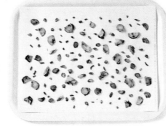

Sap and resin

Harvest from the tree in autumn when the sap is falling by making a deep incision in the bark or drilling a hole and collecting the sap in a cup tied to the tree. Sometimes a sizeable bucket is needed: a large amount of birch sap, for example, can be collected overnight at certain times of·year. Squeeze sap from latex plants such as wild lettuce and greater celandine over a bowl. Many saps can be corrosive, so wear protective gloves.

1 For aloe, carefully slice along the centre of a leaf and peel back the edges.

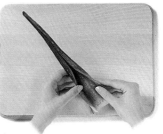

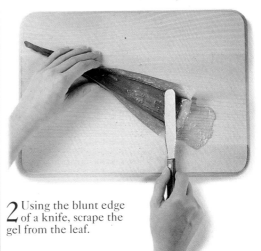

2 Using the blunt edge of a knife, scrape the gel from the leaf.

Fruit

Harvest berries and other fruits when just ripe, before the fruit becomes too soft to dry effectively. Spread on trays to dry. Turn fleshy fruit frequently to ensure even drying. Discard fruit with any signs of mould.

Bark

Harvest in autumn when the sap is falling to minimize damage to the plant. Never remove all the bark – or a band of bark completely surrounding a tree – unless you want to sacrifice the plant to herbal medicine. Dust or wipe bark to remove moss or insects: avoid over-soaking in water. Break into manageable pieces (2-5 cm square), spread on trays and leave to dry.

Bulbs

Harvest after the aerial parts have died down. Collect garlic bulbs quickly as they tend to sink downwards once the leaves have wilted and are difficult to find.

MAKING HERBAL REMEDIES

THE INSTRUCTIONS GIVEN here use standard quantities of herbs. Throughout the book, all quantities and doses are standard, unless otherwise specified. For combinations of herbs, the total amount in any given remedy should not exceed the standard quantity. For example, an infusion for colds and influenza could contain 10 g each of yarrow, elderflower and peppermint to give the required proportion of 30 g dried herb to 500 ml water.

MEASURING REMEDIES

You can use standard spoons, droppers or measuring cups for doses. Quantities for infusions and decoctions should be divided into three equal doses.

drop doses = 5-10 drops depending on age and/or condition

1 ml = 20 drops	62.5 ml = 1 sherry glass
5 ml = 1 teaspoon	150 ml = 1 tea cup or
20 ml = 1 tablespoon	wine-glass

IMPORTANT:
For children and the elderly, doses should be reduced depending on age and/or bodyweight (see pp. 172-7). If pregnant, or suffering from gastric or liver inflammation or when treating children, use non-alcoholic tinctures (see p. 125).

Infusion

A very simple way of using herbs, an infusion is made in much the same way as tea. The water should be just off the boil since vigorously boiling water disperses valuable volatile oils in the steam. Use this method for flowers and the leafy parts of plants. The standard quantity should be made fresh each day and is sufficient for three doses. Drink hot or cold.

Standard quantities
30 g dried herb or 75 g fresh herb to 500 ml water
•
Standard dose
One tea cup or wine-glassful three times a day
•
Equipment
Kettle
Teapot or tisane cup with lid
Nylon sieve or strainer
Tea cup
Covered jug for storage

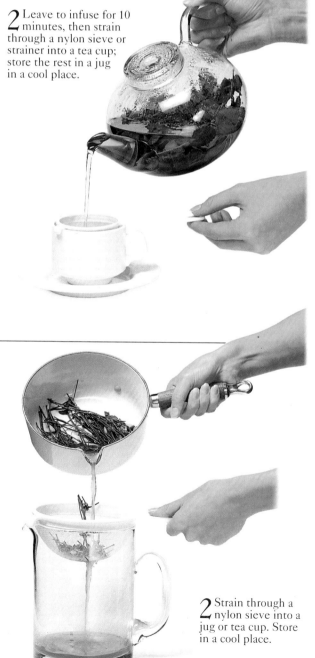

2 Leave to infuse for 10 minutes, then strain through a nylon sieve or strainer into a tea cup; store the rest in a jug in a cool place.

1 Put the herb in a pot with a close-fitting lid – a teapot is ideal. Pour hot water over the herb.

Decoction

This method involves a more vigorous extraction of a plant's active ingredients than an infusion, and is used for roots, barks, twigs and some berries. Heat the herb in cold water and simmer for up to 1 hour. As with infusions, the standard quantity should be made fresh daily and is enough for three doses. Drink hot or cold.

Standard quantities
30 g dried herb or 60 g fresh herb to 750 ml water, reduced to around 500 ml with heating
•
Standard dose
One tea cup or wine-glassful three times a day
•
Equipment
Saucepan (preferably earthenware or enamel)
Nylon sieve or strainer
Covered jug for storage

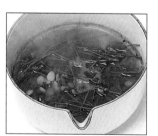

1 Place the herb in a saucepan and pour over cold water. Bring to the boil, then simmer for up to 1 hour until the volume has been reduced by one third.

2 Strain through a nylon sieve into a jug or tea cup. Store in a cool place.

Tincture

This is made by steeping the dried or fresh herb in a 25% mixture of alcohol and water (see right). Any part of the plant may be used. As well as extracting the plant's active ingredients, the alcohol acts as a preservative, and tinctures will keep for up to two years. Tinctures should be made from individual herbs; combine prepared tinctures as required. Commercial tinctures use ethyl alcohol, but diluted spirits are suitable for home use. Vodka is ideal as it contains few additives, although rum helps to disguise the flavour of less palatable herbs.

Standard quantities
200 g dried herb or 600 g fresh herb to 1 litre 25% alcohol/water mixture (e.g. dilute a 75 cl bottle of 37.5% vodka with 37.5 ml water)

•

Equipment
Large screw-top jar
Jelly bag or muslin bag
Wine press
Large jug
Dark glass bottles with screw caps for airtight storage
Funnel (optional)

Standard dose
5 ml three times a day. Tinctures should be taken diluted in water (a little honey or fruit juice can often improve the flavour); for non-alcoholic tinctures see p. 125.

CAUTION
Do not use industrial alcohol, methylated spirits (methyl alcohol) or rubbing alcohol (isopropyl alcohol) in tincture making: all are extremely toxic.

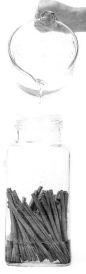

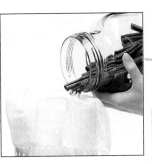

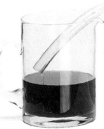

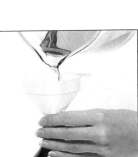

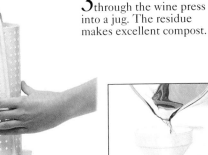

1 Put the herb into a large jar and cover with the vodka/water mixture. Seal the jar, store in a cool place for two weeks, and shake it occasionally.

2 Fit a jelly bag round the rim of a wine press (securing it if necessary). Pour the mixture through.

3 Press the mixture through the wine press into a jug. The residue makes excellent compost.

4 Pour the strained liquid into clean, dark glass bottles, using a funnel if necessary.

Syrup

Honey or unrefined sugar can be used to preserve infusions and decoctions and syrup makes an ideal cough remedy; honey is particularly soothing. The added sweetness also disguises the flavour of more unpleasant-tasting herbs, such as motherwort. Syrups can also be used to flavour medicines for children.

Standard quantities
500 ml infusion or decoction
500 g honey or unrefined sugar

•

Standard dose
5-10 ml three times a day

•

Equipment
Saucepan
Wooden spoon
Dark glass bottles with cork stoppers for storage
Funnel (optional)

1 Heat 500 ml standard infusion or decoction in a saucepan. Add 500 g honey or unrefined sugar and stir constantly until dissolved.

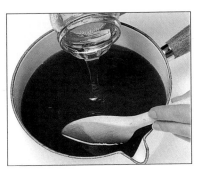

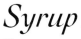

2 Allow the mixture to cool and pour into a dark glass bottle. Seal with a cork stopper (the cork is important, as syrups often ferment, and screw-topped bottles can explode).

Infused oils

Active plant ingredients can be extracted in oil, for external use in massage oils, creams and ointments. Infused oils will last up to a year if kept in a cool, dark place, although smaller amounts made fresh are more potent. There are two techniques: the hot method is suitable for comfrey, chickweed or rosemary, and the cold method for marigold and St. John's wort. If possible, repeat the process for cold infused oil using new herb and the once-infused oil, leaving to stand for a further few weeks before straining.

HOT INFUSION

Standard quantities
250 g dried herb or 750 g fresh herb to 500 ml sunflower oil

•

Equipment
Glass bowl and saucepan or double saucepan
Wine press
Jelly bag or muslin bag
Large jug
Airtight, glass storage bottles
Funnel (optional)

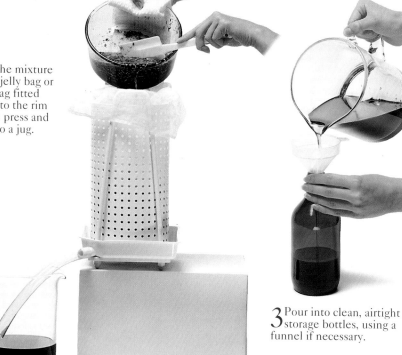

2 Pour the mixture into a jelly bag or muslin bag fitted securely to the rim of a wine press and strain into a jug.

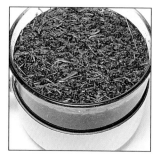

1 Put the oil and the herb in a glass bowl over a pan of boiling water or in a double saucepan and heat gently for about three hours.

3 Pour into clean, airtight storage bottles, using a funnel if necessary.

COLD INFUSION

1 Pack a large jar tightly with the herb and cover completely with oil. Put the lid on and leave on a sunny windowsill or in the greenhouse for two to three weeks.

Standard quantities
Enough flower heads to pack a storage jar
1 litre cold pressed oil depending on size of jar

Equipment
Jelly bag/muslin bag or wine press
Large jug
Airtight, glass storage bottles

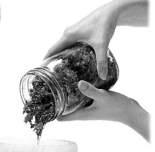

2 Pour the mixture into a jelly bag (shown here) or muslin bag, fitted securely with string or elastic band to the rim of a jug.

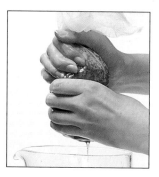

3 Squeeze the oil through the bag. Repeat steps 1 and 2 with new herb and the once-infused oil: after a few weeks, strain again and store.

Cream

A cream is a mixture of water with fats or oils, which softens and blends with the skin. It can be easily made using emulsifying ointment (available from most pharmacies), which is a mixture of oils and waxes that blends with water. Home-made creams will last for several months, but the shelf-life is prolonged by storing the mixture in a cool larder or refrigerator or adding a few drops of benzoin tincture as a preservative. Creams made from organic oils and fats deteriorate more quickly (see p. 125). The method shown below is suitable for most herbs.

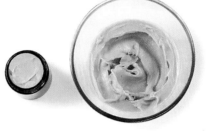

1 Melt the fats and water in a bowl over a pan of boiling water or in a double saucepan, add the herb and heat gently for three hours.

Standard quantities
150 g emulsifying ointment
70 ml glycerine
80 ml water
30 g dried herb
•
Equipment
Glass bowl and saucepan or double saucepan
Wooden spoon or spatula
Wine press
Jelly bag or muslin bag
Bowl
Small palette knife
Small, airtight storage jars

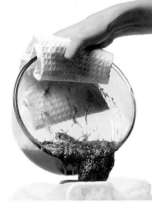

3 Use a small palette knife to fill the storage jars. Put some cream round the edge of the jar first, and then fill the middle.

2 Fit a jelly bag around the rim of a wine press. Strain the mixture into a bowl. Stir constantly until cold.

Ointment

An ointment contains only oils or fats, but no water, and unlike cream, it does not blend with the skin, but forms a separate layer over it. Ointments are suitable where the skin is already weak or soft, or where some protection is needed from additional moisture, as in nappy rash. Ointments were once made from animal fats, but petroleum jelly or paraffin wax is suitable.

Standard quantities
500 g petroleum jelly or soft paraffin wax
60 g dried herb

Equipment
Glass bowl and saucepan or double saucepan
Wooden spoon
Jelly bag or muslin bag
Jug
Glass jars with lids

3 Wearing rubber gloves, as the mixture is hot, squeeze it through the jelly bag into the jug.

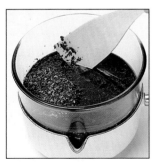

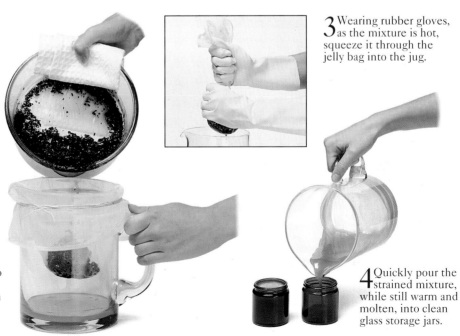

1 Melt the wax or jelly in a bowl over a pan of boiling water or in a double saucepan, stir in the herbs and heat for about two hours or until the herbs are crisp.

2 Pour the mixture into a jelly bag or muslin bag, fitted securely with string or an elastic band to the rim of a jug.

4 Quickly pour the strained mixture, while still warm and molten, into clean glass storage jars.

Powders and capsules

Herbs can be taken as powders stirred into water or sprinkled on to food, or made into capsules (these are preferable for more unpalatable herbs and are convenient for carrying around). It is best to use commercially prepared powders, which are available from specialist suppliers. Grinding herbs in a domestic grinder generates heat, which can cause chemical changes in the herbs, and hard roots can damage the grinder. Two-part gelatin or vegetarian capsule cases are available from specialist suppliers, see p. 192.

Standard quantities
Size 00 capsule case holds
200-250 mg powdered herb
•
Standard dose
Generally 2-3 capsules two
to three times a day
$^{1}/_{2}$-1 tsp powder in half
a glass of water three
times a day
•
Equipment
Saucer or flat dish
Capsule cases
Dark glass storage jars

1 To fill capsules, pour the powdered herb into a saucer, separate the two halves of a capsule case and slide them together through the powder, scooping it into the capsule.

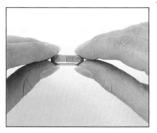

2 Fit together the two halves of the capsule. Store in dark glass jars in a cool place.

Compress

Often used to accelerate healing of wounds or muscle injuries, a compress is simply a cloth pad soaked in a hot herbal extract and applied to the painful area. A cold compress is sometimes used for headaches. Infusions, decoctions and tinctures diluted with water can all be used for a compress, and the pad can be soft cotton or linen, cotton wool or surgical gauze.

1 Soak a clean piece of soft cloth in a hot infusion or other herbal extract. Squeeze out the excess liquid.

Standard application
Use a standard infusion,
decoction or 5-20 ml tincture
in 500 ml hot water
(as specified)
•
Equipment
Cloth pad
Bowl

2 Hold the pad against the affected area. When it cools or dries, repeat the process using hot mixture.

Poultice

This has a similar action to a compress, but the whole herb rather than a liquid extract is applied. Poultices are generally applied hot (as shown below), but cold, fresh leaves can be just as suitable. Chop fresh herbs in a food processor for a few seconds or boil in a little water for 2-5 minutes. Dried herbs can be decocted or powders mixed with a little water to make a paste.

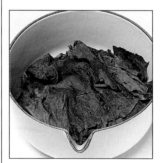

Standard application
Use sufficient herb to cover
the affected area
Replace the poultice every
2-4 hours or earlier
as need be
•
Equipment
Saucepan
Gauze/cotton strips

1 Boil the fresh herb, squeeze out any surplus liquid and spread it on to the affected area. Smooth a little oil on the skin first, to prevent the herb sticking.

2 Apply gauze or cotton strips to hold the poultice carefully in place.

OTHER HERBAL REMEDIES

Massage oils

Most essential oils irritate the skin and should be diluted before using for massage. Almond or wheatgerm is best as a carrier oil, but sunflower oil can be used if that is all you have available. In general, 5-10 drops essential oil to 20 ml (1 tbsp) carrier oil is adequate. Once diluted in this way, essential oils soon deteriorate, so prepare mixtures as required. Good massage needs skill and practice, but the oil can be suitable in home use for localized problems such as aching joints or chesty coughs. Pour about 2-5 ml massage oil on to your hand and rub gently into the affected area. An infused oil can also be suitable in some circumstances, for example, comfrey for strains and sprains, St. John's wort for inflammations and bladderwrack for arthritic conditions.

Creams and ointments from infused oils

Hot or cold infused oils can be thickened with beeswax and anhydrous lanolin to make ointments, or with beeswax, anhydrous lanolin and herbal tinctures to make creams. For a cream, melt 25 g beeswax with 25 g anhydrous lanolin, add 100 ml infused oil and 50 ml herbal tincture, then strain, stir and store as shown on p. 123. For an ointment, melt 25 g beeswax with 25 g anhydrous lanolin, then add 100 ml infused oil. Pour into clean, dark glass jars while still warm, and allow to cool.

Organic alternative to emulsifying ointment

Instead of using emulsifying ointment for making cream, a combination of organic oils and waxes can be used. Follow the instructions given on p. 123, but melt 25 g white beeswax and 25 g anhydrous lanolin instead of the emulsifying ointment and then add 100 ml sunflower oil, 25 ml glycerine, 75 ml water and 50 g dried herb. Heat and strain as before, but stir 5 drops of benzoin tincture into the cooling mixture as a preservative.

Steam inhalants

These are ideal for conditions such as catarrh, asthma or sinusitis. Place 1-2 tbsp dried herb in a bowl and pour boiling water over it. Lean over the bowl with a towel draped over your head and the bowl, and inhale for as long as you can bear the heat or until the mixture cools. Avoid going into a cold atmosphere for at least 30 minutes afterwards.

Non-alcoholic tinctures

In some cases a tincture made from ethyl alcohol is unsuitable as a herbal remedy, for example, in pregnancy, in gastric or liver inflammation, or when treating children or reformed alcoholics. Adding a small amount (25-50 ml) of almost boiling water to the tincture dose (usually 5 ml) in a cup and allowing it to cool effectively evaporates most of the alcohol.

Tincture ratios

Tinctures are sometimes recommended for use in ratio form, for example, "take 5 ml of a 1:4 tincture". When taking a tincture in ratio form, the proportion used is weight to volume. A 1:4 tincture could be made with 1 kg or 1 lb herb to 4 litres or 4 pints alcohol/water mix, or 1 g herb to 400 ml alcohol/water mix. The units used are immaterial and can be large or small accordingly.

Fluid extracts

Fluid extracts are available commercially and generally not made at home as they are measured precisely to pharmaceutical grades. They are used to increase the strength of a herbal mixture when additional action is needed.

Tonic wines

This simple method yields a mixture that is a pleasure to take. It is especially suitable for roots such as *he shou wu*, *dang gui* and ginseng. Put 500 g herb in a large jar and pour 2 litres of good quality, preferably red, wine over it. Ensure the herb is completely covered, or it will go mouldy. Cover the jar and leave for 2 weeks. Take in sherry glass doses.

Macerations

Some herbs, like valerian root, are best macerated rather than infused or decocted; use the maceration as an infusion or decoction. Pour 500 ml cold water over 25 g dried herb, and leave the mixture in a cool place overnight; strain through a nylon sieve.

Chinese decoctions

In China, herbs are mainly given in decoctions. Much larger quantities are used than in the West, with up to 150 g dried herb in 1 litre of water reduced down to 300-400 ml for three doses. The resulting mixture is very concentrated and may need to be diluted with water to suit Western palates.

Lotions

A lotion is a water-based mixture that is applied to the skin as a cooling or soothing remedy to relieve irritation or inflammation. Alcohol-based mixtures – such as tinctures – can be added to lotions to increase the cooling effect. Typically, a lotion to relieve skin irritation, for example, might include 40 ml rosewater, 20 ml borage juice, 20 ml distilled witch hazel and 20 ml chickweed tincture. Apply a little of the lotion with cotton wool or absorbent gauze two or three times a day. If treating a small local area, cover the area with a bandage afterwards.

Skin washes

Infusions or diluted tinctures can be used to bathe wounds, sores, skin rashes, ulcers or other skin conditions. Soak a pad of cotton wool in the wash and bathe the affected area from the centre outward. Alternatively, use a plastic atomizer to spray the herbal mixture on rashes or varicose ulcers.

Pessaries and suppositories

Steel moulds to make up to 24 pessaries and suppositories, as well as disposable moulds, are available from specialist suppliers. A home-made mould can be shaped from cooking foil: press it around a small object about 1 cm in diameter and 2 cm in length – a thimble is ideal. First lubricate the mould by filling it with a mixture made from 20 ml soft soap, 100 ml glycerine and 80 ml industrial alcohol or methylated spirits. After a few minutes, pour off the lubricant and drain well. Fill the mould with a pessary mixture made by melting 20 g cocoa butter in a double saucepan and stirring in 10-20 drops (0.5 -1 ml) essential oil. The unused pessary lubricant can be stored in a clean glass bottle for future use. Alternatively, heat 15 g gelatin with 20 ml glycerine and 30 ml infusion or diluted tincture. Pour the mixture into a lubricated mould and leave to set for about two hours; then open the mould and carefully remove. Store the pessaries and suppositories in a cool place.

Juices

Herb juices can be prepared using a food processor or a domestic juicer to pulp the plant. Squeeze the pulp through a nylon sieve or jelly bag to obtain the juice. Large quantities of herb are needed – a 10 litre bucket of fresh herb may yield only 100 ml or less of juice.

HERBAL FIRST AID

WE ARE MORE INCLINED to reach for patent antiseptics and painkillers in a domestic emergency than think of herbal medicines. Yet herbs can provide effective alternatives to many over-the-counter pharmacy offerings and may be available when the standard first aid kit is not – in an emergency in the countryside, for example. For home use, proprietary herbal preparations can supplement fresh herbs.

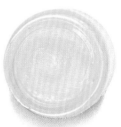

Remedies to buy

Herbal remedies can be bought ready-made in a variety of different forms, including creams, essential oils and capsules. Shown here are the most useful herbal remedies to keep at home in a first aid kit.

FIRST AID KIT
Keep herbal first aid remedies in a box in a cool place out of the reach of children.

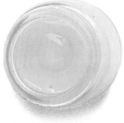

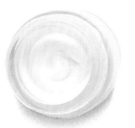

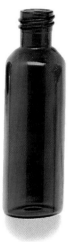

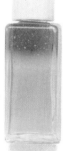

RESCUE REMEDY
The Bach Flower Remedies have a potent effect on the emotions. Rescue Remedy, also available as a cream, is good for shocks and nervous upsets.

MARIGOLD CREAM
Often sold as *Calendula*, this is antiseptic and antifungal. It is useful for all sorts of cuts and grazes.

COMFREY OINTMENT
This speeds healing of wounds by encouraging cell growth; use only on clean cuts as the rapidly healing skin may trap dirt.

CHICKWEED CREAM
A valuable first aid remedy for drawing stubborn splinters, boils, and insect stings, or for burns and scalds.

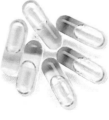

ARNICA CREAM
Effective for bruises and sprains. Do not use on broken skin as it can be irritant.

ARNICA 6X TABLETS
Essential for domestic shocks or accidents, these homeopathic tablets can be taken at 30 minute intervals until the patient feels more settled.

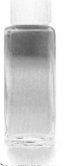

LAVENDER OIL
Add 2-3 drops to a teaspoon of carrier oil and massage into the nape of the neck and temples at the first hint of a headache or migraine. Use the same mix to relieve minor burns, scalds and sunburn.

TEA TREE OIL
Highly antiseptic and antifungal for cuts and grazes, as well as warts and cold sores.

EVENING PRIMROSE CAPSULES
A useful hangover cure. Take a large dose (2-3 g) on "the morning after" to bring rapid relief.

DISTILLED WITCH HAZEL
Use for minor burns and sunburn. Soak a swab in witch hazel to staunch the flow of blood from wounds and soothe insect bites. For bruises and sprains, keep an ice-cube tray of witch hazel in the freezer, clearly labelled.

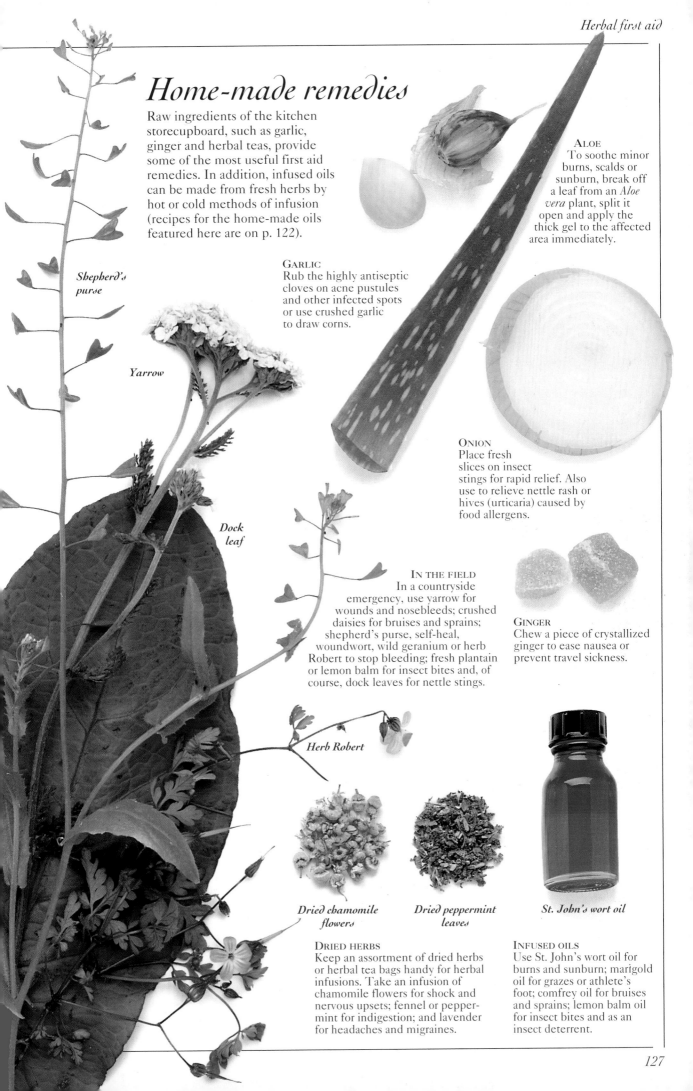

Home-made remedies

Raw ingredients of the kitchen storecupboard, such as garlic, ginger and herbal teas, provide some of the most useful first aid remedies. In addition, infused oils can be made from fresh herbs by hot or cold methods of infusion (recipes for the home-made oils featured here are on p. 122).

Shepherd's purse

Yarrow

Dock leaf

ALOE
To soothe minor burns, scalds or sunburn, break off a leaf from an *Aloe vera* plant, split it open and apply the thick gel to the affected area immediately.

GARLIC
Rub the highly antiseptic cloves on acne pustules and other infected spots or use crushed garlic to draw corns.

ONION
Place fresh slices on insect stings for rapid relief. Also use to relieve nettle rash or hives (urticaria) caused by food allergens.

IN THE FIELD
In a countryside emergency, use yarrow for wounds and nosebleeds; crushed daisies for bruises and sprains; shepherd's purse, self-heal, woundwort, wild geranium or herb Robert to stop bleeding; fresh plantain or lemon balm for insect bites and, of course, dock leaves for nettle stings.

GINGER
Chew a piece of crystallized ginger to ease nausea or prevent travel sickness.

Herb Robert

Dried chamomile flowers

Dried peppermint leaves

St. John's wort oil

DRIED HERBS
Keep an assortment of dried herbs or herbal tea bags handy for herbal infusions. Take an infusion of chamomile flowers for shock and nervous upsets; fennel or peppermint for indigestion; and lavender for headaches and migraines.

INFUSED OILS
Use St. John's wort oil for burns and sunburn; marigold oil for grazes or athlete's foot; comfrey oil for bruises and sprains; lemon balm oil for insect bites and as an insect deterrent.

HOME REMEDIES

Herbalism has always been regarded as
the "medicine of the people" – simple remedies that
can be used at home for minor ills, or to supplement more
potent remedies prescribed by professionals for chronic
and acute conditions. Herbs can be taken quite simply
as teas, although more complex preparations can
be made at home (see pp. 120-5) or are available from
health food shops and pharmacies as patent medicines.
Although most herbs are intrinsically quite safe they
should be treated with respect – do not exceed
stated doses or continue with home remedies if
conditions are persistent, are worsening or if
the true diagnosis is in doubt.

HOW TO USE THIS SECTION

In this section ailments are grouped according to body systems, life stages or action. The complaints covered here are those where home remedies are most appropriate although herbs can, of course, be used for many more ailments. The list of complaints is not intended to be comprehensive and the herbs given for each ailment represent only a small cross-section of the many plants that could be used. Selection of individual remedies will often depend on availability, but choose those which appear to have the most relevant actions: for coughs, for example, do you need an expectorant to clear phlegm, a suppressant to ease a persistent tickle, an antibacterial to combat infection or a tonic to strengthen weak lungs? Herbs can work very quickly, especially in acute conditions. However, long-standing, chronic disorders may require treatment for several months before significant results are achieved. Generally, symptoms will change as the weeks progress, so be prepared to review the remedy at least once a month, and alter it to reflect new conditions. Professional herbalists will often adjust remedies every few weeks as health and energy balance changes. For ailments not covered in this section, or for persistent conditions, consult a professional (see p. 183). Details of herbal suppliers are given on p. 192. If gathering herbs in the wild or from gardens, always consult a good plant key or field herbal to ensure plants are selected correctly.

Sample entry

Ailments

Herbs

Actions

Case history

How to use

Combinations

Cautions

Standard remedies

CASE HISTORY Based on a real life case this shows how herbs are used with other therapeutic approaches such as diet, exercise or relaxation. Names and circumstances have been changed to preserve anonymity.

AILMENTS Brief description of causes and some key symptoms.

HERB Listed in alphabetical order by botanical name, with the most widely used common name. Symbols indicate which part of the plant to use. Before using any herb refer to the pages shown in brackets.

ACTIONS Major therapeutic effects of the herb relevant to the ailments.

HOW TO USE The form in which to take each herb medicinally. Standard adult doses should be assumed unless otherwise specified. Before making or using any remedy, refer to *Making Herbal Remedies*,

pp. 120-5, which provides details of standard formulations and dosages.

COMBINATIONS Most herbs work best in combination, although the exact choice of remedies can vary enormously depending on particular individuals, their symptoms and constitution. For each ailment, additional herbs are suggested to enhance therapeutic actions. Herbalists rarely combine herbs in equal quantities, because some symptoms may be more acute and specific herbs may be considered more important for treatment. However, the herbs suggested here can be used in equal proportions unless otherwise specified.

When using a combination of herbs, the total should not exceed the standard adult dose specified in *Making Herbal Remedies*, pp.120-5. For example, a standard infusion

(enough for three doses) is made with 30g dried herb to 500 ml water. If using three herbs in combination, mix 10 g of each to 500 ml water. Tinctures are made singly and then combined for a specified dose.

CAUTIONS Many herbs contain extremely powerful chemicals and overdose can be harmful. Before taking any herbal remedy check the cautions given here and on the pages shown in brackets in the *Herb* column. Some herbs may, by law, only be prescribed by a qualified practitioner. For herbs used in combinations, check cautions on pp. 180-2 or in the A-Z section (pp. 28-115) as appropriate.

STANDARD REMEDIES All the information in the *How to use* column applies to standard formulations and dosages listed on pp. 120-5, unless otherwise stated.

IMPORTANT NOTES

- If taking medication for a particular complaint always consult your doctor or other professional medical practitioner before changing or discontinuing dosages. Some herbs will interact with orthodox drugs and care is needed. If on prescribed medication consult a professional before attempting home remedies.

- In any acute condition – fevers, coughs, digestive upsets, severe headaches – seek professional help if there is no improvement within a few days or if the condition appears to be worsening.

- Give children a fraction of an adult dose depending on age (see p. 175).

- In the elderly, metabolism gradually slows down: reduce standard adult doses with increasing frailty and loss of bodyweight.

- Essential oils are extremely potent and many can irritate mucous membranes. Unless otherwise clearly stated in the remedy charts, *do not* take essential oils internally without professional medical supervision. Before using externally, dilute essential oils in a carrier oil such as wheatgerm, almond or sunflower. Because essential oils are so expensive, many synthetic chemical substitutes are offered for sale. Always buy a reputable brand, guaranteed to be pure and unadulterated; do not be misled by low-cost products.

ACHES & PAINS

THE USUAL REACTION to muscular pain is to reach for a painkiller, such as paracetamol, which quickly lulls the body back into pain-free comfort. Pain, however, is only a symptom of an underlying problem: pulled muscles and strained tendons need restricted movement to heal, and the pain reminds us to keep movement to a minimum. Herbal remedies can do more than just deaden pain; many plants repair the damage of injury or degenerative disease, and provide symptomatic relief; some act as muscle relaxants, others as antispasmodics or anti-inflammatories. A herbal approach to

osteoarthritis, for example, may involve using comfrey ointment to help repair damaged and degenerating bone, with anti-inflammatory herbs such as willow, devil's claw or meadow-sweet to help relieve pain, and cleansing plants such as yellow dock or celery seed to eliminate toxins which can collect in the joints and contribute to discomfort. In Chinese medicine, arthritic and rheumatic pains are attributed to external "evils", such as heat, damp or cold, and are treated with "warming" or "cooling" herbs and energy tonics to combat future attacks by these "evils".

AILMENT	REMEDIES	
	Herb	*Actions*
SPRAINS & STRAINS Injuries to joints and muscles, including back strains. **KEY SYMPTOMS** • Pain following obvious injury or exertion • Swollen joints or limbs • Bruising. *IMPORTANT: If fractures are suspected or if symptoms persist for more than a few days without improvement, seek urgent professional help.*	*Arnica montana* ARNICA (see p. 180)	Promotes healing and has an antibacterial action; causes reabsorption of internal bleeding in bruises and sprains.
	Symphytum officinale COMFREY (see p. 101)	Encourages cell regrowth in connective tissues and bones; breaks down red blood cells in bruising.
	Thymus vulgaris THYME (see p. 104)	Antispasmodic; stimulates blood flow to the tissues, encouraging repair.
ARTHRITIS & RHEUMATISM There are two main types of arthritis: osteoarthritis (OA) is pain and swelling of the joints, generally due to wear and tear; rheumatoid arthritis (RA) is inflammation of many joints, and requires professional treatment. Rheumatism is a general term for any muscle pain, while lumbago is low back pain. Symptoms are often worse in damp weather. **KEY SYMPTOMS** • Stiffness and joint pain • Creaking sounds in joints • Swollen or deformed joints • Hot or burning joints (RA).	*Angelica archangelica* ANGELICA (see p. 36)	A warming and stimulating herb, good for "cold" types of osteoarthritis and for rheumatism.
	Harpagophytum procumbens DEVIL'S CLAW (see p. 180) *(Tuber)*	Potent anti-inflammatory; action has been compared with cortisone. Better for OA and degenerative conditions than for RA.
	Menyanthes trifoliata BOGBEAN (see p. 180)	Cleansing, cooling and anti-inflammatory; a useful herb for "hotter" types of arthritis and muscle pain.
	Salix alba WILLOW (see p. 94)	Rich in salicylates (anti-inflammatories that cool hot joints); useful in acute phases and for muscle pains.
GOUT Generally associated with a build-up of uric acid in the joints linked to dietary excess. **KEY SYMPTOM** • Swollen, inflamed, very painful joints; often the toes or feet.	*Apium graveolens* CELERY (see p. 37)	Clears uric acid from the joints, useful for gout and arthritic problems.
	Teucrium chamaedrys WALL GERMANDER (see p. 182)	Bitter, digestive tonic and diuretic.

CASE HISTORY
Arthritic pains

PATIENT: Mary, a retired school secretary aged 66, an enthusiastic lace-maker and gardener.

HISTORY AND COMPLAINT: For the past three years Mary had suffered from pain and stiffness in her hands, knees and hips, as well as breathlessness, palpitations and sore, irritated eyes. Hospital tests ruled out rheumatoid arthritis, but X-rays revealed wear and tear on the joints. Mary had a history of nervous problems and had taken antidepressants and sleeping pills for five years. A recent bereavement had exacerbated her symptoms.

TREATMENT: The antidepressants carried the risk of liver damage, and Mary's symptoms suggested some

liver congestion and weakness, so medication included tinctures of *bai shao yao, huai niu xi* and bogbean, as well as angelica root, willow bark and *fang feng* (total 5 ml three times a day). A few drops of the Bach flower remedy, Star of Bethlehem, were added to help her cope with her recent loss. Devil's claw (two capsules up to three times a day) helped while symptoms were acute, and a massage oil containing rosemary and juniper essence in infused bladderwrack oil was useful.

OUTCOME: A month later, Mary's painful joints and sore eyes were back to normal and her hands were no longer stiff. She switched to a herbal remedy for insomnia, and her doctor changed the antidepressants to reduce side effects.

How to use	Combinations	Cautions
Apply cream to the affected area, or soak a pad in dilute tincture and use as a compress; take homeopathic *Arnica 6x* every 1 to 2 hours.	Use as a simple.	Do not use on broken skin; use homeopathic *Arnica* only internally.
Rub cream or ointment on to the affected area as frequently as required.	Add 5-10 drops essential oils, such as thyme, lavender or juniper, to 25 ml infused oil to stimulate blood flow and ease pain.	Use only if the injury is clean; not advisable for long-term use.
Add 10 drops oil to 20 ml water and use as a compress; or add 5 drops oil to a hot bath.	Mix with 5-10 drops essential oils such as lavender, rosemary or sage, in 25 ml almond or sunflower oil as a massage oil to stimulate blood flow and ease pain.	Massage can be damaging if given too soon after injury.
Soak a pad in dilute tincture or decoction and use as a compress; take a decoction, or add 5 drops oil to a bath.	Add celery seed or a little prickly ash to decoction. Mix angelica and rosemary oil (5-10 drops of each in 25 ml carrier oil) as a massage to relieve pain.	Avoid in pregnancy.
Take 1 to 3 g powder a day in capsule form during the acute phase; take up to 15 ml tincture a day, or use in combinations.	Combine with equal amounts of tinctures of other anti-inflammatories or cleansing herbs, such as angelica, St. John's wort, bogbean or celery seed.	
Take up to 8 ml tincture three times a day; also use as an infusion or macerate 10 g herb in 100 ml red wine.	Mix black cohosh or celery seed in infusion, using 2 parts bogbean to 1 part other herbs; or add anti-inflammatories like meadowsweet to tincture.	
Take up to 5 ml fluid extract three times a day, or use in combination with other tinctures.	Add tinctures of other antirheumatics or cleansing herbs, such as angelica, black cohosh, *lignum vitae*, yellow dock or burdock.	
Take an infusion of 1 tsp to 500 ml water, or combine with other tinctures.	Add 1 part *lignum vitae* to 2 parts celery seed in an infusion; use diuretics like yarrow or gravelroot in tincture.	Use untreated seeds only; avoid in pregnancy.
Take an infusion or use up to 15 ml tincture a day.	Combine with yarrow and celery seed in an infusion to encourage uric acid excretion.	Do not exceed stated dose.

KEY

Aerial parts

Bark

Essential oil

Flowers

Leaves

Root

Seeds

STANDARD REMEDIES All recipes and doses are standard unless otherwise specified; see *Making Herbal Remedies*, pp. 120-5.

HEADACHES & MIGRAINES

HEADACHES ARE NOT illnesses in their own right, but symptoms of underlying "dis-ease". Tension headaches, for example, respond to calming herbs, but persistent ones may indicate a need for relaxation, stress-release techniques, or a radical appraisal of lifestyle. Headaches due to catarrh or sinusitis are eased by decongestant herbs, fresh air and a diet free from mucus-forming foods such as dairy produce. Migraines can be related to food intolerance or pollutants. "Hot" migraines, associated with constricted blood vessels, are relieved by ice packs and cooling remedies; "cold" ones, related to dilated blood vessels, respond to a hot towel on the forehead and warm, stimulating herbs. Some women find that migraines are linked to their menstrual cycle, and hormonal herbs may help. Digestive remedies, especially liver-cleansing herbs like agrimony, can also alleviate headaches. In Chinese medicine, the eyes are associated with the liver, and migraine can be identified with over-exuberant liver *qi* (energy).

IMPORTANT: Seek professional advice for sudden persistent headaches.

See also: sinus headaches, pp. 138-9; anxiety and tension, pp. 162-3; PMS, pp. 166-7.

AILMENT	REMEDIES	
	Herb	*Actions*
TENSION HEADACHES May be caused by tense neck muscles due to stress. Symptoms resolve with relaxation. **KEY SYMPTOM** • Pain, usually frontal.	*Scutellaria lateriflora* **SKULLCAP** (see p. 98)	Relaxant and restorative for the central nervous system; sedative; antispasmodic.
	Stachys officinalis **WOOD BETONY** (see p. 99)	Sedative; stimulates cerebral circulation; useful nervine for anxiety and worries.
MIGRAINE Severe headache, which can be linked to food sensitivity, pollutants, menstrual cycle or stress. It is associated with changes in tension within the arteries of the brain. Untreated symptoms may last for a few minutes or several days. **KEY SYMPTOMS** • Visual disturbances preceding pain • Pins and needles in limbs • Nausea and vomiting • Light sensitivity.	*Gelsemium sempervirens* **YELLOW JASMINE** (see p. 182)	Potent analgesic and sedative; useful for migraines and neuralgia.
	Lavandula spp. **LAVENDER** (see p. 73)	Sedative; analgesic with antispasmodic action; cooling, bitter remedy useful for "hot" migraines.
	Tanacetum parthenium **FEVERFEW** (see p. 102)	Anti-inflammatory; dilates the cerebral blood vessels easing "hot" migraines associated with constricted blood vessels.
NEURALGIA Severe burning or stabbing pain often felt along the course of facial nerves. Can follow injury or exposure to cold and draughts. **KEY SYMPTOMS** • Severe, very localized pain • Related areas of skin highly sensitive to touch • Regular recurrences.	*Citrus limon* **LEMON** (see p. 181)	Cooling, astringent; reputed nerve tonic; anti-inflammatory.
	Hypericum perforatum **ST. JOHN'S WORT** (see p. 68) *(Flowering tops)*	Repairs and restores the nervous system; anti-inflammatory.
	Verbena officinalis **VERVAIN** (see p. 112)	Sedative; antispasmodic; restorative for the nervous system.

CASE HISTORY
Tension headaches

PATIENT: Vera, a married secretary of 45, with two teenage daughters and a live-in mother-in-law.

HISTORY AND COMPLAINT: Vera suffered from headaches once or twice a week, for which she took patent analgesics. The pain was always localized over her right eye and often persisted for two or three days. She also complained of frequent bouts of diarrhoea. She had a tendency to depression and extreme tiredness, and never managed to find time for herself. Medical tests detected no abnormalities. She found her daughters difficult, and the constant presence of her elderly mother-in-law irksome. Shortage of money was a continual worry.

TREATMENT: A little self-indulgence was called for: lavender oil for the bath and five minutes to herself after work. Medication for stress intolerance and depression featured relaxing and tonic nervines, which also eased stomach tensions. Bach flower remedies (Impatiens, Willow and Beech) were added to encourage tolerance. Tinctures of wood betony, vervain, lemon balm, oats and pasque flower were taken in 5 ml doses three times a day, with ginseng as a general tonic.

OUTCOME: Over two months Vera's headaches became less frequent and severe. A bout of family arguments brought them back, but Vera realized how closely they were linked to stresses at home and to her emotions – when her mother-in-law went away for two weeks Vera had a pain-free fortnight. A residential home might have solved the problem, but Bach flower remedies had to do the job instead.

How to use	Combinations	Cautions
Take an infusion or tincture.	Mix 45 ml skullcap tincture and 5 ml lemon balm and take up to four 5 ml doses a day as a calming nervine.	
Take an infusion or tincture.	Add sedative nervines such as lavender, vervain, St. John's wort and skullcap to the infusion or tincture.	Avoid high doses in pregnancy.
Use restricted to professional practitioners in UK, Australia and New Zealand; maximum safe dose in UK is 5 drops 1:10 tincture in water up to 4 times. Maximum dose 5 ml per week.	Prescribed as a simple in acute phases, but can be prescribed in conjunction with drops of Jamaican dogwood tincture (up to 20 drops three times a day) and either lavender tea for "hot" migraines or rosemary for "cold" conditions.	Use only as prescribed; overdose can cause nausea and double vision.
Dilute 10 drops lavender oil in 25 ml carrier oil and massage into the temples at the first hint of symptoms; take an infusion of the flowers.	After the massage, drink an infusion of lavender flower and vervain (total of 30 g herb to 500 ml water) in wine-glass doses.	Avoid high doses in pregnancy.
Eat one leaf a day as a prophylactic, or take 5-10 drops tincture every 30 minutes while symptoms last.	Combine with other tranquillizers and analgesics, such as valerian or Jamaican dogwood tincture, taking up to 20 drops three times a day.	Avoid if taking warfarin; side effects of eating leaves can include mouth ulcers.
Gently rub a slice of fresh lemon or a little juice on the affected area, or use well-diluted lemon oil.	For symptomatic relief use as a simple.	Oil can irritate: use no more than 5 drops in 25 ml carrier oil.
Take an infusion; apply the infused oil externally to the affected area.	Add lavender and skullcap to the infusion as calming nervines.	Can cause dermatitis if skin is exposed to sunlight after taking it internally.
Soak a pad in a decoction and use as a compress; use ointment; take the infusion or 5 ml tincture.	Add lavender or St. John's wort to tincture or infusion, or up to 20 drops Jamaican dogwood tincture.	Avoid therapeutic doses in pregnancy.

KEY

Aerial parts

Essential oil

Flowers

Fruit

Root

STANDARD REMEDIES All recipes and doses are standard unless otherwise specified; see *Making Herbal Remedies*, pp. 120-5.

INFECTIONS

MODERN SCIENCE attributes infections to bacteria and viruses. Previous generations blamed flying venom, "elf-shot" or the evil eye, while Chinese medicine attributes chills and fevers to "six evils" related to climatic factors – wind, cold, heat, dampness, dryness and fire – and blames "pestilence" for severe epidemics. Many herbs traditionally used to fight infections have been identified as potent antibiotics and immune system stimulants. Unlike wide-spectrum orthodox antibiotics, they are specific in the microbes they attack, so have less impact on the friendly bacteria in the gut, making the digestive upsets that can follow orthodox medication less likely. Herbs can help to control the course of an illness as the body works to restore balance. Common colds, for example, may be "hot" or "cold" in character, or alternate between the two as the illness progresses. "Cold" conditions need warming herbs such as ginger, *gui zhi* or angelica; "hot" infections can be cooled with herbs that promote sweating, such as boneset, catmint, peppermint or mulberry leaf.

See also: catarrh, pp. 136-7; coughs, pp. 136-7; fungal infections, pp. 146-7; candidiasis, pp. 156-7.

AILMENT	REMEDIES	
	Herb	*Actions*
COLDS & INFLUENZA Generally considered to be due to viral or bacterial infections, colds and influenza are often associated with stress, fatigue, depression, and excess cold or heat. **KEY SYMPTOMS** • Fever • Muscle pain and/or headache • Nasal catarrh or stuffiness • Cough • Sore throat.	*Allium sativum* GARLIC (see p. 33) *(Bulb)*	Antimicrobial; antifungal; suitable for a wide range of infectious conditions.
	Cinnamomum cassia GUI ZHI (see p. 48)	Warms "cold" conditions; promotes sweating; antibacterial.
	Eupatorium perfoliatum BONESET (see p. 180)	Promotes sweating; reduces fever; expectorant; good for hot feverish colds and influenza with muscle pain.
	Nepeta cataria CATMINT (see p. 180)	Cools fevers, promotes sweating; astringent in catarrhal congestion.
BOILS & ABSCESSES Localized infections often due to bacteria entering a hair follicle or wound. May indicate a weakened immune system. **KEY SYMPTOMS** • Tender, inflamed area of skin • Obvious pus in boils • Pain.	*Forsythia suspensa* LIAN QIAO (see p. 181)	Antibacterial, anti-inflammatory; reduces heat; resolves abscesses and boils; cools fevers.
	Scrophularia spp. FIGWORT and XUAN SHEN (see p. 97)	Anti-inflammatory, anti-bacterial; cleansing, so good for toxic conditions.
WEAK IMMUNE SYSTEM Associated with exhaustion, food allergy or depression, this leaves the body vulnerable to infection. It could signify a more serious underlying disorder. **KEY SYMPTOMS** • Persistent colds or influenza • Frequent skin infections • Chronic fatigue.	*Astragalus membranaceus* HUANG QI (see p. 181) *(Rhizome)*	Increases production of white blood cells and strengthens the immune response; anti-bacterial; energy tonic; strengthens *wei qi*, or defence energy.
	Echinacea spp. PURPLE CONEFLOWER (see p. 53)	Antibacterial, antiviral; strengthens resistance to infections; useful for all septic or infectious conditions.

CASE HISTORY
Over-exhaustion leading to a weak immune system

PATIENT: Lucy, aged 35, the mother of an active three-year-old, was busily engaged in renovating an old farmhouse with her husband.

HISTORY AND COMPLAINT: For the past four years, Lucy had suffered constant colds and miscellaneous viruses. Problems had started during pregnancy, as Lucy exhausted her energies coping with a high-powered job in publishing and making the transition to full-time mother. Although her diet was good and she took regular exercise, repeated infections had left her exhausted, lethargic, and feeling down. For two years, her doctor had prescribed antidepressants as well as continual courses of antibiotics. The colds had increased since her daughter had started playgroup.

TREATMENT: Herbal remedies focused on immune stimulants and uplifting tonic herbs: *ling zhi*, *huang qi*, vervain, lemon balm and purple coneflower, with purple coneflower capsules as an extra boost when cold symptoms began. Supplements of *Lactobacillus acidophilus* and other friendly bacteria helped the digestive system recover from excessive antibiotics. Cold symptoms were treated with elderflower, yarrow and peppermint tea, sage gargles, and white horehound, thyme and liquorice cough syrups.

OUTCOME: After four months the recurrent colds had disappeared and Lucy began to feel more energetic and enthusiastic about life. After discussion with her doctor the antidepressants were gradually stopped.

How to use	Combinations	Cautions
Eat up to six fresh cloves a day in acute conditions, or take proprietary capsules.	Best as a simple; limit the odour by eating parsley.	If it irritates the stomach, take ginger or fennel tea. Avoid therapeutic doses during pregnancy and lactation.
Take a decoction or tincture; use bark (*rou gui*) if *gui zhi* is unavailable.	For chills, mix with a little fresh ginger root.	Avoid in pregnancy. Not suitable for "hot" feverish colds.
Take an infusion or tincture three to four times a day.	For feverish colds and influenza, combine with yarrow, elderflower and peppermint.	High doses can cause vomiting.
Take an infusion or tincture three to four times a day.	For feverish colds, can be mixed with yarrow, elderflower, boneset, ground ivy, angelica or mulberry leaf to enhance specific actions.	
Take a decoction.	Combine with cooling herbs such as *jin yin hua*, burdock seeds or *huang qin*, or antibacterials like purple coneflower in capsules.	Use before boils start to suppurate. Avoid in diarrhoea.
Make a poultice from figwort leaves; take a decoction of *xuan shen* or a tincture.	Add cooling herbs such as *lian qiao*, *jin yin hua*, goldenseal or *huang qin* to the decoction, and take antibacterials like purple coneflower in capsules.	Heart stimulant, so avoid in heartbeat abnormalities (tachycardia).
Take a decoction or tincture.	For debilitated conditions, add other energy tonics such as liquorice, *dang gui* and *bai zhu*.	Avoid if condition involves excess "heat" or *yin* deficiency.
Take 500 mg powdered root in capsules or 10 ml tincture. Repeat up to four times a day.	Use as a simple, or add anticatarrhal remedies like elderflower and catmint, or fever herbs like yarrow or boneset, depending on symptoms.	High doses can occasionally cause nausea and dizziness.

KEY

Aerial parts

Fruit

Leaves

Root

Twigs

STANDARD REMEDIES All recipes and doses are standard unless otherwise specified; see *Making Herbal Remedies*, pp. 120-5.

RESPIRATORY PROBLEMS

A HOLISTIC APPROACH to health is particularly relevant to respiratory problems. To blame chest complaints on infection, industrial pollution or an ailing heart is to address only part of the problem: emotional and spiritual factors must be considered as well. In Chinese medicine, the lungs are associated with grief, and it is notable that chest problems often follow a bereavement or other sorrow, and that chest infections tend to strike when we feel down – perhaps when in a job we dislike or unhappy at home. Herbs cannot always solve these underlying problems, but strengthening lung tonics like elecampane or cowslip, which also

act on the nervous system, can help. Breathing and breath have much greater significance in Eastern systems of medicine than they do in the mechanistic Western model. In Ayurvedic medicine, for example, breathing is regarded as the life force, and breath control is an important Yogic art. In Chinese medicine too, the breath is equated with *qi* (vital energy) and controls its flow: respiratory problems are seen not only as damaging to the vital energy, but also as signifying *qi* weakness or imbalance. The wide range of herbal respiratory remedies can relieve symptoms and restore inner balance, to tackle the underlying cause of the condition.

See also: sore throat, pp. 142-3, tonsillitis, pp. 142-3; hay fever, pp. 156-7.

AILMENT	REMEDIES	
	Herb	*Actions*
COUGHS A cough is a muscle spasm that occurs as a reaction to irritation or blockage in the bronchial tubes (the tubes from the throat to the lungs). Coughs often occur in conjunction with infections such as colds or influenza, but are sometimes associated with nervous tension and have no pathological cause. **KEY SYMPTOMS** • Productive cough may produce mucus varying from a thin, watery discharge to thick yellow or green phlegm • Unproductive cough can be very dry and irritant. **IMPORTANT:** *Seek professional help for a persistent cough of unknown cause.*	*Althaea officinalis* **MARSHMALLOW** (see p. 35)	Demulcent and expectorant; soothes inflamed respiratory mucous membranes.
	Hyssopus officinalis **HYSSOP** (see p. 69)	Warming, expectorant, antispasmodic; useful for thin, watery phlegm and coughs associated with bronchitis.
	Morus alba **SANG BAI PI** (see p. 80)	Cooling expectorant, antitussive; good for "hot" conditions.
	Pimpinella anisum **ANISE** (see p. 180)	Relaxing expectorant, antiseptic and carminative; good for irritant dry coughs and bronchial infections.
	Prunus serotina **WILD CHERRY** (see p. 182)	Cough suppressant; useful for dry, irritant or nervous coughs.
CATARRH Excessive secretions from the membranes in the respiratory system, catarrh can be "cold", with copious watery secretions, or "hot", with thick, yellow secretions. "Cold" catarrh is often linked with eating too much sweet food and a sluggish system. "Hot" catarrh can be linked to a nervous personality, and may be persistent. **KEY SYMPTOMS** • Runny nose following a cold • Irritant cough • Inflamed nasal membranes • Sinus pain in "hot" type.	*Gnaphthalium uliginosum* **MARSH CUDWEED** (see p. 181)	Anti-inflammatory; tones up the respiratory system.
	Potentilla anserina **SILVERWEED** (see p. 182)	Astringent and anticatarrhal; cooling for "hot" catarrhal conditions.
	Sambucus nigra **ELDER** (see p. 96)	Anticatarrhal, antiinflammatory and expectorant; useful for upper respiratory tract catarrh linked to colds and hay fever.
	Solidago virgaurea **GOLDEN ROD** (see p. 181)	Drying, astringent, anticatarrhal; anti-inflammatory for the mucous membranes.

CASE HISTORY
Persistent cough

PATIENT: John, 52, was an export manager with an engineering company whose work involved regular overseas travel. He was married with two teenage sons.

HISTORY AND COMPLAINT: John had suffered from a dry, irritating cough for at least seven years. It had started after a severe cold, which had trailed off into a persistent cough. His symptoms were worse at night and kept him and his wife awake. Countless hospital tests had all proved negative, and the doctor's latest theory blamed the problem on stomach acid, for which he prescribed an acid-reducing drug. However, three months of this treatment failed to bring any improvements, and John's wife persuaded him to try alternative medicine.

TREATMENT: Neither hospital tests nor medical history suggested a problem with stomach acid, but John did tend to feel hot and thirsty. Remedies included a combination of moistening herbs, such as ribwort plantain, *sang bai pi* and white horehound, with wild cherry to suppress the cough, and elecampane as a lung tonic. Wild lettuce was added to the mixture for use at night as a stronger cough suppressant.

OUTCOME: Within three weeks, the coughing bouts, which had been a nightly interruption, occurred once or twice a week. The wild cherry was dropped from the medicine as the other herbs strengthened and restored the lungs. After two further months, John's cough finally cleared.

How to use	*Combinations*	*Cautions*
Take an infusion or tincture, or take 5 ml syrup made from leaves or flowers.	Can be combined with anticatarrhals like ground ivy, or additional expectorants such as mulberry bark or white horehound.	
Take an infusion or tincture, or mix 5 ml essential oil in 20 ml carrier oil for a chest rub.	Combines well with restoratives like elecampane and white horehound in chronic conditions: use 2 parts hyssop to 1 part other herb.	
Take a decoction or tincture.	Combine with soothing and cooling herbs like marshmallow leaf or ribwort plantain, or with thyme if there is an infection.	
Take 1-2 ml tincture three times a day or dilute 10 drops essential oil in 25 ml carrier oil as a chest rub.	Combine with 1-2 ml wild lettuce for irritant coughs, or 2-3 ml thyme or hyssop tincture in infections. Add 10 drops eucalyptus oil to chest rub.	
Take an infusion, or a tincture in 2 ml doses.	Combine with astringents like mullein, tonics such as elecampane or additional cough suppressants like wild lettuce in severe cases.	Can cause drowsiness; avoid in acute infections.
Take an infusion or tincture.	Can be combined with anticatarrhals such as elderflower, *cang er zi* or golden rod, using 2 parts marsh cudweed to 1 part other herbs.	
Take an infusion or tincture.	Combine with cooling and soothing anticatarrhals like ribwort plantain, or antibacterials like garlic.	
Take an infusion or tincture.	Can be combined with other drying or astringent herbs, such as yarrow, ground ivy, golden rod, agrimony or bistort to enhance action. Use 3 parts elderflower to 1 part other herbs.	
Take an infusion or tincture.	Can be combined with other anticatarrhals, such as marsh cudweed or *xin yi*, or demulcents like ribwort plantain.	

KEY

Aerial parts

Bark

Essential oil

Flowers

Leaves

Root

Root bark

Seeds

STANDARD REMEDIES
All recipes and doses are standard unless otherwise specified; see *Making Herbal Remedies*, pp. 120-5.

AILMENT	REMEDIES	
	Herb	*Actions*
SINUSITIS Inflammation or infection of the sinus cavities in the skull. It often follows a cold but may be associated with dental problems, such as a deep-seated root abscess. It tends to affect tense people who do not express their emotions and are unwilling or find it difficult to cry. **KEY SYMPTOMS** • Pain affecting sinus areas • Headaches, which may be severe • Sinuses tender to the touch • Nasal discharge, often streaked with blood.	*Glechoma hederacea* **GROUND IVY** (see p. 181)	Anticatarrhal and astringent; suitably drying for catarrh in the sinuses and bronchi.
	Hydrastis canadensis **GOLDENSEAL** (see p. 67) *(Rhizome)*	Powerful cooling astringent and anticatarrhal.
	Myrica cerifera **BAYBERRY** (see p. 180)	Warming and astringent; stimulates the circulatory system.
	Xanthium sibiricum **CANG ER ZI** (see p. 180)	Warming anticatarrhal; useful for sinus headaches and allergic rhinitis.
BRONCHITIS Inflammation of the bronchi, which may be due to infection. Chronic conditions are often exacerbated by common colds or associated with smoking and pollution. *NOTE: All herbs listed for bronchitis are also suitable for asthmatic conditions.* **KEY SYMPTOMS** • Productive cough, often purulent phlegm • Raised temperature • Chest pains and breathlessness if the condition is chronic.	*Inula helenium* **ELECAMPANE** (see p. 70)	Lung tonic and expectorant; restorative and warming; good for weakened lungs and stubborn coughs.
	Marrubium vulgare **WHITE HOREHOUND** (see p. 182)	Antispasmodic, demulcent and expectorant; relaxes the bronchi and eases congestion.
	Primula veris **COWSLIP** (see p. 87)	Potent expectorant, good for loosening old phlegm and easing stubborn, dry coughs.
	Thymus vulgaris **THYME** (see p. 104)	Antiseptic and expectorant; useful for thick, infected phlegm and dry, difficult coughs.
ASTHMA Spasm of the bronchi (bronchospasm) leading to wheezing and breathlessness. Asthma may be associated with other allergic symptoms such as hay fever or eczema, and can run in families. Chinese medicine often associates asthma with weak kidney energy and a failure of correct *qi* circulation. Kidney tonics such as *gui zhi* could be appropriate in treatment. *NOTE: All herbs listed for bronchitis are also suitable for asthmatic conditions.* **KEY SYMPTOMS** • Wheezing on breathing out • Great difficulty in breathing. *IMPORTANT: Severe asthma can be life-threatening and requires professional medical help. Chronic asthmatics should seek professional medical advice before interrupting orthodox treatment.*	*Chamaemelum nobile* **ROMAN CHAMOMILE** (see p. 47)	Anti-allergenic, anti-inflammatory and antispasmodic; useful for allergic asthma.
	Ephedra sinica **MA HUANG** (see p. 54)	Bronchial relaxant and relaxes blood vessels; warming for all "cold" conditions of the chest.
	Eucalyptus globulus **EUCALYPTUS** (see p. 56)	Antiseptic, antispasmodic and expectorant.
	Grindelia camporum **GUMPLANT** (see p. 181)	Antispasmodic and expectorant; eases bronchospasm.

How to use	Combinations	Cautions
Take an infusion or tincture.	Can be used with other anticatarrhals like elderflower or ribwort plantain. Use 2 parts ground ivy to 1 part additional herbs.	
Take one or two 200 mg capsules of powder or 1 ml tincture three times a day.	Add eyebright powder to capsules.	Avoid in pregnancy or high blood pressure.
Use powder as a snuff, or add 5 ml tincture to 20 ml emulsifying ointment and use as a sinus massage.	Add 2-3 drops eucalyptus oil to ointment as an antiseptic and antispasmodic.	Avoid in very "hot" conditions.
Take a decoction or tincture.	Generally used in complex combinations of 10-15 other herbs to produce specific actions. For sinusitis, add herbs like *xin yi*, *lian qiao* or mulberry bark.	Very high doses can cause a dramatic fall in blood sugar.
Take a decoction, tincture or syrup.	Use as a simple, or add 10 ml horsetail juice to heal lung damage; other restorative lung herbs that can be added include hyssop, white horehound and anise.	
Take an infusion, tincture or syrup; suck horehound candy (available commercially).	Can be combined with tonics like elecampane or hyssop, or warming expectorants like angelica. Use 2 parts white horehound to 1 part additional herbs.	
Take a decoction, tincture or syrup.	Can be combined with strong expectorants like bloodroot and soothing demulcents such as ribwort plantain or liquorice. Use 2 parts cowslip to 1 part additional herbs.	Do not take high doses in pregnancy. Avoid if taking warfarin.
Take an infusion, tincture or syrup; for a chest rub, mix 10 drops essential oil in 20 ml almond oil.	Can add additional expectorants such as mulberry bark or healing herbs like horsetail for damaged lungs; the chest rub can be enhanced with 5 drops hyssop or peppermint essential oil.	Avoid therapeutic doses in pregnancy.
Add the essential oil to a chest rub or steam inhalant; immerse 1 tbsp flowers in a bowl of boiling water for a steam inhalant at the first sign of an attack.	Support with internal medication as for bronchitis, above.	Do not exceed stated dose. Do not use essential oil in pregnancy.
In UK, Australia and New Zealand use is restricted to professional practitioners. Maximum permitted dose in UK is 2.5 ml of 1:4 tincture three times a day.	Can be prescribed in combination with infusions of white horehound or hyssop; pill-bearing spurge and gumplant are often added as additional antispasmodics.	Take only as prescribed. Avoid in hypertension, glaucoma or if taking MAO inhibitors.
Mix 1-2 ml oil in 25 ml carrier oil for a chest rub; place a few drops on a pillow or handkerchief as an inhalant.	Add a total of 10-15 drops thyme, peppermint, lemon balm, anise or fennel essential oils to increase antiseptic and expectorant actions.	
Immerse 15 g in 500 ml water for an infusion and take up to 5 ml a day in doses of 1-2 ml.	Can be combined with additional antispasmodics such as pill-bearing spurge (up to 1 ml per dose of tincture), or with other expectorants and lung tonics like cowslip or elecampane.	Do not take if you have low blood pressure, since it reduces blood pressure. High doses can irritate the kidneys.

KEY

Aerial parts

Bark

Essential oil

Flowers

Fruit

Leaves

Root

Twigs

STANDARD REMEDIES All recipes and doses are standard unless otherwise specified; see *Making Herbal Remedies*, pp.120-5.

EARS, EYES, MOUTH & THROAT

ALTHOUGH MUCH OF MODERN medical practice tends to isolate sight, hearing and speech from the rest of the body, the health of the eyes, ears and mouth reflects the state of the whole body. It is now recognized that persistent problems in these organs often relate to other systemic disorders: "glue ear" in children is connected with milk allergies, and recurrent cold sores are linked to tiredness, stress and a run-down immune system. In Chinese medicine, eye problems are related to liver imbalance; hearing difficulties and tinnitus can imply kidney weakness; and persistent mouth problems or sore lips may indicate excess "heat" in the spleen. Herbal remedies are ideal for these ailments, offering symptomatic relief as well as tackling the underlying cause. In some instances, changes in diet or lifestyle are a crucial feature of the cure. Tired, strained eyes, for example, can be soothed by eyebaths of rosewater or a weak infusion of eyebright, pot marigold, cornflowers or strawberry leaves, but better lighting levels and frequent breaks from VDU screens may be the only real solution.

See also: infections, pp. 134-5; candidiasis, pp. 156-7.

AILMENT	REMEDIES	
	Herb	*Actions*
EARACHE This can be associated with catarrhal conditions or infection. **KEY SYMPTOMS** • Pain, often severe, in one or both ears • Blocked sensation in the ears • Buzzing or ringing sounds • Excessive waxy discharge • Fever • Vertigo or nausea if the inner ear is affected. *IMPORTANT: Severe infections can lead to deafness, so seek professional medical help if symptoms persist.*	*Anemone pulsatilla* **PASQUE FLOWER** (see p. 182)	Sedative, analgesic; acts directionally on ears.
	Hydrastis canadensis **GOLDENSEAL** (see p. 67)	Powerful cooling astringent with an anticatarrhal action.
	Plantago lanceolata **RIBWORT PLANTAIN** (see p. 86)	Tonifies mucous membranes and controls catarrh; useful for catarrhal conditions of the middle ear.
	Verbascum thapsus **MULLEIN** (see p. 111)	Demulcent and mildly sedative wound herb.
CONJUNCTIVITIS & BLEPHARITIS Conjunctivitis is an inflammation of the membrane that covers the eyeball (the conjunctiva). In blepharitis, the edges of the eyelid become inflamed. Both can be caused by infection, allergy, or physical or chemical irritation. **KEY SYMPTOMS:** CONJUNCTIVITIS • "Gritty" feeling in the eye • Increased sensitivity to light • Pain, soreness or swelling • Red or pink eye • Discharge that may be watery or contain pus. **KEY SYMPTOM:** BLEPHARITIS • Red, scaly eyelids.	*Agrimonia eupatoria* **AGRIMONY** (see p. 31)	Astringent and healing for mucous membranes; liver tonic that may help the eyes.
	Calendula officinalis **POT MARIGOLD** (see p. 43)	Anti-inflammatory, astringent wound herb, antiseptic; helpful for local irritation.
	Chrysanthemum morifolium **JU HUA** (see p. 181)	Antibacterial, anti-inflammatory and liver herb; good for persistent eye problems.
	Euphrasia officinalis **EYEBRIGHT** (see p. 181)	Astringent, anticatarrhal and anti-inflammatory.

CASE HISTORY
Excess catarrh causing deafness

PATIENT: Robert, an active 12-year-old, had become withdrawn and was falling behind at school.

HISTORY AND COMPLAINT: Robert had suffered from constant catarrh since babyhood. His ears were always blocked and prone to infection; as a toddler he had suffered from persistent "glue ear"; he had gone through three sets of grommets and was now into his third year of T-tubes. His hearing was getting worse, making school work and normal playground conversation difficult and he complained of a constant buzzing in his ears. Whenever he went swimming, earache and infection were sure to follow. His diet was fairly typical of a 12-year-old – too few green vegetables and more than a pint of milk a day.

TREATMENT: Herbal medicine included golden rod, purple coneflower and pasque flower in tincture form, with goldenseal capsules. For a trial month, Robert's mother replaced all milk and milk products in his diet with soya milk, and included more green vegetables and fish to boost mineral and vitamin intake.

OUTCOME: After only two weeks of herbs and a milk-free diet, Robert's hearing had improved. After three months, he had been free of ear infections and catarrh for six weeks, and could swim without getting an ear infection. The herbs were phased out and three months later, after a hospital check-up, the T-tubes were removed. He is happy with a low milk diet, and the occasional ice cream causes few problems.

How to use	*Combinations*	*Cautions*
Take 1-2 ml tincture three times a day.	Combine with anticatarrhals like goldenseal or eyebright. Use 10 drops goldenseal or up to 5 ml eyebright tinctures per dose.	
Take two 200 mg capsules or 20 drops tincture three times a day, or use 10 ml tincture in 100 ml water as eardrops (see caution for mullein below).	Add eyebright powder to capsules as an additional anticatarrhal.	Avoid in pregnancy or if you have high blood pressure; do not exceed the stated dose.
Take an infusion or tincture.	Combine tincture with elderflower tincture as an anticatarrhal, or 10 drops pasque flower tincture to focus action on the ears.	
Use cold infused oil as eardrops.	Support with antibiotic herbs such as purple coneflower in capsules, and anticatarrhals such as elderflower infusion or goldenseal capsules.	Do not use eardrops if there is a risk that the ear drum is perforated.
Bathe the eyes in an eyewash of weak, well-strained infusion (10 g herb to 500 ml water).	If there is any infection, support with antibacterials such as purple coneflower taken internally.	
Soak a pad in a well-diluted tincture and apply to the eyes as a compress; bathe styes with 5 ml tincture in 50 ml water.	Use as a simple.	
Take an infusion or tincture.	Combine with anticatarrhals like eyebright or elderflower, or liver herbs like agrimony or self-heal.	
Soak a pad in an infusion and apply to the eyes as a compress, or bathe the eyes in an eyewash of water with 5-10 drops tincture.	If there is any infection, support with antibacterials such as purple coneflower taken internally	

KEY

Aerial parts

Flowers

Leaves

Petals

Rhizome

STANDARD REMEDIES
All recipes and doses are standard unless otherwise specified; see *Making Herbal Remedies*, pp. 120-5.

AILMENT	REMEDIES	
	Herb	*Actions*
MOUTH ULCERS Painful ulcers in the mouth, often related to fungal or bacterial infection. They may be associated with excessive consumption of sugar or other foods that encourage fungal proliferation. Split or cracked lips occurring with the ulcers may indicate a vitamin deficiency. **KEY SYMPTOM** • Painful, white, raised patches, which may be very persistent.	*Commiphora molmol* **MYRRH** (see p. 50) *(Resin)*	Antimicrobial, astringent herb that heals wounds.
	Polygonum bistorta **BISTORT** (see p. 180)	Astringent, demulcent and anti-inflammatory; also suitable for other mouth inflammations.
	Salvia officinalis var. *purpurea* **PURPLE SAGE** (see p. 95)	Antiseptic and astringent. Also suitable for gingivitis and gum disorders.
COLD SORES Collections of small blisters on the face, usually around the lips. Once you are infected with the *Herpes simplex* virus, cold sores tend to recur when the immune system is weakened by infection, stress or fatigue. **KEY SYMPTOM** • Area that is painful or has a tingling sensation.	*Lavandula spp.* **LAVENDER** (see p. 73)	Topically antiseptic.
	Melaleuca alternifolia **TEA TREE** (see p. 182)	Antibiotic; stimulates the immune system.
SORE THROAT This common symptom may be associated with infection or chemical irritants. It may accompany tonsillitis, pharyngitis or laryngitis. **KEY SYMPTOMS** • Pain at the back of the mouth • Difficulty swallowing • Red, raw throat • Hoarse or croaking voice • Related fever or cold may be present or starting.	*Agrimonia eupatoria* **AGRIMONY** (see p. 31)	Astringent and healing for the mucous membranes.
	Alchemilla vulgaris **LADY'S MANTLE** (see p. 32)	Astringent; reduces inflammation; helpful for laryngitis.
	Echinacea spp. **PURPLE CONEFLOWER** (see p. 53)	Antibacterial, astringent; useful for all throat problems including tonsillitis.
	Lythrum salicaria **LOOSESTRIFE** (see p. 181)	Astringent; reduces inflammation; useful if the condition is associated with a feverish cold.
TONSILLITIS Inflammation of the tonsils is usually associated with a bacterial or viral infection. **KEY SYMPTOMS** • Very sore throat • Difficulty swallowing • Fever • Red, enlarged tonsils, which may discharge pus. *IMPORTANT: An abscess on the tonsils (quinsy) needs professional medical attention.*	*Baptisia tinctoria* **WILD INDIGO** (see p. 182)	Antimicrobial, anticatarrhal; cleanses the lymphatic system; good for persistent infections.
	Galium aparine **CLEAVERS** (see p. 62)	Alterative; cleanses the lymphatic system; good for all lymphatic problems including glandular fever and adenoids.
	Gnaphthalium uliginosum **MARSH CUDWEED** (see p. 181)	Anti-inflammatory; tonifies the mucous membranes; also good for laryngitis, pharyngitis and quinsy.
	Phytolacca americana **POKEROOT** (see p. 85)	Anticatarrhal; cleanses the lymphatic system; reduces lymphatic swellings.

How to use	Combinations	Cautions
Add 5-10 drops oil or 5 ml tincture to a glass of warm water and use as a mouthwash.	Add 5 ml sage or rosemary tincture to a mouthwash, or chew bilberries after using the mouthwash to help disguise the flavour.	Avoid in pregnancy.
For a mouthwash, use a decoction or add 5 ml tincture to a glass of water.	Add healing antibacterials like self-heal, rosemary, bilberry or wild indigo to the mouthwash. For persistent problems, take purple coneflower or garlic internally.	
For a mouthwash, use a standard infusion or add 10 ml tincture to a glass of water.	Add rosemary tincture to the mouthwash, or purple coneflower to enhance the antibacterial action.	Avoid therapeutic doses in pregnancy.
Mix 10 drops oil in 25 ml carrier oil, and dab on to the affected area.	Use as a simple; if the sore heralds a cold, take purple coneflower or garlic internally.	
Mix essential oil with 10 times its volume of carrier oil, and dab on to the affected area as soon as a developing cold sore starts to tingle.	Use as a simple. If sores recur frequently, take *huang qi* to boost the immune system or take patent Siberian ginseng tablets to increase stress tolerance.	
Gargle with an infusion or with 10 ml tincture diluted in a glass of warm water.	Use as a simple or add purple sage or rosemary tincture to the gargle.	
Gargle with an infusion or with 10 ml tincture diluted in a glass of warm water.	Add 5 ml rosemary or purple sage or up to 5 drops of cayenne tincture to the gargle for laryngitis.	Avoid in pregnancy.
Gargle with 10 ml tincture diluted in a glass of warm water, and swallow the gargle.	Use as a simple.	High doses can cause nausea and dizziness.
Gargle with an infusion or with 10 ml tincture diluted in a glass of warm water.	Can add astringent anticatarrhals such as silverweed or marsh cudweed to the gargle.	
Take 10-20 drops tincture three times a day.	Can be combined with other antibacterials such as purple coneflower, dried pokeroot or thyme, up to 5 ml tincture.	Do not exceed the stated dose; high doses may cause vomiting.
Take an infusion, or drink 10 ml fresh juice, three times a day.	Can combine with antibacterials like goldenseal (5-10 drops), purple coneflower (up to 10 ml) or dried pokeroot (10-20 drops) added to the juice in tincture form; support with gargles, as for sore throat (see above).	
Take an infusion or tincture and use as a gargle.	Combine with cleavers or purple coneflower tinctures as additional antibacterials and lymphatic cleansers.	
Take 10-20 drops tincture made from dried, not fresh, root three times a day. (Fresh root is toxic).	Can be combined with lymphatic cleansers like cleavers or cooling antibacterials like goldenseal, up to 5 ml tincture.	Do not exceed the stated dose; avoid in pregnancy.

KEY

Aerial parts

Essential oil

Leaves

Root

Stem

Whole herb

STANDARD REMEDIES
All recipes and doses are standard unless otherwise specified; see *Making Herbal Remedies*, pp. 120-5.

SKIN & HAIR

A HERBAL APPROACH to skin problems focuses on restoring internal balance, often using cleansing or cooling herbs rather than creams that may alleviate symptoms but do little to treat the cause of the problem. The same emphasis on rebalancing is found in Ayurvedic medicine: too much *pitta* (fire) causes the blood to overheat and poison the skin, too much *vata* (wind) causes dryness and itching, while excess *kapha* (damp) leads to weeping or oozing sores. Treatment is with cooling, moistening or drying herbs and an appropriate diet. The Chinese approach associates the skin with the lungs, *wei qi* (defence energy) and body fluids. Treatments based on this philosophy are being used for childhood eczema at a London hospital. Dry, flaking eczema, which is difficult to treat using modern Western medicine, has been helped by cooling Chinese herbs that increase body fluids. Trials at the hospital have produced impressive results. Fungal or parasitic skin conditions and hair problems can signify immune or energy weakness, and may be treated with tonic herbs and immunostimulants.

See also: candidiasis, pp. 156-7; warts and verrucas, pp. 160-1; vaginal thrush, pp. 168-9; nits, pp. 176-7.

AILMENT	REMEDIES	
	Herb	*Actions*
ECZEMA Skin inflammation, which may be associated with allergies, nervous stress or chemical or metal irritants. It can be highly localized if an irritant such as a metal watch strap is involved, but allergic eczema can affect all parts of the body. Creases of skin such as the folds inside the elbows or under the breasts are often affected. **KEY SYMPTOMS** • Red, inflamed patches • Itchiness • Oozing serum from raw patches • Crusts of serum forming • Lesions may bleed in acute conditions.	*Arctium lappa* **BURDOCK** (see p. 38)	Cleansing, diuretic and laxative; good for any toxic skin condition, especially scaling eczema.
	Fumaria officinalis **FUMITORY** (see p. 181)	Cleansing, diuretic and laxative; clears toxins that affect the skin from the blood.
	Oenothera biennis **EVENING PRIMROSE** (see p. 181) *(Seed oil)*	The seed oil contains essential fatty acids needed to maintain healthy tissues.
	Paeonia lactiflora **CHI SHAO YAO** (see p. 83)	Cools and stimulates blood flow; useful for "hot" conditions.
	Stellaria media **CHICKWEED** (see p. 100)	Soothing and slightly astringent; heals wounds, eases irritation and helps heal lesions.
	Urtica dioica **STINGING NETTLE** (see p. 108)	Astringent, tonic and circulatory stimulant; useful if eczema is associated with poor circulation.
	Viola tricolor **HEARTSEASE** (see p. 114)	Anti-inflammatory, diuretic and laxative; especially good for weeping eczema.
ACNE Inflammation of the sebaceous glands in the skin, which may start with blackheads. It is especially common among teenagers. **KEY SYMPTOMS** • Inflamed pustules • Excessively oily skin • Infected cysts and scarring in severe cases.	*Allium sativum* **GARLIC** (see p. 33) *(Bulb)*	Antibacterial and antifungal; good antiseptic action for infected skin conditions.
	Brassica oleracea **CABBAGE** (see p. 42)	Antibacterial and anti-inflammatory; nutritive and healing.
	Melaleuca alternifolia **TEA TREE** (see p. 182)	Potent antibacterial for infected skin conditions.

CASE HISTORY
Teenage acne

PATIENT: Edward, 17, a typical teenage schoolboy.

HISTORY AND COMPLAINT: Edward had acne with pustules around his nose and cheeks. The problem had started 18 months previously and he had also suffered from heavy catarrh and recurrent colds for the best part of a year. His diet was far from perfect, with an excess of chocolate, crisps and fizzy drinks. He admitted to a very sweet tooth, which his mother translated as at least two chocolate bars a day and as many biscuits as he could find when he got home from school.

TREATMENT: Edward did not relish the prospect of rubbing his face with garlic each evening or washing in cabbage water, so tea tree oil in rosewater was used as a lotion instead. Internal herbal remedies focused on clearing dampness and heat from the system, and improving immunity. Spots around the nose suggested excess lung heat, so *huang qin* and *sang bai pi* were included with *chi shao yao*, heartsease, yellow dock and purple coneflower. Edward also promised to try very hard to cut down on his consumption of chocolate.

OUTCOME: After six weeks, the acne was considerably reduced and the catarrh had disappeared. Then came exams. In between bouts of revision, Edward devoured chocolate bars, and before long the spots and catarrh were back. Fortunately, he realized his sweet tooth was a contributing factor, and after a further course of herbs he is managing to avoid excess chocolate.

How to use	*Combinations*	*Cautions*
Take a decoction or up to 4 ml tincture three times a day.	Can combine with other cleansing herbs such as yellow dock, figwort, cleavers, heartsease and red clover. Add flowers and leaves to the decoction for 1-2 minutes only.	
Take an infusion or up to 4 ml tincture three times a day.	Can combine with tinctures of other cleansing herbs such as burdock, yellow dock, figwort and cleavers.	
Take 3 g a day in capsule form (1-2 g a day for children).	Use as a simple.	
Best used in combinations; take a tincture or a decoction.	Combine with cooling, cleansing herbs like *sheng di huang*, heartsease, *mu dan pi*, *fang feng* and *mu tong* to enhance the effect.	
Apply ointment or cream as required; add 1 tbsp infused oil to bath water.	Use as a simple.	
Take an infusion or tincture, or use externally in cream or ointment.	Use as a simple or add other cleansing herbs like heartsease, red clover, figwort or cleavers to the infusion or tincture.	
Take an infusion or tincture, or use externally in ointment or cream.	Use as a simple externally. Can combine with cleavers, stinging nettle, red clover and fumitory as additional cleansing or tonic herbs.	Avoid high doses.
Rub the affected area with a cut clove.	Use as a simple. Add garlic to cooking. Limit the odour by eating parsley.	Because of the odour, apply at night.
Liquidize 250 g fresh leaves with 250 ml distilled witch hazel, strain, add 2 drops lemon oil and use as a lotion.	Use as a simple, but tinctures of cleavers, yellow dock and burdock can be taken as additional cleansers. Reduce sugar and acid foods in the diet.	
Add 1 ml tea tree oil to 10 ml water or equal quantities of rosewater and distilled witch hazel. Use as a lotion.	Use as a simple, but cleavers, yellow dock, burdock or purple coneflower can be taken internally as additional cleansing or anti-bacterial herbs.	

KEY

Aerial parts

Essential oil

Leaves

Root

STANDARD REMEDIES All recipes and doses are standard unless otherwise specified; see *Making Herbal Remedies*, pp. 120-5.

145

AILMENT	REMEDIES	
	Herb	*Actions*
PSORIASIS This is due to over-production of skin keratinocytes, which fail to mature into normal keratin. It can be associated with immune dysfunction, and may follow streptococcal infection or skin injury. It can be linked to a tense, isolated personality and an unwillingness to get close to other people, and may be aggravated by stress and worry. A tendency for psoriasis often runs in families. **KEY SYMPTOMS** • Patches of red skin, often with silver-coloured scales • Cycle of remission and recurrence.	*Galium aparine* **CLEAVERS** (see p. 62)	Cleansing, diuretic and astringent; useful for many types of skin problem.
	Rumex crispus **YELLOW DOCK** (see p. 182)	Cleansing, diuretic and laxative; stimulates bile flow and clears toxins.
	Scrophularia nodosa **FIGWORT** (see p. 97)	Anti-inflammatory, cleansing and circulatory stimulant; good for many chronic skin conditions.
	Solanum dulcamara **BITTERSWEET** (see p. 180)	Anti-inflammatory and liver tonic; useful where psoriasis is associated with rheumatic disorders.
	Trifolium pratense **RED CLOVER** (see p. 105)	Cleansing and diuretic; useful for many skin problems including eczema.
FUNGAL INFECTIONS Ringworm, athlete's foot and other skin infections are caused by fungi such as *microsporum*, *trichophyton* and *epidermophyton*. The toes and the scalp are the most commonly affected areas. **KEY SYMPTOMS** • Red, very irritant patches • Scaly or peeling skin.	*Aloe vera* **ALOE** (see p. 34) *(Gel)*	Demulcent, cooling for irritated skin, antiparasitic; useful for scabies.
	Calendula officinalis **POT MARIGOLD** (see p. 43)	Antifungal and astringent; heals wounds; soothing for dry or inflamed skin.
	Commiphora molmol **MYRRH** (see p. 50) *(Resin)*	Antifungal, immune stimulant, astringent.
HAIR LOSS (ALOPECIA) May be total or patchy; in men, often hereditary. Mild loss can be due to vitamin deficiency. **KEY SYMPTOM** • Bald patches or loose hairs.	*Arnica montana* **ARNICA** (see p. 180)	Stimulates blood circulation.
	Artemisia abrotanum **SOUTHERNWOOD** (see p. 182)	Traditional remedy to stimulate hair growth, although there is no scientific basis for its reputation.
PREMATURE GREYING Can be hereditary, or it may be linked to stress or premature menopause. **KEY SYMPTOM** • Hair starts to lose its colour in the 20s or 30s.	*Polygonum multiflorum* **HE SHOU WU** (see p. 181) *(Tuber)*	Kidney tonic used in China for premature menopause and early greying.
	Salvia officinalis **SAGE** (see p. 95)	Traditional remedy used to restore colour – possibly associated with its tonic and hormonal properties.
DANDRUFF Small flakes of dead skin on the scalp. It may be accompanied by seborrhoeic dermatitis and can be associated with yeast infection. **KEY SYMPTOMS** • Obvious scurf on collars • Hair dry and brittle, or greasy with yellow flakes.	*Quillaja saponaria* **SOAP BARK** (see p. 182)	Cleansing and anti-inflammatory; rich in saponins.
	Rosmarinus officinalis **ROSEMARY** (see p. 92)	Astringent, antiseptic and circulatory stimulant; also useful for psoriasis affecting the scalp.

How to use	*Combinations*	*Cautions*
Take 10 ml fresh juice or an infusion three times a day; also use externally as an ointment or cream.	Combines well with red clover to reduce over-production of cells, and with cleansing stimulants like stinging nettle or figwort. Use 3 parts cleavers to 1-2 parts other herbs.	
Take an infusion or tincture.	Combines well with burdock as a general cleanser. Add Oregon grape vine or figwort to help cleanse and cool the liver.	
Take an infusion or tincture.	Use with red clover or heartsease to help normalize skin growth, or with cleansing herbs like cleavers and yellow dock.	Heart stimulant, so avoid in heart-beat abnormalities (tachycardia).
Take a decoction of 15 g to 500 ml water in three wine-glass doses a day, or take up to 7.5 ml tincture a day.	Use as a simple or combine with cleansing herbs like yellow dock and figwort. Add nervines like skullcap if stress is a significant factor.	High doses can cause nausea and palpitations.
Take an infusion or tincture; also use externally in cream or ointment.	Can be combined with anti-inflammatory and cleansing herbs like cleavers, bittersweet, yellow dock or 10 drops *arbor vitae* tincture.	
Apply gel from a fresh leaf directly on to the affected area; ointment can also be used.	Use as a simple.	
Use as a cream or ointment, or use an infusion as a footbath or as a wash.	Add 5 ml tea tree oil to 500 ml infusion for a wash to enhance antifungal action.	
Add 10 drops oil or 10 ml tincture to 100 ml water and use as a wash; also take 1 ml tincture three times a day.	Use as a simple. Externally, add an equal amount of *arbor vitae*, or add the myrrh to pot marigold cream. Internally, take purple coneflower capsules.	Avoid taking internally in pregnancy.
Apply as a cream or ointment to affected areas, or use well-diluted tincture as a hair rinse.	Support with nervines (see pp. 162-5) and vitamin B supplements. Drink stinging nettle and burdock infusion as a cleansing stimulant.	Do not use on broken skin; do not take internally.
Take 10-20 drops tincture up to three times a day; use a standard infusion as a hair rinse.	Support with nervines and add stinging nettle, rosemary or sage to the infusion; take mineral and vitamin B supplements.	Avoid completely in pregnancy.
Take a decoction or tincture (up to 15 ml a day); patent mixtures are available.	Use as a simple or combine with tonics like *nu zhen zi*, *shu di huang* or buchu. Use 2 parts *he shou wu* and *shu di huang* to 1 part other herbs.	Avoid if also suffering from diarrhoea.
Take an infusion; use an infusion as a hair rinse.	Can add rosemary and stinging nettle to the infusion for the rinse to help darken the hair.	Avoid therapeutic doses in pregnancy or if epileptic.
Mix 500 ml decoction with 200 g soft soap and use as a shampoo.	Use as a simple.	For external use only. Do not take internally.
Use an infusion as a hair rinse; macerate 15 g herb in 250 ml ordinary shampoo for two weeks before using.	Add stinging nettle root to the rinse as a circulatory stimulant and cleansing tonic.	

Aerial parts

Essential oil

Flowers

Inner bark

Leaves

Petals

Root

Root bark

Stem

Twigs

Whole herb

STANDARD REMEDIES All recipes and doses are standard unless otherwise specified; see *Making Herbal Remedies*, pp. 120-5.

HEART, BLOOD & CIRCULATION

ANCIENT MEDICAL TRADITIONS regarded the heart as far more than just a pump to circulate the blood. In Ayurvedic medicine, it is the seat of the soul, while according to Chinese medicine, it stores *shen* (a sense of appropriateness and right behaviour). What modern Western medicine may regard as a mental or nervous disorder, Chinese medicine blames on disharmonies of *shen*, and may favour herbs such as *fu ling*, which clears "dampness" from the heart and is used as a sedative to "pacify" it. Western heart herbs boast a more orthodox set of actions. Ever since foxglove (*Digitalis purpurea*) was identified as a potent heart remedy in 1768, scientists have been investigating herbal solutions. Some are still important in modern medicine. Others are suitable for home use: hawthorn and linden tea, for example, are safe enough for use in pregnancy. Herbs can also help in controlling today's *bête noire*, cholesterol: many are very effective at lowering cholesterol and helping to prevent atherosclerosis.

See also: wounds and bleeding, pp. 126-7; haemorrhoids, pp. 154-5; varicose ulcers, pp. 160-1; varicose veins, pp. 160-1; heavy periods, pp. 168-9.

AILMENT	REMEDIES	
	Herb	*Actions*
HIGH BLOOD PRESSURE Also called hypertension, this should be regarded as a symptom of imbalance in the body, rather than as a single disease. It may be related to atherosclerosis, heart disorders and liver problems.	*Achillea millefolium* **YARROW** (see p. 30)	Relaxes the peripheral blood vessels and improves blood flow.
	Chrysanthemum morifolium **JU HUA** (see p. 181)	Dilates the coronary arteries and increases blood flow; also clears "liver heat", which can cause hypertension.
KEY SYMPTOMS • Headaches • Eye problems • Dizziness or fainting spells • Raised blood pressure reading on repeated examination • Diastolic reading (the lower of the two numbers in the reading) greater than 95-105 mm Hg.	*Crataegus spp.* **HAWTHORN** (see p. 51) *(Flowering tops)*	Improves coronary circulation, strengthens heart muscle; helps stabilize blood pressure as cardiac function improves.
	Stachys officinalis **WOOD BETONY** (see p. 99)	Circulatory tonic, relaxant and sedative; calms the heart.
IMPORTANT: Do not replace orthodox medicine with herbs without consulting your practitioner.	*Tilia europaea* **LINDEN** (see p. 181)	Relaxes and heals blood vessels; helps prevent arteriosclerosis.
	Viburnum opulus **GUELDER ROSE** (see p. 113)	Smooth muscle relaxant for the vascular system; lowers diastolic blood pressure.
LOW BLOOD PRESSURE Also called hypotension, this is often not considered serious by some doctors, but it is regarded as significant by many others.	*Convallaria majalis* **LILY-OF-THE-VALLEY** (see p. 181)	Stimulates heart contractions and improves efficiency; useful for weak, failing and elderly hearts.
KEY SYMPTOMS • General tiredness • Weak constitution • Dizziness and/or fainting spells • Palpitations and cardiac arrhythmias.	*Cytisus scoparius* **BROOM** (see p. 180) *(Flowering tops)*	Regulates heartbeat, steadying the arrhythmias that can be associated with low blood pressure and heart failure.
IMPORTANT: If the systolic reading (the higher of the two numbers) is consistently below 110 mm Hg, seek professional help.	*Leonurus cardiaca* **MOTHERWORT** (see p. 74)	Relaxing for palpitations and arrhythmias; but also has stimulating action on the heart.
	Rosmarinus officinalis **ROSEMARY** (see p. 92)	General tonic for nervous and circulatory systems; good for people who tire quickly and for the elderly and debilitated.

CASE HISTORY
Raised blood pressure with menopausal symptoms

PATIENT: Sarah, 52, divorced, with a daughter at college to support. She divided her time between caring for elderly parents and work as a musician.

HISTORY AND COMPLAINT: Sarah had been diagnosed as having slightly raised blood pressure 10 years previously. She was prescribed beta-blockers, but disliked taking drugs, and soon abandoned the tablets for various patent herbal and homeopathic remedies. Eight years later, another check revealed glaucoma and blood pressure of 180/110 mm Hg. She also had menopausal symptoms, lower back pains, dizziness, and a tendency for tinnitus, palpitations and hot flushes whenever she felt emotionally upset or did anything energetic. Her doctor urged a return to beta-blockers.

TREATMENT: Herbs to boost kidney energy and nourish the liver, rather than drugs to slow down her heart, were used. These included *shu di huang, shan zhu yu, mu dan pi* and *he shou wu*. She was also given a herbal tea containing *ju hua*, hawthorn and motherwort.

OUTCOME: Within a month, Sarah's hot flushes had vanished, she had fewer palpitations and more energy with none of the dizzy feelings. Her blood pressure was down to 155/95 mm Hg. The herbs were continued for three months, by which time her blood pressure had stabilized at 140/85 mm Hg, so she continued with only the herbal tea. Six months later at a routine check, her blood pressure was still the same and her glaucoma had improved.

How to use	Combinations	Cautions
Add 15 g herb to 500 ml water for an infusion; take up to 2.5 ml tincture 3 times a day.	Can combine with linden if arteriosclerosis is a problem, or with cardiac tonics like hawthorn.	Avoid large doses in pregnancy.
Take an infusion or tincture.	Can combine with liver herbs like *gou qi zi*, diuretics such as *fu ling* or dandelion leaf, or with sedatives, depending on the cause of hypertension.	
Take an infusion or tincture.	Can combine with linden and yarrow, or with herbs such as guelder rose to relax blood vessels.	
Take an infusion or tincture.	Can combine with linden or *fu ling*, especially if stress is contributing to the condition; use 2 parts wood betony to 1 part other herbs.	Avoid large doses in pregnancy.
Take an infusion or up to 10 ml tincture a day.	Combine with hawthorn as a cardiac tonic, or maidenhair tree if arteriosclerosis is significant.	
Take a decoction or tincture.	Combine with heart tonics such as hawthorn, or sedatives like valerian if tension is significant.	
In UK, Australia and New Zealand use is restricted to qualified practitioners. Maximum safe dose in UK is up to 1 ml tincture 3 times a day.	Should be prescribed with a diuretic such as dandelion leaf, or with tonic herbs like hawthorn or maidenhair tree, depending on the cause of the condition.	Take only as prescribed; high doses cause severe vomiting.
Take an infusion made with 15 g herb to 500 ml water, or take up to 5 ml tincture a day.	Use with tonics such as hawthorn (or lily-of-the-valley, if prescribed by a qualified practitioner), depending on the severity of the symptoms.	Avoid in pregnancy. Do not use if new to herbs; see p. 180.
Take an infusion or tincture.	Combine with rosemary and *fu ling* for both tonic and calming actions.	Avoid in pregnancy.
Take an infusion or up to 10 ml tincture a day; massage diluted oil into the chest over the heart.	Can be combined with tonics such as wood betony and motherwort.	

KEY

Aerial parts

Bark

Berries

Flowers

Leaves

STANDARD REMEDIES All recipes and doses are standard unless otherwise specified; see *Making Herbal Remedies*, pp. 120-5.

AILMENT	REMEDIES	
	Herb	*Actions*
POOR CIRCULATION This may be a sign of a more serious heart disorder, but it is often simply an inherited tendency and does not constitute a major problem. **KEY SYMPTOMS** • Exceptionally cold hands and feet • Tendency for chilblains • White or "dead" fingers (Raynaud's phenomenon).	*Capsicum frutescens* **CAYENNE** (see p. 46)	Heating, promotes sweating; a strong circulatory stimulant.
	Cinnamomum cassia **GUI ZHI** (see p. 48)	Warming, promotes sweating; encourages both blood and *qi* (energy) circulation.
	Zanthoxylum americanum **PRICKLY ASH** (see p. 182)	Circulatory stimulant, promotes sweating; warming for all "cold" conditions.
	Zingiber officinalis **GINGER** (see p. 115)	Strong circulatory stimulant, relaxes blood vessels, promotes sweating; very warming.
HARDENING ARTERIES Associated with fatty deposits accumulated in blood vessels, maybe as a protective mechanism to counter damage from smoking or other pollutants. It raises the risk of strokes. **KEY SYMPTOMS** • High blood pressure • Palpable blood vessels may feel hard and pipe-like • Eye disorders • Sudden, severe pain in the legs while walking (claudication).	*Ginkgo biloba* **MAIDENHAIR TREE** (see p. 64)	Relaxes blood vessels and improves blood flow in cerebral arteriosclerosis; eases intermittent claudication.
	Vinca major **GREATER PERIWINKLE** (see p. 181)	Contains vincamine, which improves blood flow in cerebral arteriosclerosis and can be helpful after a stroke; tonic for the cerebral arterioles.
	Viscum album **MISTLETOE** (see p. 181)	Strengthens capillary walls, reduces inflammation and encourages repair; cardiac depressant, slows heart rate.
ANAEMIA (iron-deficient type) Low haemoglobin levels, which can be due to a poor diet, heavy periods or digestive disorders. **KEY SYMPTOMS** • Breathlessness and/or palpitations • Very pale nails or inner eyelids • Rheumatic-type pains.	*Angelica sinensis* **DANG GUI** (see p. 36)	Nourishes the blood and invigorates the circulation; contains vitamin B_{12} and folic acid, so can help prevent pernicious anaemia.
	Urtica dioica **STINGING NETTLE** (see p. 108)	Rich in iron and other minerals and vitamins; highly nutritious.
HIGH CHOLESTEROL High levels of lipids (such as cholesterol) in the blood can lead to atherosclerosis and increase the risk of heart attack. They are associated with too much saturated fat in the diet, but may be hereditary. Cholesterol is needed for many body mechanisms, and is not intrinsically harmful. **KEY SYMPTOM** • Blood tests revealing high lipid levels.	*Allium sativum* **GARLIC** (see p. 33) *(Bulb)*	Reduces blood cholesterol levels; has been shown to reduce the risk of heart attacks and atherosclerosis.
	Avena sativa **OATS** (see p. 40)	Effectively reduces blood cholesterol levels, particularly low-density lipoproteins.
	Camellia sinensis **OOLONG TEA** (see p. 44)	Contains phenols, which inhibit cholesterol absorption; circulatory stimulant and tonic for blood vessels, helps to prevent atherosclerosis.
CAPILLARY FRAGILITY Weakness in blood vessel walls. **KEY SYMPTOMS** • Tendency to bruise easily • Retinal haemorrhages.	*Fagopyrum esculentum* **BUCKWHEAT** (see p. 180)	Rich in rutin (tonifies and repairs arteriole walls); specific for retinal haemorrhage.
	Viola tricolor **HEARTSEASE** (see p. 114)	Contains flavonoids, which strengthen capillary walls.

How to use	*Combinations*	*Cautions*
Add 30-50 mg herb to 500 ml water for an infusion; take up to 1 ml 1:20 tincture a dose; massage with infused oil.	Take with other warming stimulant herbs, such as a decoction of angelica root, or add 1-2 g bayberry to the infusion.	Do not exceed the stated dose; avoid large doses in pregnancy.
Take a decoction or tincture.	Combines well with a little ginger, or add maidenhair tree or rosemary.	Avoid therapeutic doses in pregnancy.
Take a decoction of 15 g herb to 600 ml water; take up to 5 ml tincture a day.	Can combine with angelica root or rosemary, or add a pinch of cinnamon powder to the decoction.	
Add up to 10 g fresh root to 600 ml water for decoctions and footbaths; take up to 10 drops 1:5 tincture per dose.	Combine with circulatory tonics such as maidenhair tree, or warming herbs like rosemary or *gui zhi*.	
Take an infusion or tincture.	Combine with wood betony as a tonic, or add linden and hawthorn for circulatory problems.	
Take an infusion or tincture.	Combine tincture with recommended mistletoe dose (below), or use linden and wood betony in infusion.	
Take 10-20 drops tincture three times a day.	Combine with greater periwinkle or maidenhair tree tinctures up to a 5 ml dose. Drink with buckwheat or linden infusion to help repair arteriole walls.	Do not use the berries, as they are toxic; avoid in pregnancy.
Take a decoction or tincture. Many proprietary preparations are available.	Can combine with *shu di huang* and *he shou wu*. Eat plenty of iron-rich foods like liver, watercress and apricots.	Avoid regular or large doses in pregnancy.
Take 10 ml juice three times a day, or take an infusion of fresh herb.	Use as a simple, but add iron-rich foods like parsley, watercress and apricots to the diet.	
Take 1 clove daily; take 2 g powdered garlic in capsules a day if there is a high risk of heart attack.	Use as a simple, but also limit the intake of saturated fats and high cholesterol foods.	Avoid therapeutic doses during pregnancy.
Add 25 g oatbran to breakfast cereal or porridge.	Use as a simple, but also limit the intake of saturated fats and high cholesterol foods.	If sensitive to gluten, see caution p. 40.
Add 1 to 2 tsp per cup of boiling water for an infusion.	Use as a simple. *Pu erh* is the most effective variety of oolong for reducing cholesterol.	Limit to 2 cups a day in hypertension and pregnancy.
Take an infusion or tincture.	Use with 10 ml horsetail juice per dose, or take rutin tablets daily.	
Take an infusion or tincture.	Can be combined with 10 ml horsetail juice per dose, or use yarrow or ribwort plantain.	

KEY

Aerial parts

Bark

Fruit

Grain

Leaves

Root

Twigs

STANDARD REMEDIES
All recipes and doses are standard unless otherwise specified; see *Making Herbal Remedies*, pp. 120-5.

DIGESTIVE PROBLEMS

GOOD DIGESTION is central to good health: dysfunction here not only starves the body of nutrients, but also leads to a build-up of toxins. Ayurvedic theory argues that these products are the source of the three humours, *pitta*, *vata* and *kapha*, which, if out of balance, can account for most diseases. In Chinese medicine, the digestive organs are associated with many other organs and bodily processes, including the blood supply, energy circulation, mental activity and muscles, and imbalances here can be linked with a wide range of physical and

emotional symptoms. In the West, too, herbal medicine has long focused on digestive function. Herbs can provide an impressive array of tonics, stimulants, carminatives and relaxants to ensure healthy function. Good digestion depends, also, on the nervous system to stimulate acid or enzyme production and gut motions, and many digestive herbs act on the nervous system and can help stress-related problems like colitis.

IMPORTANT: Seek professional advice for any change in bowel patterns that occurs suddenly or persists.

See also: mouth ulcers, pp. 142-3; threadworms, pp. 176-7.

AILMENT	REMEDIES	
	Herb	*Actions*
CONSTIPATION Generally a symptom of other health problems, this may be associated with poor diet, sluggish digestion or muscle tone, or may be due to nervous tension inhibiting bowel action. **KEY SYMPTOMS** • Lack of bowel motions for more than 24 hours • Low abdominal pain or griping • Difficulty passing stools.	*Plantago psyllium/P. ovata* **PSYLLIUM/ISPHAGULA** (see p. 86)	Mucilaginous and bulking laxatives, which lubricate the bowel; useful if stools are dry.
	Rheum palmatum **RHUBARB** (see p. 89)	Contains anthraquinones, which irritate the digestive tract, increasing gut movements.
	Viburnum opulus **GUELDER ROSE** (see p. 113)	Smooth muscle relaxant; useful if constipation is linked to visceral tension.
DIARRHOEA This is often a symptom of other imbalances in the digestive system, but can also be caused by food poisoning or bacterial infection. Suspect food may be apparent in cases of food poisoning. Bacterial infection can easily be caught by other household members. **KEY SYMPTOMS** • Loose, frequent stools • Abdominal cramps or griping pains.	*Agrimonia eupatoria* **AGRIMONY** (see p. 31)	Astringent and healing for any intestinal tract inflammation; especially suitable for children.
	Geranium maculatum **AMERICAN CRANESBILL** (see p. 180)	Astringent; gentle enough for children, the elderly and the debilitated.
	Potentilla erecta **TORMENTIL** (see p. 182)	Contains up to 20% tannins, making it very astringent and reducing the inflammation associated with diarrhoea.
GASTRITIS & **ULCERATION** Gastritis is inflammation of the stomach lining; if persistent, it can lead to ulceration. It may be due to dietary factors. **KEY SYMPTOMS** • Heartburn and acid reflux • Persistent vomiting in acute gastritis • Abdominal pain in ulcerated conditions.	*Filipendula ulmaria* **MEADOWSWEET** (see p. 58)	Anti-inflammatory; reduces stomach acid secretions and is soothing and healing for the stomach lining.
	Glycyrrhiza glabra **LIQUORICE** (see p. 65)	Anti-inflammatory; produces a viscous mucus, which coats and protects the stomach wall and limits acid production.
	Ulmus fulva **SLIPPERY ELM** (see p. 182)	Demulcent; soothes irritated mucous membranes; nutritive for debilitated conditions.

CASE HISTORY
Irritable bowel syndrome

PATIENT: Louise, a secretary aged 24; an only child still living with her parents, with an active social life.

HISTORY AND COMPLAINT: Louise had suffered from irritable bowel syndrome for three years, following a bout of food poisoning. Her main symptoms included diarrhoea (up to five times a day) and vomiting copious phlegm after each meal. A battery of hospital tests had all proved negative, and Louise had been variously prescribed antidepressants, antibiotics, tranquillizers and bulking laxatives. Her diet was far from ideal, with too much cake and milk. She sucked fruit sweets constantly to suppress nausea.

TREATMENT: A priority was to improve Louise's diet. She had recently cut out chocolate, and agreed to limit dairy products and carbohydrates, which were producing so much mucus that her system was flooded with phlegm. Soya milk and whole grain products were recommended instead. Herbs to help regulate body fluids, tonify the stomach and astringe the system were prescribed, including *ban xia*, *bai zhu*, cinnamon and agrimony. She was given *Lactobacillus acidophilus* bacteria in capsules to restore the natural gut flora. Capsules of dried ginger relieved nausea.

OUTCOME: After reducing sweet foods and milky drinks, Louise began to improve, but it took around three months before she could eat without immediately vomiting. Her stools became firmer, with motions twice a day. After six months, the herbs were phased out and dietary "lapses" are now tolerated.

How to use	*Combinations*	*Cautions*
Infuse 1 tsp seeds in a cup of boiling water, let it cool, and drink with the seeds, once or twice a day or at night.	Use either as a simple or mix one part linseed to two parts psyllium or isphagula seeds.	
Add 10-15 g herb to 600 ml water for a decoction; take 2 ml tincture up to three times a day.	Add 1-2 ml fennel, lemon balm or chamomile tincture per dose to prevent griping. Enhance with mild laxatives such as butternut or yellow dock.	Avoid in pregnancy, arthritic conditions and gout.
Take a decoction or tincture.	Add laxatives like butternut or liquorice, or additional relaxants like chamomile, depending on symptoms.	
Take an infusion or tincture.	Add soothing herbs like chamomile, ribwort plantain or marshmallow to ease gut inflammation; add bilberry or burnet to enhance astringency.	
Take an infusion or 2-3 ml tincture (made from leaves) three times a day; or take a decoction made with 20 g root to 600 ml water.	Add soothing herbs like marshmallow root, meadowsweet or ribwort plantain to ease gut inflammation; add bilberry or burnet to enhance astringency.	
Add 20 g herb to 600 ml water for a decoction; take 2-3 ml tincture up to three times a day.	Add soothing herbs like ribwort plantain or marshmallow root to ease gut inflammation.	
Take an infusion; or use a tincture or fluid extract in very hot water allowed to cool.	Increase astringency with 10 drops bistort or American cranesbill tincture or soothe with 10 drops liquorice per dose. Can also add extra anti-inflammatories, such as pot marigold.	Avoid the herb in cases of salicylate sensitivity.
Take a decoction or suck juice sticks; use a tincture or fluid extract in very hot water allowed to cool.	In severe cases can add extra soothing and healing herbs, such as 10-20 drops marshmallow or slippery elm, or add anti-inflammatories like pot marigold or meadowsweet.	Avoid in high blood pressure or if taking digoxin-based drugs.
Take up to 5 g powdered bark in capsules or mixed with water, before meals.	Combine with powdered marshmallow root in capsules if desired.	

KEY

Aerial parts

Bark

Leaves

Root

Seeds

STANDARD REMEDIES All recipes and doses are standard unless otherwise specified; see *Making Herbal Remedies*, pp.120-5.

AILMENT	REMEDIES	
	Herb	*Actions*
INFLAMED GALL BLADDER Associated with gall-stones; often caused by excess dietary fats. **KEY SYMPTOMS** • Severe colicky pain • Jaundice • Floating stools.	*Berberis vulgaris* **BARBERRY** (see p. 180)	Stimulates bile flow and eases liver congestion; bitter and laxative.
	Chionanthus virginicus **FRINGE TREE** (see p. 181)	Stimulates bile flow and liver function; laxative and cleansing.
HAEMORRHOIDS (PILES) Anal varicose veins associated with poor muscle tone and often due to straining or constipation. **KEY SYMPTOMS** • Palpable piles at anus • Bleeding on passing stools.	*Ranunculus ficaria* (see p. 182) **PILEWORT**	Astringent; tonifies blood vessels and stops bleeding.
	Sophora japonica **HUAI JIAO** (see p. 181)	Cooling, anti-inflammatory and lowers blood pressure; clears "liver heat", cools blood, stops bleeding; helps constipation.
INDIGESTION & ACIDITY Usually due to eating too much, too quickly, missing meals or to anxiety. Antacids encourage further stomach acid secretion and can worsen the condition. **KEY SYMPTOMS** • Bloating and feelings of abdominal fullness • Heartburn or acid reflux • Stomach pain.	*Foeniculum officinale* **FENNEL** (see p. 59)	Carminative and anti-inflammatory; effective for griping pains.
	Melissa officinalis **LEMON BALM** (see p. 78)	Carminative and relaxing; sedative action is useful for nervous stomach.
	Mentha piperita **PEPPERMINT** (see p. 79)	Cooling carminative; stimulates bile flow; good for nausea and nervous stomachs.
IRRITABLE BOWEL SYNDROME & COLITIS Various symptoms linked to food intolerance, anxiety or infection. **KEY SYMPTOMS** • Alternating bouts of diarrhoea and constipation • "Rabbit dropping" stools • Bloating and flatulence • Mucus in stools.	*Chamaemelum nobile* **ROMAN CHAMOMILE** (see p. 47)	Sedative, anti-inflammatory and carminative; good for nervous dyspepsia.
	Dioscorea villosa **MEXICAN WILD YAM** (see p. 52) *(Rhizome)*	Visceral relaxant, anti-spasmodic; anti-inflammatory and bile stimulant.
	Iberis amara **BITTER CANDYTUFT** (see p. 180)	Antispasmodic, relaxant, tonifies the digestive tract; carminative.
LIVER DISORDERS In our polluted society, liver congestion is very common. It can manifest itself as a pathological disorder, but often simply involves feelings of anger and stagnation. **KEY SYMPTOMS** • Tendency for constipation • Abdominal bloating • Emotional lability • Menstrual disorders • Red, itching palms • Small red abdominal spots • Sore, itching eyes.	*Bupleurum chinense* **CHAI HU** (see p. 180)	Bitter liver tonic; encourages energy flow.
	Carduus marianus **MILK THISTLE** (see p. 181)	Encourages liver cell renewal and repair in degenerative conditions, e.g. alcoholism.
	Gentiana lutea **GENTIAN** (see p. 63)	Bitter, tonic, general digestive and liver stimulant; can help anorexia nervosa.
	Taraxacum officinale **DANDELION** (see p. 103)	Restorative tonic for liver function; promotes bile flow; laxative.
NAUSEA & VOMITING Can be due to food poisoning, infections, fever or migraines. *IMPORTANT: Projectile or prolonged vomiting requires professional medical help.*	*Syzygium aromaticum* **CLOVES** (see p. 180) *(Flower buds)*	Stimulant and carminative; locally antiseptic.
	Zingiber officinalis **GINGER** (see p. 115)	Prevents vomiting; very effective for travel sickness as well as digestive upsets.

How to use	*Combinations*	*Cautions*
Add 15 g herb to 600 ml water for a decoction; or take up to 8 ml tincture a day.	Combine with anti-inflammatories such as goldenseal (5 drops tincture per dose) and liver tonics like vervain or globe artichoke.	Avoid in pregnancy.
Take a decoction in 1 tbsp doses; or take up to 5 ml tincture a day.	Combine with bitters, liver tonics or stimulants such as dandelion, milk thistle, chicory, globe artichoke or centaury, plus anti-inflammatories such as pot marigold.	
Apply ointment frequently.	Use as a simple, but take supportive liver herbs or venous tonics like king's clover.	Do not take internally.
Take a decoction or tincture; take 400 mg powder in capsules three times a day.	Use as a simple or combine with liver tonics and digestive remedies such as dandelion root, barberry, *fang feng, dang gui, zhi ke* and burnet.	Avoid in pregnancy.
Take an infusion or tincture; useful as an after-dinner tisane.	Use as a simple or add American cranesbill to reduce acidity, or peppermint, meadowsweet or chamomile to enhance carminative action.	Avoid high doses in pregnancy.
Take an infusion or tincture.	Add chamomile or meadowsweet as anti-inflammatories, or a little hops as a bitter and antispasmodic.	
Add 15 g dried herb to 500 ml water for an infusion; take up to 2.5 ml tincture per dose.	Use as a simple or add American cranesbill to help reduce acid secretions, or marshmallow root, meadowsweet and liquorice to soothe inflammation.	May reduce milk flow; use with caution if breastfeeding.
Take an infusion or tincture.	Add a few drops of peppermint or fresh ginger tincture to relieve abdominal bloating and regulate bowel activity.	Avoid excessive internal intake in pregnancy.
Add 1 tsp herb to 500 ml water for an infusion; or take as a tincture in combinations.	Add meadowsweet to soothe stomach lining; chamomile for anxiety; or a few drops fresh ginger tincture to regulate bowel activity.	Avoid in pregnancy.
Take up to 2 ml tincture per dose or an infusion made from 15 g to 500 ml water.	Add angelica root and milk thistle seed as liver tonics; or lemon balm or chamomile as relaxants.	High doses may cause nausea.
Add 10 g herb to 600 ml water for a decoction.	Combine with *bai shao yao, chuan xiong,* goldenseal and dandelion to help regulate liver function.	
Take an infusion; or take up to 10 ml tincture a day in hot water allowed to cool.	Use as a simple or add vervain, dandelion root or globe artichoke and 5 drops goldenseal as additional liver tonics.	
Add 15 g root to 600 ml water for a decoction; use 2-5 drops tincture on the tongue per dose.	Add tinctures of dandelion root, vervain, holy thistle or barberry as additional liver tonics and stimulants, up to a combined total dose of 5 ml tincture.	
Take a decoction or use a tincture or fluid extract in hot water allowed to cool.	Use as a simple or combine with vervain, barberry, wahoo or fringe tree, or add 5 drops goldenseal to improve liver function.	
Take an infusion; or take 1-2 drops essential oil on a sugar lump; add powder to food.	Use as a simple.	Do not exceed the stated dose of essential oil.
Take a tincture in drop doses while symptoms persist, or chew crystallized ginger.	Use as a simple or combine with black horehound or chamomile tincture.	Use with care in early pregnancy (see pp. 170-1).

KEY

Aerial parts

Bark

Essential oil

Flowers

Fruit

Leaves

Root

Root bark

Seeds

STANDARD REMEDIES
All recipes and doses are standard unless otherwise specified; see *Making Herbal Remedies*, pp. 120-5.

ALLERGIC CONDITIONS

A HEALTHY SYSTEM copes with allergens, but if there is tension, infection or fatigue, the arrival of an allergen tips the balance and an allergic response occurs in the form of hay fever, skin rashes or gastric upsets. Food allergies often start in babyhood, when the immature gut has to cope with unknown proteins, such as cow's milk. The immune system is triggered to repel the invader, producing inflammation, mucus and irritation. If the allergen continues to be taken, the response becomes muted with no tell-tale symptoms, merely a general weakening of the immune system. This masked allergy can manifest itself as vague arthritic pains, irritable bowel syndrome or persistent sinusitis. Herbal remedies can strengthen the respiratory and immune systems, so that the allergen does not cause the characteristic response.

See also: asthma, pp. 138-9; eczema, pp. 144-5; vaginal thrush, pp. 168-9.

AILMENT	REMEDIES	
	Herb	*Actions*
HAY FEVER & ALLERGIC RHINITIS Generally triggered by grass or tree pollens, hay fever occurs when these are prevalent. Allergies to animal fur or house dust occur throughout the year. **KEY SYMPTOMS** • Copious nasal catarrh, sneezing • Sore, irritated eyes • Asthma-like symptoms in severe cases.	*Euphrasia officinalis* **EYEBRIGHT** (see p. 181)	Decreases nasal secretions and soothes mucous membranes and conjunctiva.
	Glechoma hederacea **GROUND IVY** (see p. 181)	Astringent and anticatarrhal; good for drying secretions and inflammations.
	Plantago lanceolata **RIBWORT PLANTAIN** (see p. 86)	Good for allergic rhinitis, toning mucous membranes and healing inflammations.
FOOD INTOLERANCE Common food allergens include cow's milk, wheat and beef, and can cause a wide range of symptoms. Candidiasis can be related to food intolerance. Allergy to salicylates (aspirin) is common. Gluten intolerance can cause severe health problems. **KEY SYMPTOMS** • Digestive upsets • Stiffness and joint pain • Skin rashes and eczema • Respiratory problems • Persistent urinary infections, or vaginal thrush in candidiasis • Nervous disorders.	*Agrimonia eupatoria* **AGRIMONY** (see p. 31)	Soothes gut irritation and inflammation; heals damaged mucous membranes.
	Allium sativum **GARLIC** (see p. 33) *(Bulb)*	Antifungal; useful for excess yeasts in the gut; supports recovery of gut flora.
	Calendula officinalis **POT MARIGOLD** (see p. 43)	Antifungal; useful for excess yeasts in the gut in candidiasis.
	Hydrastis canadensis **GOLDENSEAL** (see p. 67) *(Rhizome)*	Good liver stimulant; eases gastric sensitivity; astringent and healing for mucous membranes.
HIVES (URTICARIA) Skin blisters and rashes caused by allergens, including foods, particularly those containing salicylates, or by contact with chemicals. The reaction is generally transient, but can be severe and persistent. **KEY SYMPTOM** • Irritant, red swellings on the skin.	*Brassica oleracea* **CABBAGE** (see p. 42)	Anti-inflammatory and healing; useful standby for emergencies.
	Ephedra sinica **MA HUANG** (see p. 54)	Reduces allergic response in a wide range of conditions.
	Viola tricolor **HEARTSEASE** (see p. 114)	Anti-inflammatory and soothing for any skin inflammation.

CASE HISTORY
Hay fever

PATIENT: Jonathan, aged 10, was generally healthy.

HISTORY AND COMPLAINT: Jonathan had suffered from hay fever every year since he was seven. He started sneezing in early spring and continued, with increasing severity, through summer. Antihistamines were proving less and less effective, and it was when the doctor suggested trying steroids that Jonathan's worried mother turned to alternative medicine.

TREATMENT: Jonathan started treatment in the New Year with 5 ml a day of a brew containing elderflower,

white horehound and ground ivy for the upper respiratory tract, with self-heal, dandelion and gentian to cool and cleanse the liver. This medication was continued until early spring. In the first year, symptoms were kept in check with eyebright and goldenseal capsules, supplemented by antihistamines in early summer when the oilseed rape crop peaked.

OUTCOME: In the first year, symptoms did not start until early summer. The next year, a similar regime reduced symptoms still further. Three years after starting treatment, the hay fever disappeared.

How to use	*Combinations*	*Cautions*
Take an infusion or tincture; or take two 200 mg capsules three times a day; bathe eyes with an eyewash containing water and 5 drops tincture.	Combine with goldenseal powder in capsules or with elderflower in an infusion or tincture. Often prescribed with *ma huang* (restricted herb in UK, Australia and New Zealand).	
Take an infusion or tincture.	Combine with anticatarrhals such as marsh cudweed, ribwort plantain and golden rod in tincture; take with chamomile in an infusion.	
Take an infusion or up to 4 ml tincture three times a day.	Add astringent anticatarrhals such as marsh cudweed or ground ivy. Take with chamomile in an infusion as an anti-allergenic.	
Take an infusion or up to 4 ml tincture three times a day.	Add lemon balm and chamomile to reduce stress. Combine with soothing anti-inflammatories such as marshmallow root.	
Use 1 clove a day in cooking or take two 200 mg capsules a day.	Best used as a simple, or with parsley to reduce the garlic odour.	
Take an infusion or tincture, well diluted in water.	Add antimicrobials such as purple cone-flower, nervines such as lemon balm or anti-inflammatories like elderflower or agrimony.	
Take two 200 mg capsules up to three times a day, or 2-4 ml doses of tincture up to three times a day.	Add powdered fenugreek or agrimony to capsules or liquorice to tincture, to soothe and heal mucous membranes.	Avoid in pregnancy or high blood pressure; do not exceed the stated dose.
Apply a fresh leaf directly on to the affected part, or apply juice as a lotion.	Use as a simple. Onion can be used in the same way.	
In UK, Australia and New Zealand use is restricted to professional practitioners. Maximum legal dose of herb in UK is 600 mg in a decoction or 2.5 ml of a 1:4 tincture, three times a day.	Chamomile, stinging nettle or heartsease may be added in the final minutes of decocting to help reduce the allergic response and inflammation.	Take only as prescribed. Avoid in glaucoma, very high blood pressure, or if taking MAO inhibitors (see p. 54).
Take an infusion, or up to 15 ml tincture a day; also use as a wash or in an ointment or cream.	Add 1-2 drops thyme oil to 20 ml heartsease cream, or add stinging nettle to an infusion or tincture as an additional astringent.	

KEY

Aerial parts

Leaves

Petals

Root

Twigs

STANDARD REMEDIES
All recipes and doses are standard unless otherwise specified; see *Making Herbal Remedies*, pp. 120-5.

URINARY DISORDERS

THE KIDNEYS AND URINARY system often mirror the health of an individual – persistent cystitis sufferers know well that their symptoms increase at times of stress and fatigue. Just as recurrent colds can indicate a weak immune system, so can repeated urinary infections. Tonic herbs and immune stimulant herbs are often needed after symptoms have eased. Herbal remedies generally include some sort of urinary antiseptic, which often contains volatile oils that survive the digestive process, pass into the bloodstream and are excreted via the kidneys. Soothing and softening herbs are added to help reduce inflammation and repair damage to the mucous membranes, and diuretics to increase the flow of urine and flush out toxins and dead bacteria. In Chinese medicine, urinary inflammations are regarded as problems of heat and damp rather than infections due to bacteria, and are treated with "cooling" herbs.

See also: vaginal thrush, pp. 168-9; incontinence, pp. 172-3; bedwetting, pp. 176-7.

AILMENT	REMEDIES	
	Herb	*Actions*
URINARY TRACT INFECTIONS & CYSTITIS Infections of the urinary tract usually lead to cystitis in women and urethritis in men. In some cases, the kidneys are affected. **KEY SYMPTOMS** • Frequent, painful urination • Blood, mucus or pus in urine • Fever • Pain anywhere from the groin to the mid-back. *IMPORTANT: Consult a professional practitioner if the symptoms are severe or persistent. If the infection is sexually transmitted, the case must under UK law be referred to a doctor.*	*Apium graveolens* **CELERY** (see p. 37)	Urinary antiseptic; cleanses uric acid from the system.
	Arctostaphylos uva-ursi **BEARBERRY** (see p. 180)	Produces potent antiseptic in the kidney tubules; also antiseptic and very effective for acid urine.
	Barosma betulina **BUCHU** (see p. 180)	Diuretic and urinary antiseptic; has a warming and stimulant effect on the kidneys.
	Elymus repens **COUCHGRASS** (see p. 180) *(Rhizome)*	Contains mannitol (a diuretic) and mucilages to soothe the mucous membranes; mildly antibiotic.
URINARY STONES Deposits of insoluble material – usually calcium salts – which can be associated with changes in the acidity or alkalinity of the urine. **KEY SYMPTOMS** • Sensation of "grittiness" on passing urine • Blood in urine in severe cases • Pain, which may be severe, between "loin and groin". *IMPORTANT: Consult a practitioner in severe cases.*	*Eupatorium purpureum* **GRAVELROOT** (see p. 57)	Diuretic and soothing for the urinary mucous membranes; useful for all irritations and inflammations.
	Juniperus communis **JUNIPER** (see p. 72)	Urinary antiseptic and diuretic; good for clearing acid wastes.
	Parietaria diffusa **PELLITORY-OF-THE-WALL** (see p. 182)	Diuretic and demulcent; useful for pain on urination; also for kidney stones.
PROSTATE PROBLEMS Prostatitis is associated with infection of the prostate gland; enlargement is common in older men. **KEY SYMPTOMS** • Difficulty urinating, dribbling • Urine retention in severe cases. *IMPORTANT: Any enlargement of the prostate gland requires a professional evaluation.*	*Lamium album* **WHITE DEADNETTLE** (see p. 182)	Astringent and soothing with a specific action on the reproductive system, reducing benign prostate enlargement and acting as a uterine tonic; useful after prostate surgery.
	Serenoa serrulata **SAW PALMETTO** (see p. 182)	Diuretic; urinary antiseptic with specific hormonal action on the male reproductive system, reducing benign prostate enlargement.

CASE HISTORY
Recurrent cystitis and thrush

PATIENT: Pamela, a 48-year-old sales representative, married, with a grown-up son and a daughter of 10.

HISTORY AND COMPLAINT: Pamela had had recurrent cystitis for 15 years, which was treated with regular antibiotics. Symptoms included burning on passing urine and increased frequency of urination. She was prone to thrush and tended to eat too much chocolate and yeast extract. Two weeks of antibiotics had had little effect on the latest flare-up of cystitis.

TREATMENT: Strictly curtailing sugar and yeast intake helped in long-term control of thrush, while medication

focused on the immediate symptoms with buchu, bearberry, purple coneflower, cornsilk and couchgrass. Capsules of buchu and couchgrass powder were supplied for use during the day. Tea tree pessaries were used for thrush, and *Lactobacillus acidophilus* capsules to restore the gut flora after the antibiotics.

OUTCOME: After six weeks, Pamela had been free of cystitis for a month. A "twinge" was treated with purple coneflower capsules, and she drank a weak infusion of buchu and couchgrass tea daily as a preventative. Two years later, she has only had one further bout of cystitis, again quickly treated with a similar remedy.

How to use	Combinations	Cautions
Take an infusion or up to 4 ml tincture three times a day.	Use with horsetail, cornsilk or couchgrass to soothe inflamed mucous membranes.	Avoid in pregnancy; use untreated seeds only.
Take an infusion made with 15 g herb to 500 ml water, or take up to 2 ml tincture three times a day.	Combine with couchgrass and yarrow; add horsetail or pellitory-of-the-wall to heal damaged mucous membranes.	High doses may cause nausea.
Add 15 g herb to 500 ml water for an infusion, or take up to 2 ml tincture three times a day; take up to three 200 mg capsules three times a day.	Add couchgrass and yarrow to infusion or capsules; add cornsilk if burning sensation is severe.	
Take an infusion or tincture.	Combine with buchu, bearberry or juniper as more potent antiseptics.	
Take a decoction made with 20 g herb to 600 ml water, or take up to 3 ml tincture three times a day.	Can be combined with soothing diuretics such as parsley piert, cornsilk, couchgrass or pellitory-of-the-wall for supportive healing action.	
Take an infusion made with 10 g berries to 500 ml water, or take up to 2 ml tincture three times a day; use dilute oil for a massage.	Add hydrangea or wild carrot to help clear stones and add healing diuretics like pellitory-of-the-wall, couchgrass, parsley piert or cornsilk.	Avoid in pregnancy; do not use internally for over 6 weeks without a break.
Take an infusion or tincture; take 20 ml doses of fresh juice.	Add buchu or bearberry for infections, or couchgrass or cornsilk to soothe and heal.	
Take an infusion or up to 15 ml tincture a day.	Use as a simple or with cornsilk, hydrangea or couchgrass as a healing diuretic and to enhance the action on the prostate.	
Add 10 g berries to 500 ml water for a decoction, or take up to 2 ml tincture up to three times a day.	Use as a simple or combine with hydrangea and horsetail to increase action on the prostate.	

KEY

Aerial parts

Berries

Essential oil

Flowering tops

Leaves

Root

Seeds

STANDARD REMEDIES All recipes and doses are standard unless otherwise specified; see *Making Herbal Remedies*, pp. 120-5.

LEG & FOOT PROBLEMS

OUR LEGS AND FEET tend to be neglected until something goes wrong. They bear our (often excessive) weight, and suffer generally without protest as we cram our feet into tight shoes. Herbs can help to repair these self-inflicted ills: comfrey ointment and St. John's wort oil can relieve bunions by reducing inflammation and restoring normal growth, and crushed garlic is useful for drawing corns. Varicose veins are a common problem: they can be caused by excess abdominal pressure, as in obesity, pregnancy or constipation, and often the underlying cause should be treated first. Liver herbs like goldenseal, *bai shao yao* or barberry may be useful, or general tonics for the venous system can help. Severe varicose veins can be difficult to repair, but mild damage may be helped by douching for two minutes with hot water, and two minutes with cold, twice each morning, and raising the foot of the bed by 10 cm. Varicose ulcers are related to poor venous return, but are not always accompanied by varicose veins.

See also: corns, pp. 126-7.

AILMENT	REMEDIES	
	Herb	*Actions*
VARICOSE VEINS Swollen or stretched veins in the legs, associated with poor venous return or raised abdominal pressure (as in obesity, pregnancy or persistent constipation). **KEY SYMPTOMS** • Obvious enlarged and stretched veins • Pain in the legs.	*Aesculus hippocastanum* HORSE CHESTNUT (see p. 181)	Astringent and internally strengthening to the blood vessels, possibly due to the presence of aescin.
	Hamamelis virginiana WITCH HAZEL (see p. 182)	Astringent and soothing when applied topically.
	Melilotus officinalis KING'S CLOVER (see p. 181)	A good venous tonic, rich in coumarin-like compounds; anticoagulant and anti-inflammatory.
VERRUCAS & WARTS Small, hard growths in the outer layer of skin, due to a virus. They can spread by contact and may be persistent. **KEY SYMPTOM** • Obvious growth on the skin.	*Melaleuca alternifolia* TEA TREE (see p. 182)	Extremely antibiotic; useful for fungal, bacterial and viral infections.
	Taraxacum officinale DANDELION (see p. 103) *(Sap)*	The white sap from fresh plants is corrosive, and can be effective against warts.
	Thuja occidentalis ARBOR VITAE (see p. 180) *(Leaf tips)*	Volatile oil contains thujone, which is antiseptic and effective for many topical fungal and viral infections.
VARICOSE ULCERS Slow-healing sores, associated with poor local circulation. **KEY SYMPTOM** • Spreading sores that are painful and tender to the touch.	*Symphytum officinale* COMFREY (see p. 101)	Encourages cell regrowth of connective tissues.
	Teucrium scorodonia WOOD SAGE (see p. 182)	Astringent and effective wound healer, especially for slow-healing wounds.
CRAMP Muscle spasm, which can be associated with stress, fatigue or an imbalance of body salts. **KEY SYMPTOMS** • Sharp, severe pain in the legs • Affected muscle feels rigid.	*Dioscorea villosa* MEXICAN WILD YAM (see p. 52) *(Rhizome)*	Muscle relaxant; also relaxes peripheral blood vessels.
	Viburnum opulus GUELDER ROSE (see p. 113)	Effective relaxant for both smooth and skeletal muscle; anti-inflammatory.

CASE HISTORY
Varicose ulcer

PATIENT: Joan, 69, a grandmother with three children; a keen cake-maker, leading a reasonably active retirement with her husband.

HISTORY AND COMPLAINT: Poor circulation had always been a problem for Joan, who had suffered from severe chilblains in her youth. She had spent many years in shop work, and the long hours of standing had resulted in varicose veins that, while not especially severe, were occasionally painful. In the past year she had put on weight, which had exacerbated the problem. Finally, a bad graze on her shin resulting from a fall developed into an ulcer that failed to respond to orthodox dressings after three months.

TREATMENT: Medication included internal venous tonics such as king's clover, and *san qi* as a circulatory stimulant and to help repair the damaged area. For the ulcer, comfrey powder was prescribed – made into a paste and applied night and morning – plus a wash using an infusion of wood sage and ground ivy. An infused oil of cayenne and ginger was used around the ulcer. Joan was advised to raise the end of her bed on bricks, and she agreed to diet.

OUTCOME: A month brought a weight reduction, the veins hurt much less, and the ulcer was half the size and less painful. Joan used comfrey ointment instead of paste while on holiday; a month later, it had healed.

How to use	*Combinations*	*Cautions*
Take up to 2.5 ml tincture three times a day; use a dilute tincture for compresses.	Use with liver herbs such as goldenseal or dilute with witch hazel for compresses.	Peel off seed-coating if making large quantities; it can be toxic.
Ideally, use dilute tincture rather than distilled witch hazel as a lotion or in compresses for painful veins.	Add horse chestnut or pot marigold tinctures to the lotion, to enhance astringency.	Proprietary distilled witch hazel is not as effective as dilute tincture.
Use an infusion or take up to 3 ml tincture three times a day; apply as a cream, or use 5 ml tincture in 45 ml witch hazel or rosewater as a lotion.	Use with liver herbs such as goldenseal; take internally if sluggish digestion is a contributing factor.	Do not use with warfarin or similar drugs, or if blood-clotting is a problem.
Apply drops of essential oil or cream regularly to the wart or verruca.	Can be combined with diluted lemon or garlic oils (5 drops in 25 ml almond oil) if desired.	If using lemon or garlic oil, avoid contact with surrounding skin.
Apply sap from the stem or root directly to the wart.	Use as a simple; greater celandine sap has a similar effect.	Ensure sap does not contact surrounding skin.
Apply drops of tincture frequently to the wart or verruca; can also be made into an ointment.	Use as a simple.	Avoid in pregnancy.
Apply a paste of powdered root to the ulcer and cover with gauze and a bandage.	Use as a simple, but apply a heating oil (such as cayenne) to the area *around* the ulcer (not directly to it) to help stimulate blood flow.	Can cause rapid healing: use only on clean wounds.
Use an infusion as a wash, or apply as a cream.	Add ground ivy and heartsease infusion to the wash to enhance the healing action.	
Sip a decoction or take 1 ml tincture; repeat every 15 minutes if symptoms persist.	Use as a simple or with guelder rose tincture.	Avoid in pregnancy unless under professional guidance.
Use 25 ml tincture in 75 ml rosewater as a lotion, or in a cream.	Combines well with Indian tobacco in cramp creams – use 10 ml Indian tobacco tincture in 60 ml guelder rose cream.	Internal use of Indian tobacco is restricted.

KEY

Aerial parts

Bark

Essential oil

Leaves

Root

Seeds

Whole herb

STANDARD REMEDIES All recipes and doses are standard unless otherwise specified; see *Making Herbal Remedies*, pp. 120-5.

NERVOUS DISORDERS

HOLISTIC MEDICINE FOCUSES on the needs of body, mind and spirit, and this is especially true of any condition labelled as "nerves". Physical manifestations of nervous disorders may include insomnia, palpitations or headaches; emotional aspects include irritability, depression, anger or guilt, while lack of determination or emptiness can typify a spiritual vacuum. Herbs can operate on the same three levels. Vervain is a good example: it is an effective liver tonic and relaxing nervine; taken in Bach flower remedy form, it is good for the perfectionist, slightly obsessional person who tries to do too many jobs at once; on a spiritual level, it can increase understanding and psychic awareness. Herbs affect the mind and emotions in ways that we are only beginning to understand. There are reports of aromatic chemicals from essential oils reaching the part of the brain that acts as a centre for the emotions and has a role in memory. Small wonder, then, that scents are so evocative of past events, or that aromatic herbs can affect our emotions. In Eastern medicine, emotional imbalance is accepted as a possible cause of physical disease and herbs are used to strengthen spiritual centres such as the *chakras*, which are located at points from the crown of the head to the base of the spine.

See also: tension headaches, pp. 132-3; neuralgia, pp. 132-3; forgetfulness or confusion in the elderly, pp. 172-3; Parkinsonism, pp. 172-3; hyperactivity, pp. 176-7.

AILMENT	REMEDIES	
	Herb	*Actions*
ANXIETY & TENSION Excessive life-stresses can lead to a variety of health problems, which are not always obviously linked to tension. **KEY SYMPTOMS** • Inability to relax • Emotional lability – tendency to cry or be irritable for no obvious cause • Headaches • Sleeplessness.	*Anemone pulsatilla* PASQUE FLOWER (see p. 182)	Nervine and anodyne with sedative action; useful for nervous tension and sexual problems.
	Scutellaria lateriflora SKULLCAP (see p. 98)	Relaxant and restorative for the central nervous system; good for nervous debility.
	Stachys officinalis WOOD BETONY (see p. 99)	Sedative and calming for the nervous system; good for nervous debility, fearfulness and exhaustion.
	Tilia europaea LINDEN (see p. 181)	Reduces nervous tension and helps prevent arteriosclerosis.
	Verbena officinalis VERVAIN (see p. 112)	Relaxing nervine with a tonic effect on the liver.
PANIC ATTACKS These can be associated with excessive stress, but may also be linked to food intolerance. Severe cases may need psychiatric counselling. **KEY SYMPTOMS** • Palpitations • Intense feelings of fear • Feelings of impending doom.	*Citrus aurantium* NEROLI OIL (see p. 49)	Sedative and antidepressant, traditionally used for hysteria, panic and fearfulness; eases palpitations and cardiac spasm.
	Cypripedium calceolus LADY'S SLIPPER (see p. 181)	Increasingly rare herb, but very effective as a sedative, nervous tonic and hypnotic for over-active systems.
	Piscidia erythrina JAMAICAN DOGWOOD (see p. 181)	Sedative and anodyne, useful for severe nervous tension, insomnia or nervous migraine.
	Rosa damascena DAMASK ROSE (see pp. 90-1)	Very soothing for the nerves; antidepressant and prevents vomiting; gentle sedative.

CASE HISTORY
Lack of self-determination

PATIENT: Rosemary, 52, a reformed alcoholic in an unhappy marriage with a domineering husband.

HISTORY AND COMPLAINT: After years of finding solace in the bottle, Rosemary had started to take control of her own life again with the support of her friends, her church and Alcoholics Anonymous. But she felt unable to leave her husband, largely because of financial considerations, and was concerned that his constant nagging would force her to start drinking again. Physical symptoms included rheumatic-type pains in her legs and lower back, persistent colds, sleeplessness and general lack of enthusiasm for life. A hysterectomy three years earlier had been followed by hormone replacement therapy, which she had recently stopped, leading to hot flushes and night sweats. Rosemary had also had a brief affair with a friend's husband, which left her feeling lonely and guilt-ridden.

TREATMENT: A massage oil of lavender, basil and rosemary was suggested to ease aches and pains and nervous problems, while chaste-berry and goldenseal capsules were given for menopausal symptoms. Wood betony, *gotu kola* and skullcap helped counter depression, sense of loss and a lingering need for addiction, with *ling zhi* to provide a spiritual boost and help self-determination. Herbs were taken as powders or teas, as tinctures are unsuitable for reformed alcoholics.

OUTCOME: The aches and pains disappeared within a week. Rosemary became more cheerful and her sleep improved. She began to feel that the alcohol problem was under control, and took a part-time job in a local shop, focusing her attention on outside activities. She now feels less threatened by her husband's behaviour, and acknowledges that she might consider leaving him in the future. She continues to drink wood betony tea and takes *ling zhi* periodically.

How to use	Combinations	Cautions
Take up to 1 ml tincture three times a day, or add 5 g to 500 ml water for infusion.	Can be combined with Jamaican dogwood and/or passionflower for over-excited states.	Use only the dried plant.
Take an infusion or tincture, or take powdered herb in capsules.	Use as a simple, or combine with wood betony, lavender and lemon balm to increase calming, sedating action.	
Take an infusion or tincture, or take powdered herb in capsules.	Good as a simple or combine with chamomile, vervain, skullcap or lavender to enhance tonic or sedating action.	Large doses can cause vomiting. Avoid high doses in pregnancy.
Take an infusion or up to 10 ml tincture a day.	Add lemon balm and chamomile to infusion for a generally relaxing tea.	
Take an infusion or tincture.	Use as a simple or combine with wood betony, linden, chamomile or *gotu kola* to enhance sedating effects.	Avoid in pregnancy.
Mix 1 ml oil in 20 ml carrier oil for a massage; add 10 drops to a bath; take up to 5 ml orange flower water a day or use in cooking.	Can be combined with 5-10 drops lavender or benzoin oil to enhance calming action.	Use with caution in pregnancy.
Add up to 10 g to 500 ml water for infusion, or take up to 2 ml tincture three times a day.	Add up to 20 g skullcap, passionflower or valerian to infusion to enhance sedating action if desired.	
Take a decoction or up to 5 ml tincture a day.	Add pasque flower, valerian or hops to the tincture up to a combined total of 5 ml per dose for additional sedating action.	Do not exceed the stated dose.
Mix 2 ml rose oil in 20 ml carrier oil for a massage; add oil to baths; use rosewater as a lotion and in cooking.	Can combine with a few drops of sandalwood or patchouli oil, to increase calming effect.	Use only good quality, genuine rose oil medicinally.

KEY

Aerial parts

Essential oil

Flowers

Rhizome

Root bark

STANDARD REMEDIES All recipes and doses are standard unless otherwise specified; see *Making Herbal Remedies*, pp. 120-5.

AILMENT	REMEDIES	
	Herb	*Actions*
DEPRESSION Deficiency of the nervous system traditionally associated with a surfeit of the "melancholic" humour in Galenical medicine. **KEY SYMPTOMS** • Misery, feeling down • Inability to concentrate • Lack of interest in the present • Withdrawn, silent demeanour • Poor digestive function with constipation.	*Avena sativa* OATS (see p. 40)	Antidepressant and restorative nerve tonic.
	Borago officinalis BORAGE (see p. 41)	Restorative for the adrenal cortex; eases depression.
	Ocimum basilicum BASIL (see p. 82)	Antidepressant and spiritually uplifting, especially effective for the lower *chakras*; useful to encourage earthing or "groundedness".
	Turnera diffusa DAMIANA (see p. 179)	Stimulating nervine, good for the male hormonal system; antidepressant.
INSOMNIA Can be associated with over-excitement, anxiety and worries, or some physical cause, such as pain, which needs treating. In Chinese medicine it can signify excessive "heart fire". **KEY SYMPTOMS** • Inability to fall asleep • Frequent wakefulness during the night • Restlessness, vivid dreamy sleep.	*Eschscholzia californica* CALIFORNIAN POPPY (see p. 180)	Gentle and non-addictive hypnotic; tranquillizer and anodyne; safe for children.
	Humulus lupulus HOPS (see p. 66) (Strobiles)	Sedative, hypnotic and anodyne; calms excess excitability.
	Lactuca virosa WILD LETTUCE (see p. 182)	Sedative – the latex was once known as "poor man's opium"; fresh herb is especially potent when it goes to seed; garden lettuce has a milder effect.
	Passiflora incarnata PASSIONFLOWER (see p. 182)	Sedative, hypnotic and anodyne; calms the nervous system and promotes sleep.
INABILITY TO RELAX Herbs have long been used to induce a state of relaxation, with "mind-enhancing" herbs used in many shamanistic traditions to induce deep trance-like states with altered levels of awareness. In Western society, tobacco and cannabis (although illegal) are two herbs that still fulfil this role.	*Artemisia vulgaris* MUGWORT (see p. 39)	Gentle nervine; useful for menopausal tension, mild depression and stress.
	Chamaemelum nobile ROMAN CHAMOMILE (see p. 47)	Sedative, carminative and antispasmodic; good for excitement and nervous stomach.
	Hydrocotyle asiatica GOTU KOLA (see p. 181)	Relaxing and restorative for the nervous system; good for neurotic disturbances.
	Lavandula spp. LAVENDER (see p. 73)	Sedative and analgesic; antispasmodic action.
	Melissa officinalis LEMON BALM (see p. 78)	Antidepressant and restorative for the nervous system.
	Valeriana officinalis VALERIAN (see p. 110)	Very potent tranquillizer; antispasmodic and mild anodyne.

How to use	*Combinations*	*Cautions*
Take a decoction or 2-3 ml fluid extract; eat oatmeal as porridge.	Combines well with vervain in tincture or add 10 drops lemon balm to the dose to enhance antidepressant action.	If sensitive to gluten, see caution p. 40.
Take 10 ml juice three times a day.	Use as a simple.	Restricted herb in Australia and New Zealand.
Eat fresh leaves; add 5 drops essential oil to bath water, or mix 1 ml in 20 ml carrier oil for massage; take up to 3 ml tincture three times a day or take an infusion.	Combine leaves with lemon balm or rose petals in an infusion; add a few drops of geranium or rose oil to massage oil to increase uplifting effects.	Do not use the oil in pregnancy.
Take up to 2.5 ml tincture three times a day, or add 20 g herb to 500 ml for an infusion.	Combine with oats for general depression; if anxiety is a problem, combine with skullcap or wood betony using equal amounts of tincture up to a total of 5 ml per dose.	
Take an infusion or tincture at night.	Use as a simple or combine with passionflower, lavender or cowslip flowers if over-excitability is a problem.	
Take up to 5 ml tincture a day, or add 10 g herb to 500 ml water for an infusion. Take at night.	Can be combined with additional calming herbs such as valerian or passionflower up to 5 ml tincture per dose.	Avoid in depression. Do not exceed stated dose.
Take an infusion or tincture before going to bed; the fresh leaves can also be eaten in salads.	Use as a simple, or add a few drops of cowslip flower tincture per dose if over-excitability is a problem; valerian and passionflower can be added to increase tranquillizing action.	Excess can lead to insomnia and increased sexual activity; lower doses can cause sleepiness, so avoid if driving.
Take 5 ml tincture half an hour before bed, or drink a tea with 2-3 tsp herb per cup.	Add lavender and chamomile to infusion if desired.	Avoid high doses in pregnancy.
Take up to 2 ml tincture three times a day, or drink a weak infusion.	Combine with wood betony, skullcap or vervain for menopausal tension with emotional stress; combine tinctures up to a total of 5 ml per dose.	Avoid in pregnancy and when breastfeeding.
Add 2-3 drops essential oil or 500 ml infusion to baths; take tincture or drink chamomile tea regularly.	Use as a simple, or add lemon balm, skullcap or *gotu kola* to tincture as a restorative; combine with 2-3 drops lavender oil in baths as an additional sedative.	Avoid internal use in pregnancy. Do not exceed stated dose.
Take an infusion or tincture.	Use as a simple or mix with a little lavender or chamomile to enhance calming action.	Do not use for more than 4 weeks without a break.
Take infusion or up to 4 ml tincture per dose; massage dilute oil into temples.	Use as a simple or combine with wood betony, linden or vervain to ease tensions and stress.	Avoid high doses in pregnancy.
Drink fresh herb as tea, or take up to 5 ml tincture a day (more effective in low doses).	Use as a simple in tea or combine with wood betony, skullcap, or vervain tincture for sedating or restorative action.	
Take maceration, infusion or tincture; also available in 200 mg capsules or tablets.	Use as a simple or add a small amount of hops if there is excitability.	Can lead to over-excitedness; try a small dose first (see p. 110).

Aerial parts

Essential oil

Flowers

Leaves

Root

STANDARD REMEDIES All recipes and doses are standard unless otherwise specified; see *Making Herbal Remedies*, pp. 120-5.

GYNAECOLOGICAL PROBLEMS

THE HOLISTIC APPROACH of herbal medicine is particularly relevant to the common disorders of a woman's reproductive cycle: pre-menstrual syndrome (PMS), period pain, menopausal problems and so on. Emotions and spiritual disharmonies can be even more significant than physical disorders. Modern Western medicine, however, all too often delivers a verdict of "no abnormalities detected" after a battery of tests, and relies on repeat prescriptions for tranquillizers, hormone replacement therapy or even a hysterectomy. Traditional Chinese medicine closely associates the female reproductive system with the liver which, among other functions, "stores blood" and controls the flow of *qi*, or energy, around the body. Common PMS symptoms can be explained in terms of liver disharmony: irritability – the liver is

associated with anger; abdominal bloating – stagnation of *qi* in the lower abdomen; digestive upsets and sweet cravings – excess liver energy "invading the spleen" and causing deficiency and weakness. Treatment therefore often centres on herbs to stimulate and move liver energy. Modern Western herbal treatments, too, can adopt a multidimensional holistic approach; for example, hormone regulators like chaste-tree can be combined with uterine tonics such as motherwort or black cohosh to ease menstrual disorders. In Chinese medicine, menopausal symptoms are also explained in energy terms – as a "rundown" in kidney energy. The kidney is considered to store the body's "vital essence" or *jing*. This can be considered the body's life force – a combination of creative and repro-

AILMENT	REMEDIES	
	Herb	*Actions*
PRE-MENSTRUAL SYNDROME This can be associated with hormonal imbalance or stagnant *qi* levels. **KEY SYMPTOMS** • Irritability or anger • Depression and emotional upsets • Abdominal bloating • Breast swelling and tenderness • Food cravings (especially for sweet foods) • Constipation and/or diarrhoea.	*Alchemilla vulgaris* LADY'S MANTLE (see p. 32)	Regulates menstrual cycle with gentle hormonal action; astringent.
	Oenothera biennis EVENING PRIMROSE (see p. 181)	Contains γ-linolenic acid for prostaglandin production; eases breast tenderness.
	Paeonia lactiflora BAI SHAO YAO (see p. 83)	Balances liver function and soothes liver energy; nourishes blood and *yin*.
	Vitex agnus-castus CHASTE-TREE (see p. 180)	Acts on the pituitary gland to stimulate and normalize hormonal function.
PERIOD PAIN Also known as dysmenorrhoea, this may be due to blood stagnation before bleeding starts, or to uterine cramps once the flow begins. **KEY SYMPTOMS** • Lower abdominal pain either before or at the start of a period • Pain spreading to thighs or legs • Abdominal bloating • Flow may be scanty or have excessive clots.	*Anemone pulsatilla* PASQUE FLOWER (see p. 182)	Nervine and anodyne, good for all pains involving reproductive organs.
	Angelica sinensis DANG GUI (see p. 36)	Regulates menstrual function, nourishes the blood, liver *qi* stimulant.
	Caulophyllum thalictroides BLUE COHOSH (see p. 180) *(Rhizome)*	Antispasmodic with steroidal component that stimulates the uterus; good for pain due to blood stagnation.
	Viburnum prunifolium BLACK HAW (see p. 113)	Antispasmodic for uterine muscle; symptomatic remedy for cramping pain.

ductive energies – and menopausal syndrome can be explained in terms of kidney energy weakness affecting both liver and heart functions (see pp. 14-15) and causing symptoms such as night sweats, hot flushes, palpitations, back pain and irritability. Treatments therefore generally focus on kidney or liver tonics or calming heart herbs. In Ayurvedic medicine, sexual energy is seen as an aspect of creative and spiritual force and should be respected as such. Ayurveda also sees the reproductive organs as linked to some of the *chakras* or energy centres within the body, the root *chakra* being associated with our sense of belonging, or "groundedness": women who are unhappy with their role in life may suffer from reproductive disorders as a physical aspect of this disharmony. A hysterectomy can also unsettle the root *chakra*, leaving some women unable to concentrate, settle or relax. They seem to have a restless, rootless quality that can be difficult to ease.

CASE HISTORY
Pre-menstrual syndrome

PATIENT: Lucy, a 29-year-old marketing manager, found her work very stressful. She faced pressure from her mother to start a family, and from her live-in boyfriend to fulfil a domestic role.

HISTORY AND COMPLAINT: Lucy suffered from classic PMS symptoms: mood swings with extremes of irritability, abdominal bloating and tender, swollen breasts, plus painful, heavy periods.

TREATMENT: She was advised to spend at least ten minutes relaxing every day to help her unwind, and was also given a prescription for liver *qi* stagnation, which included *chai hu, bai shao yao, bai zhu, fu ling,* peppermint, ginger and liquorice.

OUTCOME: Within six weeks, Lucy's PMS was greatly reduced, with little fluid retention and much less irritability. Over the next two months, her irregular menstrual cycle returned to normal, menstrual cramps lessened and breast tenderness gradually disappeared.

KEY
Aerial parts
Berries
Seed oil
Root
Root bark

How to use	Combinations	Cautions
Take a tincture or use an infusion with other herbs.	Combine with 10-20 drops black cohosh, pasque flower, mugwort or *dang gui* tinctures per dose, or add white deadnettle or wood betony to the infusion.	Avoid in pregnancy.
Take 250-500 mg in capsules a day.	Use as a simple, but can be combined with other PMS strategies such as vitamin B supplements.	
Best used in combinations; or take a decoction of 40 g to 500 ml water in three doses.	Mix 10 g *bai shao yao* with 5 g each of *bai zhu, dang gui, chai hu,* liquorice, *fu ling* and 1 g ginger. Add 5 g *chen pi* for breast tenderness.	Avoid if symptoms include diarrhoea and stomach chills.
Take 10 drops tincture in water each morning in the second half of the cycle.	Use as a simple, but can be combined with other PMS strategies such as evening primrose oil and vitamin B supplements.	High doses can cause a sensation of ants creeping over the skin.
Take up to 20 drops tincture three times a day for symptomatic relief, or add 5 g herb to 500 ml water for an infusion.	Add 10-15 g St. John's wort to the infusion.	Use only the dried plant.
Best used in combinations; add 30 g herb to 500 ml water for a decoction and take in three doses.	Combine with 5-10 g *chai hu,* mugwort, *bai shao yao* or *chuan xiong* in a decoction. Available in many patent remedy forms in Chinese herb shops.	Avoid regular or large doses in pregnancy.
Use a tincture or decoction; best used in combinations.	Add 1-2 ml skullcap, motherwort, yarrow, false unicorn root, *mu dan pi* or *chi shao yao* tinctures per dose.	Avoid in early pregnancy.
Take 20 ml tincture in water, repeat up to three times if necessary.	Use as a simple or with 20-30 drops Jamaican dogwood tincture per dose.	

STANDARD REMEDIES All recipes and doses are standard unless otherwise specified; see *Making Herbal Remedies*, pp. 120-5.

AILMENT	REMEDIES	
	Herb	*Actions*
HEAVY PERIODS Also known as menorrhagia, this condition often appears to have no pathological cause and herbs can help. Heavy periods increase the risk of anaemia. **KEY SYMPTOMS** • Flooding • Excessive clots • Prolonged bleeding – more than seven days • Shortened menstrual cycle. *IMPORTANT: Seek professional advice if there is a sudden or unusual change in menstrual flow.*	*Artemisia vulgaris* var. *indicus* **AI YE** (see p. 39)	Styptic and warming herb for the meridians; useful if bleeding is prolonged.
	Calendula officinalis **POT MARIGOLD** (see p. 43)	Astringent with wide-ranging action for regulating menstrual cycle.
	Capsella bursa-pastoris **SHEPHERD'S PURSE** (see p. 45)	Astringent and anti-haemorrhagic herb specific for urogenital bleeding; eases root *chakra*.
	Lamium album **WHITE DEADNETTLE** (see p. 182)	Astringent and anti-spasmodic; regulates uterine blood flow and acts on reproductive organs.
MENOPAUSAL SYNDROME This is associated with hormonal changes and, in Chinese medicine, with kidney *qi* weakness. **KEY SYMPTOMS** • Irregular menstruation • Hot flushes and night sweats • Mood swings and depression • Vaginal dryness (eyes may also be dry) • Palpitations • Possible hypertension • Forgetfulness.	*Chamaelirium luteum* **FALSE UNICORN ROOT** (see p. 181) *(Rhizome)*	Stimulates ovarian hormones, and can be helpful for early menopause after hysterectomy, or to restart the system after years of contraceptives.
	Leonurus cardiaca **MOTHERWORT** (see p. 74)	Sedative, heart tonic and uterine stimulant; good for palpitations and anxiety.
	Polygonum multiflorum **HE SHOU WU** (see p. 181) *(Tuber)*	Kidney *qi* tonic, nourishes the blood; useful for early menopause.
	Vitex agnus-castus **CHASTE-TREE** (see p. 180)	Acts on the pituitary gland to stimulate and normalize hormonal function; can be helpful after hysterectomy.
VAGINAL THRUSH Often related to general systemic weakness allowing opportunist yeasts to proliferate. **KEY SYMPTOMS** • Milky discharge • Itching.	*Calendula officinalis* **POT MARIGOLD** (see p. 43)	Antifungal, astringent and healing.
	Melaleuca alternifolia **TEA TREE** (see p. 182)	Effective antifungal that does not irritate the vaginal membranes.
VAGINAL ITCHING Irritation that can be associated with menopausal syndrome, psychological factors or infection. **KEY SYMPTOMS** • Itching and dryness • Possible pain on intercourse.	*Rosa damascena* **DAMASK ROSE** (see pp. 90-1)	Cooling, soothing, astringent and anti-inflammatory with an uplifting effect to drive away melancholy.
	Verbena officinalis **VERVAIN** (see p. 112)	Gentle nervine, stimulating for liver and uterus; anti-depressant and energizing.
HYSTERECTOMY Post-operative help can relieve symptoms of premature meno-pause or disordered root *chakra*. **KEY SYMPTOMS** • Menopausal syndrome • Difficulty concentrating, forgetfulness • Irritability and excitability • Lack of calm contentment.	*Ligustrum lucidum* **NU ZHEN ZI** (see p. 181)	Stimulates kidney energy and alleviates symptoms of early menopause.
	Ocimum basilicum **BASIL** (see p. 82)	Antidepressant; tonic for root *chakra*; stimulates adrenal cortex and kidney *yang*.
	Stachys officinalis **WOOD BETONY** (see p. 99)	Sedative, stimulant for cerebral circulation and root *chakra*; eases fears and worry.

How to use	Combinations	Cautions
Add 15 g herb to 500 ml water for an infusion, or take up to 2.5 ml tincture three times a day.	Add shepherd's purse, self-heal or *han lian cao* to tincture or infusion, or combine with *dang gui* in a decoction.	Do not use in pregnancy without professional advice.
Take an infusion or tincture.	Add 1 ml shepherd's purse, lady's mantle, greater periwinkle or American cranesbill tincture per dose as additional astringents.	
Take an infusion or tincture.	Add 5 drops goldenseal tincture per dose or add white deadnettle to infusion.	
Take an infusion or tincture.	Combine with American cranesbill or greater periwinkle.	
Take 5-10 drops tincture four to six times a day.	Use as a simple or combine with 5 drops lady's mantle, or 2-3 ml black cohosh or Mexican wild yam tincture per dose.	
Take an infusion or tincture.	Combine with other sedative nervines like lavender or vervain, or with sage and mugwort to ease night sweats.	Avoid in pregnancy.
Best used in combinations in a decoction of 50 g herb to 750 ml water, or tonic wine.	Combine with *nu zhen zhi*, *gou qi zi*, *shu di huang* or cinnamon in a decoction.	Avoid if symptoms include diarrhoea.
Take 10 drops tincture in water each morning, or take two 200 mg capsules of powdered herb.	Use as a simple or combine 15 g powder with 5 g goldenseal powder in capsules to relieve hot flushes and other symptoms.	High doses can cause a sensation of ants creeping over the skin.
Use an infusion as a douche; apply cream or use infused oil as a lotion.	Add 5 drops purple coneflower to the douche or take garlic internally.	
Dilute 5 ml oil in 15 ml carrier oil and put 5 drops on a tampon and insert for 4 hours; use in pessaries or cream.	Use as a simple, or combine with infused marigold oil on a tampon, or add 20 drops tea tree oil and 10 drops thyme oil to 20 g cocoa butter for 12 pessaries.	
Use rosewater as a lotion, or add 2 drops essential oil to cream.	Make a cream with 10 ml pasque flower tincture, 20 ml lady's mantle tincture and 20 ml rosewater in 50-70 ml emulsifying ointment.	Use only the best quality, genuine rose oil medicinally.
Take an infusion or up to 5 ml tincture three times a day.	Combine with lavender, oats or lady's mantle; useful for itching of nervous origin.	Avoid in pregnancy.
Take a tincture or use in combination with other herbs in a decoction.	Add tonics such as *he shou wu*, *wu wei zi* or *ling zhi*; add 1-2 ml rose or wood betony tincture for additional support.	
Eat 2-3 fresh leaves with salads; take a tincture or use dilute oil for a massage.	Add 2 drops rose oil to 5 ml basil oil in 45 ml carrier oil for a massage; add 10-20 drops pasque flower tincture per dose.	
Take an infusion or tincture.	Combine with lavender, vervain or basil in tincture and infusion or add 10-20 drops chaste-tree tincture to the morning dose.	

KEY

Aerial parts

Berries

Essential oil

Flowering tops

Leaves

Petals

Root

STANDARD REMEDIES
All recipes and doses are standard unless otherwise specified; see *Making Herbal Remedies*, pp. 120-5.

PREGNANCY & CHILDBIRTH

FOR GENERATIONS OF WOMEN, herbal remedies were the only option for easing the ills of pregnancy and the trials of childbirth. Although nowadays we are far more cautious about using herbs during pregnancy, they still have an important role to play. They provide a safe alternative to orthodox drugs which can be harmful: butternut, for example, is a suitably gentle laxative; nettle tea, watercress or burdock can help anaemia, while powdered slippery elm or marshmallow root will ease heartburn. Morning sickness is often best

treated with a variety of remedies; women who feel sick much of the time may find that a regular repeated remedy may increase nausea. A selection of tinctures in drop doses is the best solution. The uterus can be prepared for the exertions of childbirth with tonic herbs or dilute sage oil massaged into the abdomen during the last three weeks. After the birth, basil and motherwort tea can help clear the placenta, and new mothers should take homeopathic *Arnica 6x* tablets every 15-30 minutes for a few hours to help repair stressed tissues.

See also: anaemia, pp. 150-1; constipation, pp. 152-3; heartburn, pp. 154-5; cramp, pp. 160-1; varicose veins, pp 160-1.

AILMENT	REMEDIES	
	Herb	*Actions*
MORNING SICKNESS Nausea and vomiting (during the first three months of pregnancy), often on rising, but may last all day. Severe cases (*hyperemesis gravidarum*) may require hospital treatment because of the risk of liver disease and dehydration. **KEY SYMPTOMS** • Vomiting on rising • Feelings of nausea.	*Ballota nigra* **BLACK HOREHOUND** (see p. 180)	Prevents vomiting, sedative; useful for nervous dyspepsia.
	Chamaemelum nobile **ROMAN CHAMOMILE** (see p. 47)	Reduces feelings of nausea and calms the stomach; suitably relaxing nervine in stressful situations.
	Zingiber officinalis **GINGER** (see p. 115)	Prevents vomiting; has been used successfully in hospital trials involving *hyperemesis gravidarum* patients.
PREPARING FOR THE BIRTH Herbs have long been used to help the body prepare for childbirth by tonifying the uterine muscles.	*Mitchella repens* **SQUAW VINE** (see p. 182)	Uterine tonic and stimulant; astringent and restorative for the nervous system.
	Rubus idaeus **RASPBERRY** (see p. 93)	Tonifies the uterus.
PERINEAL TEARS Tears in the perineum can be painful and slow to heal. These herbs also help bruising and soreness. **KEY SYMPTOM** • Tears in the perineum during birth, which may require stitches.	*Hypericum perforatum* **ST. JOHN'S WORT** (see p. 68) *(Flowering tops)*	Anti-inflammatory, healing and astringent.
	Ranunculus ficaria **PILEWORT** (see p. 182)	Very astringent.
	Symphytum officinale **COMFREY** (see p. 101)	Healing – encourages cell growth and can help limit scar tissue.
BREASTFEEDING PROBLEMS Women can be deterred from breastfeeding for many reasons: the baby may have difficulty latching on to the nipple or there may be soreness and lack of milk. **KEY SYMPTOMS** • Sore nipples • Lack of milk • Excessive milk/engorgement.	*Brassica oleracea* **CABBAGE** (see p. 42)	Anti-inflammatory and healing; relieves both engorgement and mastitis.
	Calendula officinalis **POT MARIGOLD** (see p. 43)	Antiseptic, anti-inflammatory and soothing for dry skin.
	Galega officinalis **GOAT'S RUE** (see p. 181)	Increases milk flow and encourages development of breasts.

CASE HISTORY
Bleeding in pregnancy

PATIENT: Julie, 32, happily married with two daughters aged 2 and 4, and starting her third pregnancy.

HISTORY AND COMPLAINT: Julie had suffered from continuous bleeding throughout her first two pregnancies, and spent much of the nine months confined to bed. With two lively under-fives, she was worried that the third pregnancy would be the same, leading to severe disruption for the entire family. This time, light spotting started during the sixth week of her pregnancy. In traditional Chinese medicine, many uterine bleeding disorders can be attributed to a weakness in the *chong* (vital) and *ren* (responsibility) channels – what we regard in the West as acupuncture meridians. The *ren* channel is regarded as being closely related to all the *yin* channels in the body, and is also called the "conception vessel", as it starts in the uterus. The *chong* channel communicates with all the other channels and also starts in the uterus. These channels are associated with childbirth, and any "coldness" and deficiency here can lead to bleeding during or after pregnancy.

TREATMENT: Herbal capsules containing *dang gui, shu di huang, ai ye, bai shao yao*, liquorice and *chuan xiong* were used to warm and nourish the deficient channels.

OUTCOME: Within two weeks, the uterine bleeding had stopped. Julie continued with a normal pregnancy, and produced a healthy daughter at term.

How to use	*Combinations*	*Cautions*
Take up to 2 ml tincture in hot water up to three times a day, or sip a weak infusion.	Alternate with other remedies if symptoms persist.	
Drink one cup infusion before rising or take 5-10 drop doses tincture as required (up to 5 ml a day).	Best as a simple, but can alternate with lemon balm, fennel, basil, ginger or peppermint if need be.	Do not exceed stated dose.
Take up to 1 g powdered herb in capsules per dose, or take 2-5 drops tincture as required (up to 1 ml a day).	Best as a simple, but alternate with other remedies as required.	Do not exceed stated dose; use with respect in early pregnancy.
Take one cup infusion a day in the last two months of pregnancy.	Use as a simple or combine with raspberry leaves.	
Take one cup infusion a day in the last two months of pregnancy; drink plenty during labour.	Use as a simple during pregnancy; add rose petals and wood betony to infusion during labour.	
Apply the infused oil or add a strong infusion to a hip bath.	Add lavender and marigold oils to infused oil, or add the dried herbs to infusion for baths.	
Apply cream to affected areas.	Combines well with witch hazel.	Do not take internally.
Apply cream, infused oil or ointment to affected areas, or add an infusion to a hip bath.	Mix 2 ml lavender oil in 20 ml infused oil base.	Can cause rapid healing: use only on clean wounds.
Place a slightly softened fresh leaf between the breast and the bra.	Use as a simple; drink sage tea to reduce milk flow, if weaning.	
Apply cream to sore nipples after every feed.	Use as a simple, or combine with squaw vine in cream.	
Add 15 g herb to 500 ml water for an infusion, or take up to 2 ml tincture per dose.	Can combine with other herbs to promote milk flow, such as fennel, dill, fenugreek and milk thistle.	

KEY

Aerial parts

Flowers

Leaves

Petals

Root

STANDARD REMEDIES
All recipes and doses are standard unless otherwise specified; see *Making Herbal Remedies*, pp. 120-5.

PROBLEMS OF THE ELDERLY

FOR THOSE WHO REGARD the body as a machine, the problems of old age are associated with mechanical decay – joints suffer from wear and tear, leading to osteoarthritis; the digestive system rebels against a lifetime of low-fibre foods and laxatives, leading to constipation or diverticulosis; and mental acuity is blunted. In Chinese medicine, the problems of old age are more likely to be associated with a run-down in vital energy: declining kidney essence – a key factor in menopausal syndrome (see pp. 166-9) – can account for the incontinence, tinnitus and deafness that affect so many old people. Strengthening tonic herbs like *he shou wu, nu zhen zi* or *han lian cao* can often help with these problems. The Chinese also use *qi*, or energy,

weakness to explain some of the constipation problems of the elderly – a specific herb for this is *huo ma ren*, the seeds of *Cannabis sativa* or marijuana. (In the West, these are generally supplied pre-boiled, to prevent illicit cultivation.) Depending on precise symptoms, these may be prescribed in combination with herbs like apricot seeds (*xing ren*), bitter orange, *bai shao yao*, rhubarb root or *dang gui*. Herbal tonics can also counter symptoms of mental confusion: in China, ginseng has always been popular among those wealthy enough to afford it, while in Ayurvedic medicine *Chyavan Prash*, a mixture of around 20 herbs, sometimes with silver or gold foil added, has a similar role. Such *qi* tonics may not prevent dementia, but they

See also: arthritis, pp. 130-1; constipation, pp. 152-3; prostate problems, pp. 158-9; tonic herbs, pp. 178-9.

AILMENT	REMEDIES	
	Herb	*Actions*
LATE-ONSET DIABETES Caused by lack of insulin, leading to high blood sugar levels. It is often associated with obesity and poor diet, and is generally non-insulin dependent. **KEY SYMPTOMS** • Excessive thirst and urination • Mental confusion • Weight loss • Lethargy.	*Galega officinalis* **GOAT'S RUE** (see p. 181)	Enlarges the islets of Langerhans in the pancreas, which are responsible for insulin production.
	Trigonella foenum-graecum **FENUGREEK** (see p. 106)	Hypoglycaemic herb – in trials, it has reduced urine sugar levels by 50%.
	Vaccinium myrtillus **BILBERRY** (see p. 109)	Hypoglycaemic and increases insulin production.
INCONTINENCE Involuntary urination, which may be associated with weakened pelvic floor muscles, obstruction to the bladder outflow, or lack of kidney *qi*. **KEY SYMPTOMS** • Urgent and frequent urination • Bedwetting • Leakage with coughing or laughing.	*Astragalus membranaceus* **HUANG QI** (see p. 181)	Replenishes vital energy and helps to regulate water metabolism.
	Cupressus sempervirens **CYPRESS** (see p. 180)	Astringent and relaxing oil, good for all types of excess fluid production.
	Equisetum arvense **HORSETAIL** (see p. 55)	Healing and tonic for the urinary mucous membranes.
FORGETFULNESS OR CONFUSION This is common in old age, and can be helped by tonic herbs to strengthen the kidney *qi*, *yin* or *yang* energies, as appropriate (see pp. 178-9).	*Emblica officinalis* **AMALAKI** (see p. 180)	*Yin* tonic; widely used in Ayurvedic medicine for senility.
	Hydrocotyle asiatica **GOTU KOLA** (see p. 181)	Nerve tonic used in Ayurvedic medicine to promote mental calm and clarity.
	Salvia officinalis var. *purpurea* **PURPLE SAGE** (see p. 95)	Traditional ingredient of many medieval longevity tonics; good *qi* tonic.

can certainly improve energy levels and increase alertness. Herbs can also help in distressing conditions like Parkinson's disease. Deadly nightshade, a highly toxic remedy unsuitable for home use, was the main treatment for Parkinsonism until recently. As well as reducing salivation, this antispasmodic herb helps to control tremors, and is the original source of atropine, which is still prescribed by orthodox practitioners for the disease. The related plants henbane and thorn apple can also be effective, but are not for home use. Some argue that the whole plants are considerably more effective for controlling Parkinsonism than synthetic atropine or other artificially derived drugs.

IMPORTANT: *The metabolism of the elderly is often slow, and doses for old people may need to be lower than for adults in their prime.*

CASE HISTORY
Late-onset diabetes mellitus

PATIENT: Henry, 72, overweight, averse to exercise.

HISTORY AND COMPLAINT: Henry had been feeling very lethargic, and complained of persistent thirst. A blood test by his doctor indicated abnormally high sugar levels and suggested late-onset diabetes. Henry was given a diet sheet and instructed to lose weight. Urine tests over a month regularly showed raised glucose levels.

TREATMENT: Henry disliked taking medication, so the emphasis of treatment was on diet. He was happy to eat plenty of garlic, onions and cinnamon toast, which can all help reduce blood sugar levels. He took doses of fenugreek powder after meals, and tolerated goat's rue and bilberry leaf tea.

OUTCOME: Within a few days, fasting urinary sugar levels were lower, with normal levels recorded occasionally after another week. His doctor was satisfied after a month, and deferred medication.

How to use	Combinations	Cautions
Take an infusion or tincture before meals.	Use as a simple or combine with stinging nettle or bilberry leaf in an infusion; add 2-4 ml sweet sumach tincture per dose. Eat a high fibre diet with plenty of garlic.	Blood sugar levels need careful monitoring.
Take up to 1 g powdered herb after meals, or make a decoction.	Eat a high fibre diet with plenty of garlic; add powdered cloves or cinnamon to capsules if desired.	Blood sugar levels need careful monitoring.
Drink an infusion before meals.	Add goat's rue or stinging nettle to infusion; eat a high fibre diet with plenty of garlic.	Blood sugar levels need careful monitoring.
Take a decoction with other herbs, or 1-2 g doses powdered herb in capsules, or a tincture.	Combine with *dang gui, chuan xiong* and *chi shao yao* in a decoction.	Avoid herb if condition involves excess "heat" or *yin* deficiency.
Add 50 drops to 25 ml almond oil and massage into the lower abdomen twice a day.	Use as a simple or add 10-25 drops pine oil to 25 ml of the diluted cypress oil massage mixture.	
Take 10 ml juice twice a day.	Use as a simple or with 2-5 ml St. John's wort or sweet sumach tincture per dose.	
Eat fresh, dried (Indian gooseberry) or stewed fruit.	Generally taken in *Chyavan Prash* (a herb jelly sold in Indian markets and restaurants).	
Take an infusion or tincture in 5-10 ml doses.	Take as a simple or combine with *han lian cao* in infusion or tincture.	
Take one tea cup of infusion or 10 ml tincture a day.	Use as a simple or combine with rosemary.	Can trigger fits in epileptics, who should avoid the herb.

KEY

Aerial parts

Essential oil

Fruit

Leaves

Rhizome

Seeds

STANDARD REMEDIES
All recipes and doses are standard unless otherwise specified; see *Making Herbal Remedies*, pp. 120-5.

CHILDREN'S COMPLAINTS

GENTLE HERBS can be ideal for many children's ailments: soothing and relaxing remedies like chamomile or linden can ease over-excitement and encourage sleep. In fevers, cooling herbs such as elderflower, yarrow and catmint can be freely given, while purple coneflower is an ideal antibiotic. For coughs try hyssop, liquorice or white horehound in syrup; for persistent catarrh try replacing milk products with soya-based preparations and using herbs like ground ivy and eyebright in capsules or tinctures. Soya is a good source of calcium, so eliminating dairy products from a child's diet is unlikely to cause any deficiencies. Hyperactivity can be related to food allergy – avoid colorants (E102 and E110 in particular). Constipation needs to be treated with gentle laxatives rather than stimulating purgatives – try psyllium seeds disguised in breakfast cereal, or butternut, rather than rhubarb root or senna. Unfortunately, many

See also: infections and fevers, pp. 134-5; catarrh, pp. 136-7; earache, pp. 140-1; eczema, acne and ringworm, pp. 144-7; hay fever, pp. 156-7.

AILMENT	REMEDIES	
	Herb	*Actions*
NAPPY RASH & CRADLE CAP A painful, raw area of nappy rash around the anus and on the buttocks may be due to irritant stools or wet nappies; it can be related to yeast infections, especially if the mother is breast-feeding while on antibiotics. Cradle cap is a scaly dermatitis affecting the scalp, and is often due to over-active sweat glands; it is not serious or contagious. **KEY SYMPTOMS** • Nappy rash: sore, red, painful inflammation around the anus or anywhere in the nappy area • Cradle cap: scaly crust over the scalp.	*Arctium lappa* **BURDOCK** (see p. 38)	Cleansing and tonifying for the sweat and oil glands of the scalp in cradle cap.
	Plantago major **PLANTAIN** (see p. 86)	Locally healing and soothing.
	Symphytum officinale **COMFREY** (see p. 101)	Encourages cell regrowth; demulcent and soothing.
	Viola tricolor **HEARTSEASE** (see p. 114)	Soothing and anti-inflammatory; useful for a wide range of skin disorders.
COLIC Colic is caused by spasmodic contractions of the intestines associated with gas and tension, and often follows rushed or tense feeding times. **KEY SYMPTOMS** • Pain causing small babies to scream loudly • Tense, bloated abdomen • Wind and flatulence.	*Chamaemelum nobile* **ROMAN CHAMOMILE** (see p. 47)	Sedative, carminative and antispasmodic; good for excitement and nervous stomach.
	Foeniculum officinale **FENNEL** (see p. 59)	Carminative; reduces griping pains.
	Nepeta cataria **CATMINT** (see p. 180)	Carminative and anti-spasmodic; can encourage sleep in restless babies.
GASTRIC UPSETS Bilious attacks in children can be a type of migraine, and may be linked to food intolerance. **KEY SYMPTOMS** • Sudden diarrhoea and vomiting • Stomach ache.	*Agrimonia eupatoria* **AGRIMONY** (see p. 31)	Astringent and healing for stomach lining; stimulates bile flow; helpful in food allergies; ideal for diarrhoea.
	Geranium maculatum **AMERICAN CRANESBILL** (see p. 180)	Astringent and tonifying for diarrhoea and gastritis.

herbs taste unpleasant, so persuading children to swallow them can be a problem. Babies may be coaxed to take weak infusions of chamomile or linden from a bottle, while breastfeeding mothers can take the remedy themselves, as it will pass into their milk; this is especially useful with colic remedies like dill or fenugreek. Toddlers will generally accept powders or tinctures in half a teaspoon of honey, while capsules are ideal as soon as the child is old enough to swallow them. Dilute tinctures given in drop doses on the tongue are acceptable, or they may be flavoured with peppermint, liquorice or raspberry vinegar, as appropriate. For infants or long-term use, it is best to give non-alcoholic tinctures (see p. 125).

IMPORTANT NOTE

Children's doses need to be reduced depending on age. All doses in the tables below and overleaf are the full adult dose unless otherwise specified. For children use the following proportions:

AGE	DOSE (*expressed as a fraction of an adult dose*)
0 - 1 yr	one-twentieth
1 - 2 yrs	one-tenth
3 - 4 yrs	one-fifth
5 - 6 yrs	three-tenths
7 - 8 yrs	two-fifths
9 - 10 yrs	half
11 - 12 yrs	three-fifths
13 - 14 yrs	four-fifths
15 plus	full dose

How to use	Combinations	Cautions
Add 5 drops tincture to a bottle for babies under 10 kg; add 10 drops tincture for babies over 10 kg.	Can combine with heartsease for cradle cap.	
Apply ointment or infused oil frequently as required; put fresh, washed, crushed leaves in the nappy at each change.	Add 1-2 drops tea tree oil to 5 ml infused oil if fungal infection develops.	
Apply ointment or infused oil frequently as required; use a paste of powdered root as a poultice for nappy rash.	Use arrowroot powder instead of baby talcum powder when changing nappies.	Can cause rapid healing; ensure affected area is clean.
Use an infusion as a wash on affected areas; apply infused oil or ointment to nappy rash, or use cream for cradle cap.	Add lemon balm or ground ivy to a wash or cream, if desired. The hard crusts of cradle cap can be softened with vegetable oil left overnight.	
Use homeopathic *Chamomilla 3x*: for babies, give 5-10 drops or 1-5 crushed pillules up to three times a day.	Use as a simple; breastfeeding mothers can drink chamomile tea to relax themselves and soothe the baby's colic.	Do not exceed stated dose.
Give babies 5-10 drops tincture in a bottle of water or add to feeds; breastfeeding mothers should drink a cup of infusion before feeds.	As an alternative, dill can be used in the same way.	
Add 5-10 drops tincture to a baby's bottle of water or to feeds, or give a dilute infusion.	Use as a simple.	
Give an infusion or tincture (see dosage chart above).	Can combine with chamomile, catmint or lemon balm for nervous stomach; combine with a little marshmallow for inflammations.	Avoid in constipation.
Give an infusion or tincture (see dosage chart above).	Can combine with agrimony, meadowsweet, marshmallow or chamomile to enhance action.	

KEY

Aerial parts

Flowers

Leaves

Root

Seeds

STANDARD REMEDIES
All recipes and doses are standard; all doses in the table here and overleaf are the full adult dose unless otherwise specified; see *Making Herbal Remedies*, pp. 120-5.

AILMENT	REMEDIES	
	Herb	*Actions*
SLEEPLESSNESS Sleepless babies increase tension in the entire household. Check the room temperature and, as the problem may associated with insecurity, be very loving.	*Chamaemelum nobile* ROMAN CHAMOMILE (see p. 47)	Sedative, carminative and antispasmodic; ideal for over-excitement.
	Eschscholzia californica CALIFORNIAN POPPY (see p. 180)	Sedative, mild hypnotic and antispasmodic; good for over-excitement.
THREADWORMS Parasitic worms are common in children, and can be due to poor hygiene. Cases are generally mild. KEY SYMPTOMS • Anal itching • White, threadlike worms in the stools.	*Allium ursinum* RAMSOMS (see p. 182) *(Bulb)*	Potent antiseptic, similar to garlic.
	Brassica oleracea CABBAGE (see p. 42)	Traditional remedy for intestinal worms; antibacterial and healing.
NITS The eggs of head lice on the hair. KEY SYMPTOM • Itching head.	*Melaleuca alternifolia* TEA TREE (see p. 182)	Effective antiseptic; also antibacterial and antifungal.
TEETHING Teething pains can affect babies from the age of 4 or 5 months.	*Chamaemelum nobile* ROMAN CHAMOMILE (see p. 47)	Sedative, carminative, antispasmodic.
HYPERACTIVITY Excessive over-activity can be related to food intolerance, "liver fire" or excess liver *qi*.	*Prunella vulgaris* XIA KU CAO (see p. 88) *(Flower spikes)*	Used in Chinese medicine to calm "liver fire" associated with over-excitability.
BEDWETTING Can be a congenital disorder, or due to insecurity, emotional upsets or minor urinary tract infections.	*Rhus aromatica* SWEET SUMACH (see p. 182)	Astringent and tonic for the urinary system; traditionally used for bedwetting in childhood, although scientific evidence for efficacy is scant.
TRAVEL SICKNESS Nausea and vomiting related to motion, as on car journeys or sea voyages, is common in childhood.	*Mentha piperita* PEPPERMINT (see p. 79)	Prevents vomiting, antispasmodic.
	Zingiber officinalis GINGER (GAN JIANG) (see p. 115)	Prevents vomiting, carminative.
CHILDHOOD INFECTIONS & FEVERS Sudden swings in body temperature to abnormally high levels are common in childhood illnesses, and cooling fever herbs can help. Professional medical help is needed in many childhood infections, although herbs can be used as alternatives to orthodox antibiotics to relieve specific symptoms of mumps, measles, chicken pox and other infections.	*Echinacea spp.* PURPLE CONEFLOWER (see p. 53)	Antibacterial and antiviral; also strengthens resistance to infections; useful for all septic or infectious conditions.
	Hyssopus officinalis HYSSOP (see p. 69)	Relaxing expectorant, particularly suitable for children's coughs and respiratory infections.
	Lonicera japonica JIN YIN HUA (see p. 76) *(Flower buds)*	Cooling for feverish conditions; antibacterial and anti-inflammatory.

How to use	*Combinations*	*Cautions*
For babies, add 100-500 ml infusion or 2-3 drops essential oil to bath water.	Use as a simple; breastfeeding mothers can drink chamomile tea to relax both themselves and their babies.	Do not exceed stated dose.
Give an infusion or tincture about 30 minutes before bed (see dosage chart on p. 175).	Add a little honey to make it more palatable for children; can add chamomile or a little skullcap to increase soothing action.	
Give an infusion or 10 ml juice; also use as an enema once a week.	Use as a simple, or use garlic instead for older children.	
Give a glass of juice each morning for three days.	Can combine with carrot juice. An alternative traditional cure is to feed the child nothing but grated carrot for two days.	
Put a few drops of oil on a fine comb and comb the hair well, or add 5-10 drops to shampoo or hair rinse; repeat daily.	Use as a simple or combine with well diluted lemon oil (no more than 5 drops in 25 ml carrier oil – it can irritate).	
Use *Chamomilla 3x* (see colic on p. 174) or put 1-2 drops oil on a wet swab and apply to the gum.	Add 1 drop clove essential oil to the swab. Give a weak linden infusion by bottle.	Do not exceed stated dose of essential oil.
Give an infusion or tincture (see dosage chart on p. 175).	Can be combined with calming nervines like chamomile or wood betony. Add a small amount of vervain or *bai shao yao* to soothe the liver; add agrimony for food allergies.	
Give 10-15 drops tincture up to three times a day.	Combine with cornsilk or horsetail if urinary infection is suspected; combine with St. John's wort or wood betony for related nervous problems.	
Give drop doses of tincture while travelling.	Older children can be given peppermint sweets.	Do not use for babies.
Give one to two 200 mg capsules before travelling.	Best as a simple; ginger sweets and biscuits can be useful for younger children or give crystallized ginger to chew.	
Give two 200-250 mg capsules of powdered root three times a day or 10 ml tincture (see dosage chart on p. 175).	Effective as a simple, or add elderflower, catmint or yarrow in feverish conditions. Add 5-10 drops pokeroot or 2-5 ml cleavers tincture for mumps. Add 2-5 drops fresh ginger tincture if nausea is a problem in measles.	High doses can occasionally cause nausea and vomiting.
Give up to 10 ml tincture a day or give an infusion (see dosage chart on p. 175).	Can be combined with elderflower, catmint or purple coneflower in infections and fevers, or add white horehound to soothe the mucous membranes in irritable coughs.	
Give an infusion or tincture (see dosage chart on p. 175).	In hot, feverish conditions, can add elderflower, peppermint, catmint or a little *lian qiao*. Use cooling lotions such as rosewater with borage juice (restricted herb in Australia and New Zealand) or chickweed cream to ease irritation of skin rashes in chicken pox.	

KEY

Aerial parts

Essential oil

Flowers

Leaves

Root

Root bark

STANDARD REMEDIES All recipes and doses are standard; all doses in the table here and on pp. 174-5 are the full adult dose unless otherwise specified; see *Making Herbal Remedies*, pp. 120-5.

TONIC HERBS

HERBS HAVE BEEN USED for millennia to restore energy, strengthen the spirit and tonify particular body organs. Today, fashionable Eastern tonics, such as ginseng and *dang gui*, are more popularly used than traditional Western tonics, like rosemary and sage. Tonic herbs can be classified in numerous ways: as boosting energy or *qi*, nourishing blood or body fluids, balancing the "humours" of Ayurvedic medicine (see pp. 12-13), strengthening immunity, or stimulating *jing* – the "vital essence", which in Chinese medicine is stored in the kidneys and is the source of our creative and reproductive energies. Herbalists also associate tonics with particular organs and meridians of the body: *bai zhu*, for example, is especially good for digestive weaknesses, elecampane for the lungs and St. John's wort as a restorative for the nerves. Tonic herbs are also used to strengthen the spirit: the Taoists used herbs like *ling zhi* and *he shou wu* to increase mental acuity, while in India *amalaki* and *shatavari* play a similar role.

IMPORTANT: Tonic herbs should not be taken during acute illness without professional guidance.

ENERGY & QI TONICS

In the East, illness is often defined in terms of energy deficiency – either *yin* or *yang* – and is treated with a variety of energy or *qi* tonics. Deficiency can lead to stagnation and symptoms of stagnant *qi* can include gastric fullness, chest pains or headaches. Herbs to help "move" energy, such as *chen pi* or ginger, are often added to the tonic mixture. Energy tonics can be useful in exhaustion or convalescence, for example after influenza.

SYMPTOMS OF YANG DEFICIENCY
• Frequent colds or infections; fatigue
• Fluid retention; coldness and pallor
• Pale, puffy tongue; slow, tired pulse.

SYMPTOMS OF YIN DEFICIENCY
• Feverishness and night sweats; thirst and dry mouth
• Debility following a long illness
• Red, shiny tongue; fast pulse.

IMPORTANT: A correct diagnosis is important because the use of inappropriate tonic remedies – such as a yang *tonic when* yang *energies are already in excess – can make the condition worse. Seek professional help for severe or persistent problems.*

BAI ZHU
Atractylodes macrocephala

Parts used: rhizome.
Actions: energy tonic for spleen and stomach; diuretic and carminative; helps to regulate *qi* and strengthen the lower limbs.
How to use: take a decoction or tincture.
Combinations: can be combined with *ban xia* and *chen pi* for stomach weakness or with cinnamon and *fu ling* for lung problems.

DA ZAO
Ziziphus jujuba

Parts used: fruit (Chinese date).
Actions: energy tonic for spleen and stomach; nourishes blood, nutritive, sedative, calms the spirit; moderates toxic herbs.
How to use: use 3-10 fruits per dose in decoctions or eat fresh.
Combinations: use with ginseng or *dang gui* as appropriate.

OTHER ENERGY & QI TONICS

AMERICAN GINSENG (*Panax qinquefolius*) p. 84.
ELECAMPANE (*Inula helenium*) p. 70; pp. 138-9.
GOTU KOLA (*Hydrocotyle asiatica*) pp. 164-5; 172-3; p. 181.
HE SHOU WU (*Polygonum multiflorum*) pp. 146-7; 168-9; p. 181.
HUANG QI (*Astragalus membranaceus*) pp. 172-3; p. 181.
ROSEMARY (*Rosmarinus officinalis*) p. 92; pp. 146-9.
SHAN YAO (*Dioscorea opposita*) p. 52.

DANG SHEN
Codonopsis pilosula

Parts used: root.
Actions: demulcent and expectorant, acting on lungs and spleen; widely used as a substitute for ginseng, it is milder and more *yin* in character; it is particularly good for nourishing stomach *yin*.
How to use: take a decoction or tincture; drink as a tonic wine.
Combinations: use with *fu ling*, *bai zhu* and liquorice.

FU LING
Poria cocos

Parts used: dormant fungus.
Actions: diuretic, sedative and energy tonic; acts on the heart to calm the spirit; strengthens the spleen and moves *qi*; also tonifies *yin* functions and regulates body fluids.
How to use: take a tincture or up to 15 g per dose in decoctions.
Combinations: use with *bai zhu*, *dang shen* and liquorice for debility.

KOREAN or CHINESE GINSENG
Panax ginseng (see p. 84)

Parts used: root.
Actions: energy stimulant with a tonic effect on all body organs, especially lungs and spleen; demulcent.
How to use: take a decoction or tincture; or take 500 mg-4 g powdered root in capsules a day; use as a general tonic for three to four weeks in autumn to strengthen the body for winter.
Combinations: can be combined with *huang qi* for debility or ginger for asthma and chronic coughs.
Caution: avoid high doses or prolonged use in pregnancy and hypertension, see p. 84.

LING ZHI
Ganoderma lucidum

Parts used: fruiting body.
Actions: immune stimulant, nervine, strengthens the spirit, heart tonic, antibacterial, anti-allergenic and anti-tussive; Taoist herb said to increase spiritual awareness, determination and longevity.
How to use: take a tincture or up to 600 mg powder in capsules a day.
Combinations: take as a simple or combine with *shiitake*.

SIBERIAN GINSENG
Eleutherococcus senticosus

Parts used: root.
Actions: antispasmodic and antirheumatic; increases stamina and ability to cope with stress; less heating than Korean ginseng and suitable for those who find it too stimulating.
How to use: take a tincture or 500 mg-2 g in capsules or patent tablets.
Combinations: use as a simple.

WU WEI ZI
Schisandra chinensis

Parts used: fruit.
Actions: astringent, sedative and aphrodisiac; effective kidney and skin tonic; take for insomnia and anxiety; an all-round tonic, known as "five-taste fruit", which acts on all organs; good for allergic skin conditions.
How to use: take an infusion or tincture; or take 200-250 mg powdered herb in capsules three times a day.

KIDNEY TONICS

In Chinese medicine the kidneys store the *jing*, or "vital essence", and are associated with reproduction and creativity. In Western medicine, the hormones produced by the adrenal cortex can be said to play a similar role, and many traditional kidney tonics support the adrenal glands as well.

SYMPTOMS OF KIDNEY ENERGY WEAKNESS
• Lower back pain
• Tinnitus or deafness
• Premature greying of the hair
• Exhaustion; impotence or frigidity
• Excess urination
• Wheezing/asthma-like symptoms
• Morning diarrhoea.

BORAGE
Borago officinalis
(see p. 41; pp. 164-5)

Parts used: flowers, leaves.
Actions: stimulates the adrenal cortex, anti-inflammatory, diuretic, cooling *yin* tonic, antidepressive; a cleansing and stimulating herb for the kidneys; also strengthens lung and heart *yin*.
How to use: take an infusion; or take 10 ml juice three times a day or 10 ml tincture three times a day.
Combinations: take the juice as a simple or combine with *he shou wu* or *nu zhen zi*.
Caution: restricted herb in Australia and New Zealand.

BU GU ZHI
Psoralea corylifolia

Parts used: fruit.
Actions: strengthens kidney *yang*, diuretic, astringent, anti-bacterial.
How to use: take a decoction.
Combinations: can be combined with *wu zhu yu*, *wu wei zi*, nutmeg and ginger for early morning diarrhoea associated with kidney weakness.
Caution: can cause photo-sensitivity of the skin.

CINNAMON
Cinnamomum spp. (see p. 48)

Parts used: bark, twigs.
Actions: warming tonic for kidney *yang* and spleen; strengthens digestion.
How to use: take a tincture, decoction, or capsules.
Combinations: use with ginseng or *huang qi* as an energy tonic or *shu di huang* for menstrual irregularities.

DAMIANA
Turnera diffusa
(see pp. 164-5)

Parts used: aerial parts.
Actions: *yang* tonic, aphrodisiac, diuretic, stimulating nervine, mild laxative, urinary antiseptic; good for impotence in men and frigidity in women.
How to use: take 3 ml tincture three times a day or 18 g powdered herb in 500 ml infusion.
Combinations: use with oats as a nerve tonic or *buchu* to warm the kidneys.

HAN LIAN CAO
Eclipta prostrata

Parts used: aerial parts.
Actions: antibacterial, astringent, a *yin* tonic which nourishes the kidneys and liver and stops bleeding; take for heavy menstrual or postpartum bleeding.
How to use: take an infusion or up to 10 ml tincture a day.
Combinations: use with *gotu kola* as a general tonic.

SHI HU
Dendrobium officinale

Parts used: stems.
Actions: *yin* tonic particularly good for the kidney; also strengthens lung and stomach and increases body fluids; cooling; used to nourish *jing* and for dry coughs and fevers; reputedly increases sexual vigour.
How to use: take a tincture or decoction made with 60 g herb to 750 ml water.
Combinations: traditionally Taoists used *shi hu* with liquorice as a general tonic.

TONICS FOR BLOOD & BODY FLUIDS

In Chinese medicine, blood and body fluids are closely linked to *yin* energy and are nourished by herbs that are *yin* in character. Blood deficiency can, of course, be due to anaemia, although Chinese medicine also cites liver disharmony, heart weakness or psychological factors. In Ayurveda, these herbs may be classified as encouraging *kapha* (dampness) and easing symptoms of excess *pitta* (fire) and *vata* (wind), see pp. 12-13.

SYMPTOMS OF BLOOD DEFICIENCY
• Dizziness, vertigo; poor eyesight
• Lethargy, palpitations
• Dry skin, thirst
• Menstrual irregularities
• Pale tongue; pallid face and lips.

DANG GUI
Angelica sinensis
(see p. 36; pp. 150-1; 166-7).

Parts used: root.
Actions: sedative, analgesic, laxative, reduces blood pressure, circulatory stimulant and blood tonic; possibly the single most important tonic herb for women; good for all gynaecological disorders and during the menopause; also a good tonic for men.
How to use: take a tincture or patent tablets; take up to 15 g per dose in a decoction.
Caution: avoid regular or large doses in pregnancy and diabetes.

DI HUANG
Rehmannia glutinosa

Parts used: root.
Actions: demulcent, laxative, stops bleeding; the raw herb (*sheng di huang*) is used as a nourishing and cooling *yin* remedy, while the cooked herb (*shu di huang*) is better to nourish blood and *jing*.
How to use: take up to 10 ml tincture three times a day or up to 15 g per dose in a decoction.
Combinations: use *shu di huang* with *shan zhu yu*, *shan yao* and *gou qi zi* for menopausal problems; *sheng di huang* combines with *qing hao* and *mu dan pi* for *yin* deficiency.

GOU QI ZI
Lycium chinense

Parts used: berries.
Actions: good tonic for the kidneys; stops bleeding and lowers blood sugar.
How to use: take a decoction or tincture; eat dried berries as currants or use in cooking.
Combinations: can be combined with *ju hua* for high blood pressure associated with liver disharmony; use with *he shou wu*, *shu di huang* and *chen pi* for kidney exhaustion linked to overwork or old age.

SHATAVARI
Asparagus racemosus

Parts used: root.
Actions: diuretic, expectorant, demulcent, strengthens the female reproductive system, promotes milk flow; an important *yin* tonic in Eastern medicine used to increase fertility, spiritual awareness and compassion; also strengthens kidney *yin*.
How to use: take a decoction or 200-250 mg powdered root in capsules.

STANDARD REMEDIES
All recipes and doses are standard unless otherwise specified; see *Making Herbal Remedies*, pp. 120-5.

OTHER KIDNEY TONICS

BUCHU (*Barosma betulina*) pp. 158-9; p. 180.
FENUGREEK (*Trigonella foenum-graecum*) p. 106.
HE SHOU WU (*Polygonum multiflorum*) pp. 146-7; 168-9; p. 181.
NU ZHEN ZI (*Ligustrum lucidum*) pp. 168-9; p. 181.
SAW PALMETTO (*Serenoa serrulata*) pp. 158-9; p. 182.

OTHER TONICS FOR BLOOD & BODY FLUIDS

AMALAKI (*Emblica officinalis*) pp. 172-3; p. 180.
BAI SHAO YAO (*Paeonia lactiflora*) p. 83; pp. 166-7.
DA ZAO (*Ziziphus jujuba*) p. 178.
HE SHOU WU (*Polygonum multiflorum*) p. 181.
LING ZHI (*Ganoderma lucidum*) p. 178.
MAI MEN DONG (*Ophiopogon japonicus*) p. 181.
NU ZHEN ZI (*Ligustrum lucidum*) pp. 168-9; p. 181.
PURPLE CONEFLOWER (*Echinacea spp.*) p. 53.
SAN QI (*Panax notoginseng*) p. 84.
SANG SHEN (*Morus alba*) p. 80.
STINGING NETTLE (*Urticaria dioica*) p. 108.

OTHER MEDICINAL HERBS

AMALAKI: *Emblica officinalis*
Parts used: fruit.
Actions: tonic, laxative.

AMERICAN CRANESBILL: *Geranium maculatum*
Parts used: leaves, root.
Actions: astringent, stops external bleeding, tonic.

ANISE: *Pimpinella anisum*
Parts used: essential oil, seeds.
Actions: expectorant, carminative, antiseptic, antispasmodic.

ARBOR VITAE: *Thuja occidentalis*
Parts used: leaf tips.
Actions: astringent, antimicrobial, expels worms, anti-inflammatory, muscle stimulant.
Caution: avoid in pregnancy.

ARNICA: *Arnica montana*
Parts used: flowers.
Actions: heals wounds, immunostimulant.
Caution: do not use on broken skin; use homeopathic *Arnica* internally only.

BAI XIAN PI: *Dictamnus dasycarpus*
Parts used: bark.
Actions: cooling, antibacterial.

BAI ZHU: *Atractylodes macrocephala*
(see **Tonic herbs** pp. 178-9).

BAN XIA: *Pinellia ternata*
Parts used: tuber.
Actions: anti-tussive, expectorant, prevents vomiting, anticatarrhal.

BARBERRY: *Berberis vulgaris*
Parts used: bark, berries, root.
Actions: cooling, antiseptic, anti-inflammatory, bitter.
Caution: avoid in pregnancy.

BAYBERRY: *Myrica cerifera*
Parts used: bark.
Actions: stimulant, astringent, promotes sweating.
Caution: avoid in very "hot" conditions.

BEARBERRY: *Arctostaphylos uva-ursi*
Parts used: leaves.
Actions: urinary antiseptic, astringent.
Caution: high doses may cause nausea.

BENZOIN: *Styrax benzoin*
Parts used: essential oil, gum.
Actions: expectorant, astringent, antispasmodic.

BIRCH: *Betula verrucosa*
Parts used: bark, leaves, sap.
Actions: bitter, astringent, antirheumatic.

BISTORT: *Polygonum bistorta*
Parts used: root.
Actions: astringent, stops diarrhoea and bleeding, anticatarrhal.

BITTER CANDYTUFT: *Iberis amara*
Parts used: aerial parts.
Actions: antispasmodic, relaxant, tonifies the digestive tract, carminative; traditionally used for gout and rheumatism.

BITTERSWEET: *Solanum dulcamara*
Parts used: root bark, twigs.
Actions: antirheumatic, diuretic.
Caution: high doses may cause nausea and palpitations.

BLACK COHOSH: *Cimicifuga racemosa*
Parts used: rhizome.
Actions: diuretic, antirheumatic, anti-inflammatory, sedative, anti-tussive, uterine stimulant.
Caution: avoid in early pregnancy.

BLACK HOREHOUND: *Ballota nigra*
Parts used: aerial parts.
Actions: prevents vomiting, stimulant, antispasmodic.

BLOODROOT: *Sanguinaria canadensis*
Parts used: rhizome.
Actions: expectorant, tonic, antibacterial.
Caution: avoid in pregnancy.

BLUE COHOSH: *Caulophyllum thalictroides*
Parts used: rhizome.
Actions: tonic, antispasmodic, anti-inflammatory, uterine stimulant, diuretic, antirheumatic.
Caution: avoid in early pregnancy.

BLUE FLAG: *Iris versicolor*
Parts used: rhizome.
Actions: anti-inflammatory, diuretic, stimulant, cathartic.

BOGBEAN: *Menyanthes trifoliata*
Parts used: leaves.
Actions: antirheumatic, bitter, tonic.

BOLDO: *Peumus boldo*
Parts used: leaves.
Actions: liver stimulant, diuretic.

BONESET: *Eupatorium perfoliatum*
Parts used: aerial parts.
Actions: promotes sweating, relaxes peripheral blood vessels, laxative, antispasmodic, expectorant, promotes bile flow.
Caution: high doses can cause vomiting.

BROOM: *Cytisus scoparius*
Parts used: flowering tops.
Actions: diuretic, laxative, increases blood pressure, uterine stimulant.
Caution: avoid in pregnancy or if blood pressure is already high; prolonged use can result in liver damage.

BU GU ZHI: *Psoralea corylifolia*
(see **Tonic herbs** pp. 178-9).

BUCHU: *Barosma betulina*
Parts used: leaves.
Actions: diuretic, tonic, urinary antiseptic, promotes sweating.

BUCKWHEAT: *Fagopyrum esculentum*
Parts used: leaves.
Actions: reduces blood pressure, relaxes blood vessels, repairs blood vessel walls.

BURNET: *Sanguisorba officinalis*
Parts used: leaves, root.
Actions: astringent, stops external bleeding, antibacterial, healing.

CALIFORNIAN POPPY: *Eschscholzia californica*
Parts used: aerial parts.
Actions: analgesic, hypnotic, sedative.

CALUMBA: *Jateorhiza palmata*
Parts used: root.
Actions: bitter, carminative, reduces blood pressure.

CANG ER ZI: *Xanthium sibiricum*
Parts used: fruit.
Actions: anticatarrhal, analgesic, antibacterial, antifungal, antispasmodic.
Caution: very high doses can cause a dramatic fall in blood sugar.

CARDAMOM: *Elettaria cardamomum*
Parts used: seeds.
Actions: antispasmodic, carminative, digestive stimulant.

CASCARA SAGRADA: *Rhamnus purshiana*
Parts used: bark.
Actions: digestive tonic, purgative.

CATMINT: *Nepeta cataria*
Parts used: aerial parts.
Actions: antispasmodic, carminative, digestive stimulant, promotes sweating, cooling.

CENTAURY: *Centaurium erythraea*
Parts used: aerial parts.
Actions: bitter, liver stimulant.

CHAI HU: *Bupleurum chinense*
Parts used: root.
Actions: energy tonic, liver stimulant, cooling, antibacterial, anti-inflammatory, analgesic, stimulates bile flow, reduces blood cholesterol levels.

CHASTE-TREE: *Vitex agnus-castus*
Parts used: berries.
Actions: stimulates pituitary gland and hormone production.
Caution: high doses may cause a sensation of ants creeping over the skin (formication).

CHICORY: *Cichorium intybus*
Parts used: root.
Actions: diuretic, laxative, tonic.

CHUAN XIONG: *Ligusticum wallichii*
Parts used: rhizome.
Actions: circulatory stimulant, reduces blood pressure, sedative.

CI JI LI: *Tribulus terrestris*
Parts used: fruit.
Actions: diuretic, reduces blood pressure, liver stimulant.

CLOVES: *Syzygium aromaticum*
Parts used: essential oil, flower buds.
Actions: antiseptic, anodyne, antispasmodic, carminative, stimulant, prevents vomiting.

CORNFLOWER: *Centaurea cyanus*
Parts used: flowers.
Actions: anti-inflammatory, stimulant, tonic.

CORNSILK: *Zea mays*
Parts used: stamens.
Actions: demulcent, diuretic, specifically healing for urinary mucous membranes, tonic.

COUCHGRASS: *Elymus repens*
Parts used: rhizome.
Actions: cleansing diuretic, healing and demulcent.

CYPRESS: *Cupressus sempervirens*
Parts used: essential oil.
Actions: antiseptic, anti-spasmodic, diuretic, sedative.

DA ZAO: *Ziziphus jujuba*
(see **Tonic herbs** pp. 178-9).

DAMIANA: *Turnera diffusa*
(see **Tonic herbs** pp. 178-9).

DANG SHEN: *Codonopsis pilosula*
(see **Tonic herbs** pp. 178-9).

DAN ZHU YE: *Lophatherum gracile*
Parts used: aerial parts.
Actions: diuretic, cooling.

DEVIL'S CLAW: *Harpagophytum procumbens*
Parts used: tuber.
Actions: anti-inflammatory, antirheumatic, analgesic, sedative, diuretic, liver stimulant.

DI GU PI: *Lycium chinense*
Parts used: root bark.
Actions: tonic, lowers blood cholesterol, decreases blood sugar levels.

DI HUANG: *Rehmannia glutinosa*
(see **Tonic herbs** pp. 178-9).

DILL: *Anethum graveolens*
Parts used: seeds.
Actions: carminative.

DU HUO: *Angelica pubescens*
Parts used: root.
Actions: analgesic, anti-inflammatory, antirheumatic.

EVENING PRIMROSE: *Oenothera biennis*
Parts used: seed oil.
Actions: important source of γ-linolenic acid needed for prostaglandin production.

EYEBRIGHT: *Euphrasia officinalis*
Parts used: aerial parts.
Actions: antiseptic, anticatarrhal, anti-inflammatory.

FALSE UNICORN ROOT: *Chamaelirium luteum*
Parts used: rhizome.
Actions: diuretic, causes vomiting, uterine tonic.

FANG FENG: *Ledebouriella seseloides*
Parts used: root.
Actions: antibacterial, promotes sweating, cooling.

FRINGE TREE: *Chionanthus virginicus*
Parts used: root bark.
Actions: promotes bile flow, liver stimulant, diuretic, tonic.

FU LING: *Poria cocos*
(see *Tonic herbs* pp. 178-9).

FUMITORY: *Fumaria officinalis*
Parts used: aerial parts.
Actions: antispasmodic, liver and gall bladder stimulant. ·

GERANIUM: *Pelargonium odorantissimum*
Parts used: essential oil.
Actions: antidepressant, tonic, analgesic, diuretic, sedative.

GLOBE ARTICHOKE: *Cynara scolymus*
Parts used: aerial parts.
Actions: liver tonic and restorative, promotes bile flow.

GOAT'S RUE: *Galega officinalis*
Parts used: aerial parts.
Actions: decreases blood sugar levels, insulin stimulant, promotes milk flow.

GOLDEN ROD: *Solidago virgaurea*
Parts used: aerial parts.
Actions: anticatarrhal, anti-inflammatory, healing, urinary antiseptic, sedative, reduces blood pressure, promotes sweating.

GOTU KOLA: *Hydrocotyle asiatica*
Parts used: aerial parts.
Actions: diuretic, sedating nervine, cooling, tonic.
Caution: high doses can cause headaches or aggravate itching.

GOU QI ZI: *Lycium chinense*
(see *Tonic herbs* pp. 178-9).

GREATER CELANDINE: *Chelidonium majus*
Parts used: aerial parts.
Actions: anti-inflammatory, liver stimulant, diuretic, cleansing.
Caution: avoid in pregnancy.

GREATER PERIWINKLE: *Vinca major*
Parts used: aerial parts.
Actions: astringent, sedative.

GROUND IVY: *Glechoma hederacea*
Parts used: leaves.
Actions: astringent, anticatarrhal.

GUMPLANT: *Grindelia camporum*
Parts used: aerial parts.
Actions: expectorant, antispasmodic, reduces heart rate.
Caution: avoid in low blood pressure; high doses can irritate kidneys.

HAN LIAN CAO: *Eclipta prostrata*
(see *Tonic herbs* p. 178-9).

HE SHOU WU: *Polygonum multiflorum*
Parts used: tuber.
Actions: tonic, antispasmodic, antibacterial, laxative.

HERB ROBERT: *Geranium robertianum*
Parts used: leaves.
Actions: astringent, stops external bleeding.

HOLY THISTLE: *Cnicus benedictus*
Parts used: aerial parts.
Actions: bitter, antiseptic, expectorant, heals wounds.

HORSE CHESTNUT: *Aesculus hippocastanum*
Parts used: bark, seeds.
Actions: astringent, anti-inflammatory.
Caution: seed coating can be toxic, so peel if making large quantities of herbal remedies.

HUAI JIAO: *Sophora japonica*
Parts used: fruit.
Actions: laxative, stops bleeding.
Caution: avoid in pregnancy.

HUAI NIU XI: *Achyranthes bidentata*
Parts used: root.
Actions: circulatory stimulant, analgesic, liver tonic.

HUANG LIAN: *Coptis chinensis*
Parts used: root.
Actions: antibacterial, analgesic, anti-inflammatory, promotes bile flow, sedative.

HUANG QI: *Astragalus membranaceus*
Parts used: rhizome.
Actions: immunostimulant, antimicrobial, cardiotonic, diuretic.
Caution: avoid if condition involves excessive "heat" or *yin* deficiency (see pp. 178-9).

HUO MA REN: *Cannabis sativa*
Parts used: seeds.
Actions: stimulating laxative.

HYDRANGEA: *Hydrangea arborescens*
Parts used: rhizome/root.
Actions: diuretic, kidney stimulant, laxative.

ICELAND MOSS: *Chondrus crispus*
Parts used: lichen.
Actions: demulcent, expectorant, prevents vomiting, nutritive.

INDIAN TOBACCO: *Lobelia inflata*
Parts used: aerial parts.
Actions: relaxant, antispasmodic, causes vomiting, expectorant, promotes sweating, anti-asthmatic.
Caution: Indian tobacco is restricted in the UK; use only under the guidance of a qualified practitioner. Available from pharmacies only in Australia and New Zealand.

JAMAICAN DOGWOOD: *Piscidia erythrina*
Parts used: root bark.
Actions: anodyne, sedative.
Caution: do not exceed stated dose.

JIE GENG: *Platycodon grandiflorus*
Parts used: root.
Actions: antibacterial, antifungal, expectorant, lowers blood sugar.

JU HUA: *Chrysanthemum morifolium*
Parts used: flowers.
Actions: anti-inflammatory, antimicrobial, cooling, reduces blood pressure.

KING'S CLOVER: *Melilotus officinalis*
Parts used: flowering aerial parts.
Actions: antispasmodic, anticoagulant, demulcent, diuretic.
Caution: do not use with warfarin or other blood-thinning drugs, or with any blood-clotting problem.

LADY'S SLIPPER: *Cypripedium calceolus*
Parts used: rhizome.
Actions: analgesic, restoring nervine, sedative.

LEMON: *Citrus limon*
Parts used: essential oil, fruit.
Actions: antihistaminic, anti-inflammatory, diuretic, venous tonic.
Caution: ensure essential oil is well diluted before use – it can irritate the skin.

LIAN QIAO: *Forsythia suspensa*
Parts used: fruit.
Actions: antibacterial, anti-inflammatory, cooling.
Caution: avoid in diarrhoea or *yin* deficiency.

LIGNUM VITAE: *Guaiacum officinalis*
Parts used: heartwood.
Actions: anti-inflammatory, antirheumatic, circulatory stimulant.

LILY-OF-THE-VALLEY: *Convallaria majalis*
Parts used: aerial parts, leaves.
Actions: heart tonic, diuretic, purgative, causes vomiting.
Caution: restricted in the UK, Australia and New Zealand; use only under the guidance of a qualified practitioner.

LINDEN: *Tilia europaea*
Parts used: flowers.
Actions: sedating nervine, promotes sweating, relaxes blood vessels, healing for blood vessel walls.

LING ZHI: *Ganoderma lucidum*
(see *Tonic herbs* pp. 178-9).

LOOSESTRIFE: *Lythrum salicaria*
Parts used: aerial parts.
Actions: astringent, antibacterial, lymphatic cleanser, heals wounds.

LOVAGE: *Levisticum officinale*
Parts used: root, seeds.
Actions: carminative, promotes sweating, warming digestive tonic, expectorant, anticatarrhal, diuretic.

LUO SHI TENG: *Trachelospermum jasminoides*
Parts used: leafy stems.
Actions: anti-rheumatic, antibacterial, antispasmodic, cooling.

MADDER: *Rubia tinctorum*
Parts used: root.
Actions: antispasmodic, diuretic.

MAI MEN DONG: *Ophiopogon japonicus*
Parts used: tuber.
Actions: promotes secretion of body fluids, tonic, sedative, antitussive, lowers blood sugar levels, antibacterial.

MARSH CUDWEED: *Gnaphthalium uliginosum*
Parts used: aerial parts.
Actions: anticatarrhal, anti-inflammatory, astringent, tonifying to mucous membranes.

MILK THISTLE: *Carduus marianus*
Parts used: aerial parts, seeds.
Actions: liver tonic and stimulant, promotes milk flow, demulcent, antidepressant.

MISTLETOE: *Viscum album*
Parts used: young leafy twigs.
Actions: reduces blood pressure, slows heart rate, anti-tumour.
Caution: do not use berries, which are toxic and restricted in the UK; avoid in pregnancy.

MOUSE-EAR HAWKWEED: *Hieracium pilosella*
Parts used: aerial parts.
Actions: anticatarrhal, antispasmodic, diuretic, expectorant, heals wounds.

MU TONG: *Akebia trifoliata*
Parts used: stems.
Actions: diuretic, promotes milk flow, anti-inflammatory.

NU ZHEN ZI: *Ligustrum lucidum*
Parts used: berries.
Actions: tonic, immunostimulant, diuretic.

OAK: *Quercus robur*
Parts used: bark.
Actions: strong astringent.

OREGON GRAPE: *Berberis aquifolium*
Parts used: rhizome, root.
Actions: cleansing, stops diarrhoea, promotes bile flow, tonic.
Caution: avoid in pregnancy.

PARSLEY PIERT: *Aphanes arvensis*
Parts used: aerial parts.
Actions: demulcent, diuretic.

PASQUE FLOWER: *Anemone pulsatilla*
Parts used: aerial parts.
Actions: antispasmodic, sedating nervine.
Caution: use only the dried plant.

PASSIONFLOWER: *Passiflora incarnata*
Parts used: leaves.
Actions: sedative, anodyne, hypnotic, antispasmodic.
Caution: avoid high doses in pregnancy.

PATCHOULI: *Pogostemon patchouli*
Parts used: essential oil.
Actions: antidepressant, aphrodisiac, sedative, tonic.

PELLITORY-OF-THE-WALL: *Parietaria diffusa*
Parts used: aerial parts.
Actions: demulcent, diuretic, soothing for urinary mucous membranes.

PILEWORT: *Ranunculus ficaria*
Parts used: root, leaves.
Actions: astringent, used for haemorrhoids.
Caution: do not take internally.

PILL-BEARING SPURGE: *Euphorbia pilulifera*
Parts used: aerial parts.
Actions: anti-asthmatic, anticatarrhal, antispasmodic, expectorant.
Caution: do not combine with liquorice.

PRICKLY ASH: *Zanthoxylum americanum*
Parts used: bark.
Actions: carminative, circulatory stimulant, promotes sweating, tonic.

QING HAO: *Artemisia annua*
Parts used: aerial parts.
Actions: anti-malarial, cooling, antimicrobial.

QUASSIA: *Picrasma excelsa*
Parts used: wood.
Actions: expels worms, bitter.

RAMSOMS: *Allium ursinum*
Parts used: aerial parts, bulbs.
Actions: decreases blood sugar levels, lowers serum cholesterol, antimicrobial.

RUE: *Ruta graveolens*
Parts used: leaves.
Actions: antispasmodic, anti-tussive, promotes menstrual flow, lowers blood pressure, circulatory tonic.
Caution: avoid in pregnancy.

SAFFLOWER: *Carthamus tinctorius*
Parts used: flowers.
Actions: laxative, diuretic, anti-inflammatory.

SANDALWOOD: *Santalum album*
Parts used: essential oil.
Actions: antidepressant, antiseptic, antispasmodic, carminative, expectorant, sedative, tonic.

SAW PALMETTO: *Serenoa serrulata*
Parts used: berries.
Actions: aphrodisiac, tonic, diuretic, urinary antiseptic.

SENNA: *Cassia senna*
Parts used: leaves.
Actions: stimulating laxative.

SHAN ZHU YU: *Cornus officinalis*
Parts used: fruit.
Actions: tonic, diuretic, reduces blood pressure, antimicrobial.

SHATAVARI: *Asparagus racemosus*
(see *Tonic herbs* pp. 178-9).

SHENG DI HUANG: (see *Di huang* p. 179).

SHI HU: *Dendrobium officinale*
(see *Tonic herbs* pp. 178-9).

SHU DI HUANG: (see *Di huang* p. 179).

SIBERIAN GINSENG: *Eleutherococcus senticosus*
(see *Tonic herbs* pp. 178-9).

SILVERWEED: *Potentilla anserina*
Parts used: aerial parts.
Actions: anticatarrhal, anti-inflammatory, astringent, diuretic.

SLIPPERY ELM: *Ulmus fulva*
Parts used: bark.
Actions: demulcent, nutritive, astringent.

SOAP BARK: *Quillaja saponaria*
Parts used: inner bark.
Actions: detergent, expectorant, anti-inflammatory.
Caution: do not take internally.

SOUTHERNWOOD: *Artemisia abrotanum*
Parts used: aerial parts.
Actions: expels worms, antiseptic, bitter, uterine stimulant.
Caution: avoid in pregnancy.

SPINY RESTHARROW: *Ononis spinosa*
Parts used: root.
Actions: diuretic, expectorant, metabolic stimulant, sedative.

SQUAW VINE: *Mitchella repens*
Parts used: aerial parts.
Actions: astringent, diuretic, tonic, restorative, uterine stimulant.

SWEET FLAG: *Acorus calamus*
Parts used: rhizome.
Actions: carminative, antispasmodic, promotes sweating.
Caution: use restricted in Australia and New Zealand.

SWEET SUMACH: *Rhus aromatica*
Parts used: root bark.
Actions: astringent, diuretic, tonic, antidiabetic.

TEA TREE: *Melaleuca alternifolia*
Parts used: essential oil.
Actions: antibacterial, antifungal, antiseptic.

TORMENTIL: *Potentilla erecta*
Parts used: root.
Actions: astringent – especially for gut wall.

TRUE UNICORN ROOT: *Aletris farinosa*
Parts used: rhizome.
Actions: digestive stimulant, tonic.

WAHOO: *Euonymus atropurpureus*
Parts used: bark/root bark.
Actions: liver stimulant, promotes bile flow.

WALL GERMANDER: *Teucrium chamaedrys*
Parts used: aerial parts.
Actions: anticatarrhal, antimicrobial, digestive stimulant, anti-inflammatory.
Caution: recent research suggests that long term use may cause liver damage; do not exceed stated dose.

WEI LING XIAN: *Clematis chinensis*
Parts used: rhizome/root.
Actions: analgesic, antibacterial, antirheumatic.

WHITE BRYONY: *Bryonia alba*
Parts used: root.
Actions: antirheumatic, cathartic.

WHITE DEADNETTLE: *Lamium album*
Parts used: flowering tops.
Actions: astringent, tonic for reproductive organs, antispasmodic.

WHITE HOREHOUND: *Marrubium vulgare*
Parts used: aerial parts.
Actions: antispasmodic, stimulating expectorant, bitter, soothing tonic for the mucous membranes.

WILD CARROT: *Daucus carota*
Parts used: aerial parts.
Actions: carminative, diuretic, urinary antiseptic.

WILD CHERRY: *Prunus serotina*
Parts used: bark.
Actions: anti-tussive, digestive stimulant, sedative.
Caution: avoid in acute infections; can cause drowsiness.

WILD INDIGO: *Baptisia tinctoria*
Parts used: leaves, root.
Actions: antibacterial, antiseptic, laxative, cooling.
Caution: do not exceed stated dose; high doses may cause vomiting.

WILD LETTUCE: *Lactuca virosa*
Parts used: leaves.
Actions: hypnotic, sedative, decreases blood sugar levels.
Caution: may cause drowsiness; do not drive or operate machinery; excess doses may cause insomnia or increased sex drive.

WITCH HAZEL: *Hamamelis virginiana*
Parts used: bark, leaves.
Actions: astringent, sedative, tonic.

WOOD SAGE: *Teucrium scorodonia*
Parts used: aerial parts.
Actions: astringent, antirheumatic, carminative, heals wounds, promotes sweating, promotes bile flow.

WOUNDWORT: *Stachys palustris*
Parts used: aerial parts.
Actions: antispasmodic, antiseptic, heals wounds.

WU WEI ZI: *Schisandra chinensis*
(see *Tonic herbs*, pp. 178-9).

WU ZHU YU: *Evodia rutaecarpa*
Parts used: fruit.
Actions: analgesic, antibacterial, warming, stimulant.

XIANG FU: *Cyperus rotundus*
Parts used: tuber.
Actions: carminative, analgesic, uterine antispasmodic, encourages *qi* (energy) flow.

XIN YI: *Magnolia liliflora*
Parts used: flowers, flowerbuds.
Actions: anticatarrhal, antifungal, analgesic, anti-inflammatory for the nasal mucous membranes, warming.
Caution: high doses can cause dizziness.

XING REN: *Prunus armeniaca*
Parts used: seeds, nuts.
Actions: anti-tussive, expectorant, laxative.

YELLOW DOCK: *Rumex crispus*
Parts used: root.
Actions: cleansing, promotes bile flow, strong laxative.

YELLOW JASMINE: *Gelsemium sempervirens*
Parts used: root.
Actions: analgesic, reduces blood pressure, sedative, eases neuralgia.
Caution: use is restricted in the UK, Australia and New Zealand; use only as prescribed – overdose can cause nausea and double vision.

ZE XIE: *Alisma plantago*
Parts used: rhizome.
Actions: diuretic, reduces blood pressure, antibacterial, liver cleanser.

ZHI ZI: *Gardenia jasminoides*
Parts used: fruit.
Actions: cooling, reduces blood pressure, sedative, antibacterial.

CONSULTING A HERBALIST

MANY PEOPLE REGULARLY use herbs as safe and effective home remedies for minor ailments, but persistent or serious problems need professional help from a qualified herbal practitioner. Choosing someone with whom you feel empathy and whom you can trust can be just as important in treatment as taking the most appropriate herbs. The best way to find a practitioner is through personal recommendation from a like-minded friend. Alternatively,

ask the national regulatory body (see p. 192) for a list of herbalists practising in your area. You can consult a herbalist about a wide range of health problems: aches and pains, high blood pressure, urinary dysfunction, digestive ailments, menstrual disorders, asthma or bronchitis, skin complaints, nervous disorders, even chronic conditions for which herbalism is often seen as the last resort, such as rheumatoid arthritis, ME or emphysema.

WHO ARE THE HERBALISTS?
National practices and regulations vary dramatically. In China, traditional herbal medicine is available in special hospitals as an alternative to Western medicine, while in Japan herbal remedies are available as part of the mainstream health system.

In France, herbal practitioners are almost always medical doctors or phytotherapists who have studied plant medicine at postgraduate level. In Germany, alternative practitioners qualify as *Heilpraktiker* (licensed naturopathic healers) and have comparable status to orthodox medical practitioners; even orthodox practitioners are just as likely to prescribe a plant remedy as they are a pharmaceutical drug. In many eastern European medical schools the study of herbal remedies remains an important part of the student curriculum.

Britain has a well-established system for training herbal practitioners, who have not necessarily obtained any other medical qualification. The National Institute of Medical Herbalists was founded in 1864. Members qualify by examination after four or five years of specialist study. Students from many countries attend courses run by the School of Phytotherapy in Britain and Institute members are now spread – albeit thinly – around the globe. Members use the initials MNIMH or FNIMH after their names.

In Australia, trained herbalists become full members of the National Herbalists Association of Australia and use the initials NHAA after their names. They are classified as Health Care

Professionals by the Commonwealth government.

In other parts of the world, including some states in the USA, it is illegal for anyone to prescribe herbal remedies or set themselves up as a herbal practitioner; yet self-medication with herbs is permitted. Elsewhere, just about anyone, trained or not, can set up in business as a medical herbalist and dispense all manner of "cures", whether or not they might be appropriate.

WHAT THE HERBALIST DOES
Consulting a herbalist is not all that different from consulting a family doctor – or rather, as visiting a doctor might have been forty or fifty years ago. Indeed, many herbalists compare their approach to that of an old-fashioned physician: they listen patiently, ask questions to uncover relevant symptoms and use time-honoured diagnostic techniques such as feeling the pulse, looking at the tongue, looking at the retina, listening to chest wheezes, palpating the abdomen to identify causes of pain, or checking reflexes. Simple on-site clinical tests may include urine analysis or measuring haemoglobin levels from a tiny drop of blood. They look into a patient's medical history as well as reviewing the current illness, asking about family tendencies, allergies, diet, lifestyle, stresses and worries.

If a patient is already taking orthodox medication the herbalist needs to know. Herbalists would certainly not recommend ceasing to take vital drugs, but any incompatibility with herbal remedies must be considered. Indeed, many

patients turn to herbs because they wish to phase out pharmaceutical drugs, for whatever reason, and a safe programme of replacing them with gentler herbal remedies needs to be devised (preferably with the support and cooperation of the patient's regular doctor). Herbal remedies can be helpful for sufferers trying to break an addiction to tranquillizers or sleeping pills, for example, or can be an alternative for those suffering side effects from non-steroidal anti-inflammatory drugs for arthritis.

Some herbalists follow a semi-orthodox path, prescribing herbal remedies to ease symptoms just as modern drugs do, while others focus on holistic treatments urging major lifestyle changes. There may be advice about foods to avoid or eat more of, recommended relaxation routines, or Bach flower remedies to help emotional factors affecting physical well-being.

The first consultation generally takes at least an hour, and subsequent ones about 20 minutes or so. Herbalists like to see patients soon after the first consultation to check on progress – perhaps after a few weeks – then follow this up with regular meetings every four to six weeks for three months, or more in chronic cases. The herbal medication is likely to be altered slightly after each consultation to reflect changes in the condition.

At the end of the consultation, the herbalist makes up a prescription, based on tinctures, creams, oils, powders, capsules or dried herbs. Whatever the remedy, healing is a two-way process and patients must take responsibility for their own health and actively participate in any cure.

GLOSSARY

ADRENAL CORTEX Part of the adrenal gland, which produces corticosteroid hormones.

ALKALOID Highly active plant constituent, containing nitrogen atoms usually in a ring-shaped molecule.

ALTERATIVE Cleansing, stimulating efficient removal of waste products.

ANALGESIC Relieves pain.

ANODYNE Allays pain.

ANTIBIOTIC Destroys or inhibits the growth of micro-organisms.

ANTICOAGULANT Hinders blood-clotting.

ANTIHYDROTIC Limits the production of water-based fluids including sweat.

ANTIMICROBIAL Destroys micro-organisms.

ANTISPASMODIC Reduces muscle spasm and tension.

ANTI-TUSSIVE Inhibits the cough reflex helping to stop coughing.

APERIENT Mild laxative.

ASTRINGENT Precipitates proteins from the surface of cells or mucous membranes, producing a protective coating; has a binding and contracting effect.

AYURVEDIC Traditional system of Indian medicine, which literally means "a science of life".

BITTER Stimulates secretion of digestive juices and encourages appetite.

BLACK BILE One of the four Galenical (*q.v.*) humours (*q.v.*) associated with the earth element and considered cold and dry.

BLOOD Apart from the familiar substance, "blood" was one of the four Galenical (*q.v.*) humours (*q.v.*) associated with the air element and considered hot and damp.

BLOOD STAGNATION Concept in traditional Chinese medicine where the blood circulation is retarded or where blood vessels become blocked for any reason. Considered to interfere with the normal flow of *qi* (*q.v.*) through the body.

BULK LAXATIVE Increases the volume of faeces, producing larger, softer stools.

CARDIOACTIVE Affecting heart function.

CARMINATIVE Relieves flatulence, digestive colic and gastric discomfort.

CATHARTIC Drastic purgative (*q.v.*).

CHAKRA Centre or point of spiritual power and energy in the body.

CHANNEL See *meridian*.

CHOLAGOGUE Stimulates bile flow from the gall bladder and bile ducts into the duodenum.

CHOLERETIC Increases secretion of bile by the liver.

CHOLERIC Galenical (*q.v.*) temperament related to yellow bile (*q.v.*).

CIRCULATORY STIMULANT Increases blood flow.

COLD CONDITIONS Concept in traditional Chinese medicine associated with chills, poor circulation, thirst for hot drinks, feeling cold, fatigue, sharp pain, frequent urination or *yang* (*q.v.*) deficiency.

COLIC Spasmodic pain affecting smooth muscle, for example in the guts, gall bladder or urinary tract.

COUMARIN Active plant constituent, generally smelling of new mown hay, which encourages blood-clotting.

DEMULCENT Softens and soothes damaged or inflamed surfaces, such as the gastric mucous membranes.

DIURETIC Encourages urine flow.

DOCTRINE OF SIGNATURES Theory that the appearance of a plant indicates its inherent medicinal properties.

ECLECTIC System of herbal medicine developed in the United States in the 19th century.

EMETIC Causes vomiting.

EMOLLIENT Softens and soothes the skin.

ESSENTIAL OIL Commercially available volatile oil extracted from plants by steam distillation and containing a mixture of active constituents; highly aromatic.

EXPECTORANT Encourages the loosening and removal of phlegm from the respiratory tract.

FEBRIFUGE Reduces fever.

GALENICAL Traditional system of Western medicine based on the four humours (*q.v.*) theory of Ancient Greece.

GLYCOSIDE Active plant constituent containing one or more sugar groups.

HOT CONDITIONS Concept in traditional Chinese medicine associated with fevers, increased metabolic rate, thirst for cold drinks, increased heat sensitivity, irritability, burning pains, thick catarrh or *yin* (*q.v.*) deficiency.

HUMOUR Theoretical body fluid important in Galenical (*q.v.*) and Ayurvedic (*q.v.*) medicine.

HYPERTENSION High blood pressure.

HYPOTENSION Low blood pressure.

IMMUNOSTIMULANT Enhances and increases the body's immune (defence) mechanism.

JING The "vital essence" of traditional Chinese medicine responsible for creative and reproductive energies and stored in the kidneys.

KAPHA Ayurvedic (*q.v.*) humour (*q.v.*) associated with dampness or phlegm (*q.v.*).

LAXATIVE Encourages bowel motions.

MELANCHOLIC Galenical (*q.v.*) state related to black bile (*q.v.*).

MERIDIAN In Chinese medicine, a conduit which can be compared to an imaginary line (or channel) linking points on the body's surface with internal organs in which *qi* (*q.v.*) flows. Traditional Chinese medicine defines 14 main channels and eight extra channels. The surface points are used in acupuncture.

MUCILAGE Complex sugar molecules that are soft and slippery and protect mucous membranes and inflamed tissues.

NARCOTIC Causes stupor and numbness.

NERVINE Affects the nervous system – may be stimulating, sedating or relaxing.

NEURALGIA Pain along a nerve.

PERIPHERAL CIRCULATION Blood supply to limbs, skin and muscles (including heart muscle).

PHLEGM In modern Western medicine similar to catarrh or sputum; Galenical (*q.v.*) humour (*q.v.*) associated with the water element and considered cold and damp; *kapha* (*q.v.*); associated with spleen deficiency in traditional Chinese medicine.

PHLEGMATIC Galenical (*q.v.*) state related to phlegm (*q.v.*).

PHYSIOMEDICALISM System of herbal medicine developed in the United States in the 19th century.

PITTA Ayurvedic (*q.v.*) humour (*q.v.*) associated with fire or bile.

PROSTAGLANDINS Hormone-like substances that have a wide range of functions, including acting as chemical messengers and causing uterine contractions.

PURGATIVE Drastic laxative.

QI (CH'I) In Chinese medicine the body's vital energy.

RUBEFACIENT Stimulates blood flow to the skin, causing local reddening.

SANGUINE Galenical (*q.v.*) state related to blood (*q.v.*).

SAPONINS Active plant constituents, similar to soap, producing a lather in water; can irritate the digestive tract; expectorant; some chemically resemble steroidal hormones.

SEDATIVE Soothing and calming.

SIMPLE A single herb used on its own.

STEROIDS Group of chemicals with a characteristic multi-ring molecular structure. Naturally-occurring steroids include the sex hormones and adrenaline.

STYPTIC Stops external bleeding.

SYSTEMIC Affecting the entire body.

TANNIN Active plant constituents which combine with proteins; originally derived from plants used for tanning leather; astringent (*q.v.*).

TERPENE Complex active plant constituents with a carbon ring structure, generally highly aromatic and included in essential oil (*q.v.*).

TONIC Restoring, nourishing and supporting for the entire body.

TONIFY Strengthen and restore.

TOPICAL Local administration of herbal remedy, e.g. to the skin or eye; effect herb has in local treatment.

VASOCONSTRICTOR Reduces the diameter of blood vessels.

VASODILATOR Increases the diameter of blood vessels.

VATA Ayurvedic (*q.v.*) humour (*q.v.*) associated with wind or air.

VENOUS RETURN Blood flow from the extremities through the veins back to the heart.

VULNERARY Heals wounds.

WEI QI Concept in Chinese medicine of defence energy, comparable with the immune system.

YANG Aspect of being equated with male energy – dry, hot, ascending, exterior.

YELLOW BILE Galenical (*q.v.*) humour (*q.v.*) associated with the fire element and considered hot and dry; *pitta* (*q.v.*).

YIN Aspect of being equated with female energy – damp, cold, descending, interior.

BIBLIOGRAPHY

HERBS PAST & PRESENT

ORIGINS OF WESTERN HERBALISM:
Dioscorides: *De Materia Medica*, ed. R T Gunther, Oxford University Press, 1934.
Gerard, John: *The Herball or Generall Historie of Plantes*, John Norton, London, 1597.
Grieve, Maud: *A Modern Herbal*, Jonathan Cape, 1931.
Griggs, Barbara: *Green Pharmacy*, Jill Norman & Hobhouse, London, 1981.
The Herbal Remedies of the Physicians of Myddfai (*Meddygon Myddfai*) trans. John Pughe, Llanerch Enterprises, Lampeter, 1987.
Paracelsus: *Paracelsus – Selected Writings*, ed. Jolande Jacobi, Princeton University Press, 1988.
Manniche, Lise: *An Ancient Egyptian Herbal*, British Museum Publications, London, 1989.
Mills, Simon Y: *Out of the Earth*, Viking, London, 1991.
Morris, Brian: "The rise and fall of Victorian herbalism" in *Herbs*, 15(3), 1990.
Pliny: *Natural History*, Harvard University Press, 1956.
Rohde, Eleanour Sinclair: *The Old English Herbals*, Longmans Green & Co, London, 1922.
Siraisi, Nancy: *Medieval and Early Renaissance Medicine*, University of Chicago Press, 1990.
Theophrastus: *Enquiry into Plants*, 2 vols, Harvard University Press, 1916.
Tierra, Michael: *Planetary Herbology*, Lotus Press, Santa Fe, 1988.
Turner, William: *A New Herball*, 1551; facsimile ed. George Chapman and Marilyn Tweddle, Carcanet Press, 1989.
Valnet, Jean: *Se Soigner par les Légumes, les Fruits et les Céréales*, Librairie Maloine, Paris, 1967.

A SCIENCE OF LIFE: Donden, Yeshi: *Health through Balance*, Snow Lion, Ithaca, 1986.
Frawley, David: *Ayurvedic Healing*, Passage Press, Salt Lake City, 1989.
Frawley, David & Lad, Vasant: *The Yoga of Herbs: An Ayurvedic Guide to Herbal Medicine*, Lotus Press, Santa Fe, 1988.
Heyn, Birgit: *Ayurvedic Medicine*, Thorsons, London, 1987.
Svoboda, Robert E: *Ayurveda – Life, Health and Longevity*, Arkana, London, 1992.

CHINESE HERBAL MEDICINE: Beinfield, Harriet & Korngold, Efrem: *Between Heaven and Earth: A Guide to Chinese Medicine*, Ballantine Books, New York, 1991.
Kaptchuk, Ted: *Chinese Medicine – the Web that has no Weaver*, Rider, London, 1983.
Lu, Henry C: *Chinese System of Food Cures*, Sterling, New York, 1986.
Teeguarden, Ron: *Chinese Tonic Herbs*, Japan Publications, Tokyo, 1984.
The Yellow Emperor's Classic of Internal Medicine, trans. Ilza Veith, University of California Press, 1966.

NORTH AMERICAN TRADITIONS: Coffin, Albert: *A Botanic Guide to Health*, London, 1866.
Moerman, Daniel E: *Medicinal Plants of North America*, University of Michigan, Museum of Anthropology.
Thomson, Samuel: *A Narrative of the Life and Medical Discoveries of Samuel Thomson*, Boston, 1825.
Vogel, Virgil: *American Indian Medicine*, University of Oklahoma Press, 1970.

A–Z OF MEDICINAL HERBS

Bensky, Dan & Gamble, Andrew: *Chinese Herbal Medicine Materia Medica*, Eastland Press, Seattle, 1986.
Hoffman, David: *The Holistic Herbal*, Findhorn Press, 1983.
Holmes, Peter: *The Energetics of Western Herbs*, Artemis Press, Boulder, 1989.
Leung, Albert: *Chinese Herbal Remedies*, Wildwood House, London, 1985.
Mills, Simon Y: *A Dictionary of Modern Herbalism*, Thorsons, Wellingborough, 1985.
Priest, A W & Priest, L R: *Herbal Medication: a Clinical and Dispensary Handbook*, Fowler, London, 1982.
Stuart, Malcolm: *The Encyclopaedia of Herbs and Herbalism*, Orbis, London, 1979.
Valnet, Jean: *Phytotherapy*, Librairie Maloine, Paris, 1972.
Weiss, R F: *Herbal Medicine*, Beaconsfield Publishers, Beaconsfield, 1988.
Wren, R C: *Potter's New Cyclopaedia of Botanical Drugs and Preparations*, C W Daniel, Saffron Walden, 1988.
Yeung, Him-che: *Handbook of Chinese Herbs and Formulas*, Institute of Chinese Medicine, Los Angeles, 1985.

ALLIUM SATIVUM: review, 2nd International Garlic Symposium, in *Cardiology in Practice*, supplement, June 1991; Abdullah, T H et al: *Journal of the National Medical Association*, 80(4), 1988: 439-45.

AVENA SATIVA: Journal of the American Medical Association, 265(14), 1991: 1833-9.

CAMELLIA SINENSIS: Muramatsu, K, Fukuyo, M & Hara, Y: *Journal of Nutrition, Science and Vitaminology*, 32, 1986: 613-22; Chow, Kit & Kramer, Ione: *All the Tea in China*, China Books, 1990.

EUCALYPTUS GLOBULUS: Russian 1973 research, quoted in Tisserand, Robert: *The Art of Aromatherapy*, 2nd ed., C W Daniel, Saffron Walden, 1985.

EUPATORIUM CANNABIUM: Archivum Immunologine et Therapiae Experimentalis, 23, 1975: 846; "Anti-tumour properties of eupatoriopicrin", in *Planta Medica*, 1986: 430, quoted in Rombi, M: *Phytotherapy: A practical handbook of herbal medicine for the practitioner*, Herbal Health Publishers.

GINKGO BILOBA: European Journal of Pharmacy, 164, 1989: 293-302; *Herbalgram*, No 7, 1985: 5; ibid. No 15, 1988: 12; ibid. No 22, 1990: 21.

LINUM SPP: Erasmus, Udo: *Fats and Oils*, Alive Books, Vancouver, 1986.

PANAX GINSENG: "Ginseng caused androgynous baby", in *General Practitioner* 1991, Jan 11: 20; Fulder, S: *The Tao of Medicine*, Destiny Books, New York, 1982.

SALVIA OFFICINALIS: Svoboda, K P & Deans, S G: review, 21st International Symposium on Essential Oils, Lahti, Finland, 1990.

SYMPHYTUM OFFICINALIS: Furuya, T & Asaki, K: *Chemical & Pharmacology Bulletin*, 16(12), 1968: 2512-16; Taylor, A & Taylor, N C: *Proceedings of the Society of Experimental and Biological Medicine*, 114, 1963: 772-4.

TRIGONELLA FOENUM-GRAECUM: Hepper, F Nigel: *Pharaoh's Herbs*, HMSO, London, 1990; Atiya, Nayra: *Khul-Khaal: Five Egyptian Women Tell Their Stories*, American University in Cairo Press, 1984; *European Journal of Clinical Nutrition* 44, 1990: 301-6;

Bailey, C J & Day, C: *Diabetes Care*, 12(8), 1989: 553-64.

TUSSILAGO FARFARA: Flock, A et al: Department of Pharmacognosy, University of Uppsala, 1976, quoted in Mabey, R: *The Complete New Herbal*, Elm Tree Books, London, 1988; Kerry, Bone: "Coltsfoot – is it safe?" in *British Journal of Phytotherapy*, 1(3/4), 1990: 32-5.

HERBAL REMEDIES

ACHES & PAINS: Pinget, M & Lecomte, A: "The effects of *Harpagophytum* arkocelules in degenerative rheumatology", Arkopharma, France, 1988.

RESPIRATORY PROBLEMS: For research on *cang er zi*, see: Wang, Xindong: *Journal of Beijing College of TCM*, 10(2), 1987: 26. Translated abstract in *Traditional Chinese Medicine Digest*, II(3/4), 1987: 100-1.

SKIN: For Chinese herbal remedies in childhood eczema, see: *The Lancet*, 1990, 31 Mar: 335, 795.

EARS, EYES, MOUTH & THROAT: For milk allergy and otitis media, see: *Journal of Allergy and Clinical Immunology* 83(1), 1989: 239.

HEART: For oat bran and cholesterol, see: *Journal of the American Medical Association*, 1991, Jul-Aug: 20; *American Journal of Clinical Nutrition*, 52(3), 1990: 495-9; For other herbs and cholesterol see: *European Journal of Clinical Nutrition*, 44, 1990: 79-88.

DIGESTIVE PROBLEMS: Okpanyi, S N et al: "Gastrointestinal motility modulation with Iberogast", paper presented at First World Conference on Medicinal and Aromatic Plants for Human Welfare, Maastricht, 19-25 July 1992, in press.

GYNAECOLOGICAL PROBLEMS: Parvati, Jeannine: *Hygieia: A Woman's Herbal*, Wildwood House, London, 1979.
Shuttle, Penelope & Redgrave, Peter: *The Wise Wound: Menstruation and Everywoman*, Paladin Grafton Books, London, 1986; For use of the "free and easy" formula for moving liver *qi* in treating PMS, see: Jiang, Zhaojun: *Journal of Shandong College of TCM*, 10(1), 1986: 22, translated in *Traditional Chinese Medicine Digest* 1(3), 1986: 54, and *The Handbook of Traditional Chinese Gynecology*, Blue Poppy Press, 1987: 47.

PREGNANCY & CHILDBIRTH: McIntyre, Anne: *Herbs for Pregnancy and Childbirth*, Sheldon Press, London, 1988.
Weed, Susan S: *Wise Woman Herbal for the Childbearing Year*, Ash Tree Publishing, New York, 1986.

URINARY SYSTEM: Murray, Michael T: "Serenoa repens treatment of benign prostatic hyperplasia", in *Journal of the American Quack Association*, 4(4), 1989: J2-3.

NERVOUS SYSTEM: For aromatic chemicals and the olfactory nerve, see: Forster, H, Niklas, H & Lutz, S, in *Planta Medica*, 40 (4), 1980: 309.

HERBS FOR THE ELDERLY: For herbs in late-onset diabetes, see Khan, A et al: "Insulin potentiating factors and chromium content of selected foods and spices", in *Biological Trace Elements Research*, 24, 1990.

TONIC HERBS: Willard, Terry: *Reishi Mushroom – Herb of Spiritual Potency and Medical Wonder*, Sylvan Press, Washington, 1990.

INDEX

USEFUL ADDRESSES

KEY • = postal supplier (mail order)
✻ = retail supplier

PROFESSIONAL AND TRADE ASSOCIATIONS

Ayurvedic Living, PO Box 188, Exeter, Devon EX4 5AB.
British Herbal Medicine Association, Field House, Lyle Hole Lane, Redhill, Avon BS18 7TB.
The British Herb Growers Association, c/o NFU, Agriculture House, London SW1X 7NJ.
The General Council and Register of Consultant Herbalists, Marlborough House, Swanpool, Falmouth, Cornwall TR11 4HW.
The National Institute of Herbal Medicine, 9 Palace Gate, Exeter, Devon EX1 1JA.
The National Medicines Group Secretariat, PO Box 5, Ilkeston, Derbyshire DE7 8LX.
The Register of Chinese Herbal Medicine, 98b Hazelville Road, London N19 3NA.

TRAINING COURSES

The School of Phytotherapy/Herbal Medicine, Bucksteep Manor, Bodle Street Green, Hailsham, East Sussex BN27 4RJ.

HERBAL SUPPLIERS

WESTERN HERBS
• ✻ **Baldwin, G & Co**, 171-173 Walworth Road, London SE17 1RW.
• **Brome & Schimmer Ltd**, Unit 3, Romsey Industrial Estate, Romsey, Hants S051 0HR.
✻ **Culpeper Ltd** (Head Office), Hadstock Road, Linton, Cambridge CB1 6NJ.

• **East-West Herbs Ltd**, Langston Priory Mews, Kingham, Oxon 0X7 6UW.
✻ **East West Herb Shop**, 2 Neal's Yard, Covent Garden, London WC2H 9DP.
• **Gerard House**, 3 Wickham Road, Boscomb, Bournemouth BH7 6JX.
• ✻ **Granary Herbs**, The Granary, Bearsted, Kent ME14 4NN.
• **Hambledon Herbs**, Hambledon, Henley-on-Thames, Oxon RG9 6SX.
• **The Herbal Apothecary**, 120 High Street, Syston, Leics IE7 8GC.
✻ **Neal's Yard Remedies** (Head Office), 1A Rossiter Road, London SW12 9RY.
✻ **Pepper Alley Herbs**, The Spice Warehouse, Pepper Alley, Banbury, Oxon OX16 8JB.
• **Phytoproducts**, 3 Kings Mill Way, Hermitage Lane, Mansfield, Notts NG18 5ER.
• **Potters Herbal Supplies**, Leyland Mill Lane, Wigan, Lancs WN1 2SB.
• **Power Health Products**, 10 Central Avenue, Airfield Estate, Pocklington, York YO4 2NR.
✻ **Selsley Herb Shop**, 4 George Street, Nailsworth, Stroud, Glos GL5 OAG.

EASTERN HERBS
• ✻ **AcuMedic Centre**, 101-103 Camden High Street, London NW1 7JN.
• **East-West Herbs Ltd** (see *Western herbs*)
✻ **East West Herb Shop** (see *Western herbs*)
• **Mayway Herbal Emporium**, 34 Greek Street, London W1V 5LN.

ESSENTIAL OIL SUPPLIERS

• **Butterbur & Sage**, 101 Highgrove Street, Reading RG1 5EJ.
• **Hartwood Aromatics**, Hartwood House, 12 Station Road, Hatton, Warwicks CV35 7LG.

• **Norman & Germaine Rich**, 2 Coval Gardens, London SW14 7DG.
• **Shirley Price Aromatherapy**, Wesley House, Stockwell Road, Hinckley, Leics LE10 1RD.

EQUIPMENT SUPPLIERS

CAPSULES AND CAPSULE-MAKING MACHINES
• **Dav-Caps**, PO Box 11, Monmouth, Gwent NP5 3NX.
• **The Herbal Apothecary** (see *Western herbs*)

JELLY BAGS, WINE PRESSES, ETC.
Available from chemists, department stores, wine-making specialists and hardware shops.

STORAGE BOTTLES, JARS, AND OTHER CONTAINERS
• ✻ **Baldwin, G & Co** (see *Western herbs*)
• **Bristol Bottle Co**, Unit 1, Ashmead Trading Estate, Ashmead Road, Keynsham, Avon BS18 1T2.
• **The Homoeopathic Supply Co**, Fairview, 4 Nelson Road, Sheringham, Norfolk NR26 8BU.
Also available from good chemists and medicinal supplies companies.

OINTMENT BASES, ANHYDROUS LANOLIN, GLYCERINE, COCOA BUTTER, FIXED OILS, PARAFFIN WAXES, AND OTHER PHARMACY SUPPLIES
• **Butterbur & Sage** (see *Essential Oil Suppliers*)
• **Potters Herbal Suppliers** (see *Western herbs*)

PESSARY MOULDS
• **The Herbal Apothecary** (see *Western herbs*)
• **Quaestus**, The Studio, Llanbedr, Crickhowell, Powys, Wales NP8 1SR.

ACKNOWLEDGMENTS

Dorling Kindersley would like to thank Rosie Pearson and Claire Le Bas for their editorial help, as well as Louise Abbott, Diana Craig and Carolyn Ryden; Helen Gatward for picture research; Nicholas Jackson for DTP; Sarah Ponder and Gill Shaw for assisting with design; Sarah Ashun for assisting Steve Gorton at photography; Hilary Guy for styling pages 8-9; Diana Mitchell for finding herbs; Sue Bosanko for the index; Iris and Victor Hill, Lauren and Mark Holyoake, Colin Neville, Molly and Ken Neville, and Niki Sarluis for their kind help in finding and providing herbs.

The following companies and individuals also provided herbs and herbal preparations: Andrew Wickens and Marion Brown of Iden Croft Herbs; East-West Herbs Ltd; Hollington Nurseries; Arne Herbs; Tony Carter of The Herbal Apothecary; Fiona Crumley of the Chelsea Physic Garden; Christopher Hedley; Allen Coombes of The Sir Harold Hillier Gardens and Arboretum; Sally Gardens.

ILLUSTRATORS
Colette Cheng: 14,15,16; Tina Hill: 10, 14-15, 27; Gillie Newman: 32, 34, 37, 44, 46, 50, 52, 53, 54, 56, 57, 61, 64, 65, 67, 69, 74, 75, 78, 79, 81, 82, 84, 85, 88, 92, 98, 113; Sarah Ponder: symbols throughout book.

KEY TO PICTURE POSITIONS
t = top; c = centre; b = bottom; l = left; r = right

PICTURE CREDITS
All photography by Steve Gorton except for: Bodleian Library (L.1.5. MED): 19br; The British Library: 13tr; The Mansell Collection: 11cr, 19tr, 23tr; Mary Evans Picture Library: 11br, 17tr, 20bl, 20cl, 22bl; Book of Tibetan Medicine - Teaching Material Produced by the Traditional Medical School in Lhasa, Tibet: 13br; Salus-Haus: 23br; Science Photo Library: 18bl; University of Durham Oriental Museum: 12b; Wellcome Institute Library, London: 21tr; Werner Forman Archive: 11tr; Martin Cameron: 118-124; Martin Norris 126-127 except for: Peter Anderson: 126cr, 127bl.

THE HERB SOCIETY
The Herb Society was founded as "The Society of Herbalists" in 1927 by Hilda Leyel who ran the organization as a mixture of medical practice and herbal product retailing, under the name of *Culpeper*.

Practical medical herbalism remained an important aspect of the Society's work until the 1960s, when changing legislation made this alternative therapy once more freely available to all. In 1974, The Society of Herbalists became a registered educational charity and later the name was changed to "The Herb Society" to reflect more accurately the organization's aims, purposes and ambitions. The brand name *Culpeper* was franchised to a private company which continues trade as the *Culpeper* retail chain.

Today The Herb Society has about 2,000 members and encourages interest in and knowledge of all aspects of herbs: gardening, cookery, folklore, cosmetics, dyeing and history, as well as herbal medicine. Its publications include the magazine *Herbs*, a newsletter for members, *Herbarium*, as well as information sheets and occasional booklets. The Society also organizes lectures and nursery open days, and has recently founded the annual Culpeper Seminar.

For more information contact: The Secretary, The Herb Society, PO Box 599, London SW11 4RW.

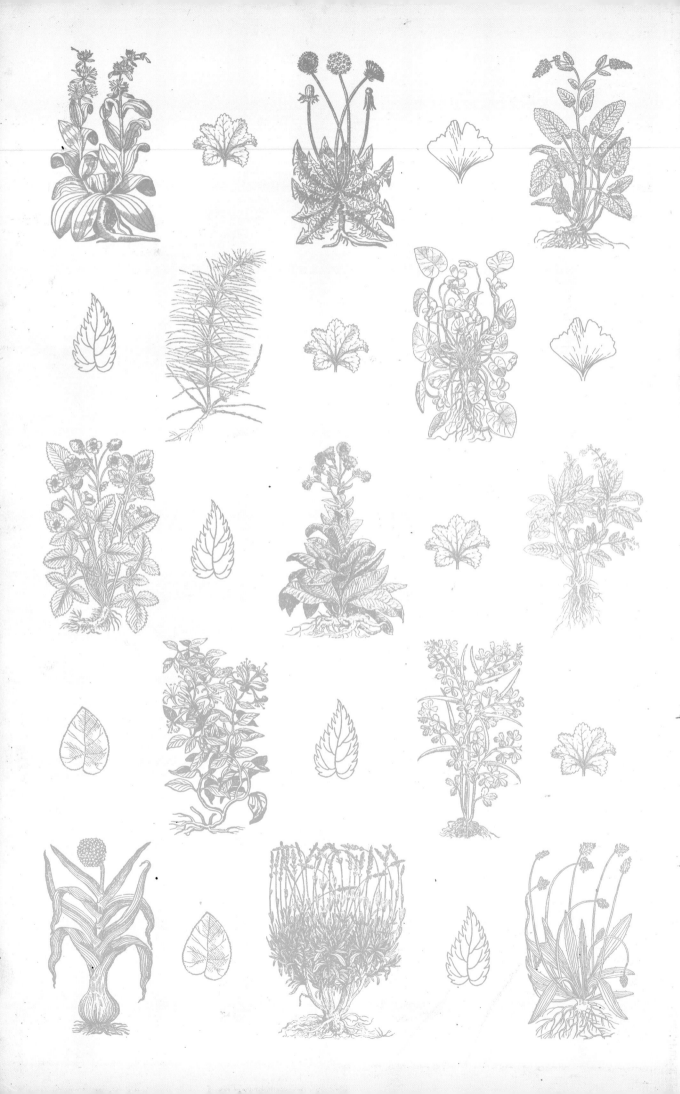